rev. Plumbinga

75 Arguments

risala.

Pg. 296
Position Essay

75 Arguments

An Anthology

Alan Ainsworth
Houston Community College—Central

Boston Burr Ridge, IL Dubuque, IA Madison, WI New York
San Francisco St. Louis Bangkok Bogotá Caracas Kuala Lumpur
Lisbon London Madrid Mexico City Milan Montreal New Delhi
Santiago Seoul Singapore Sydney Taipei Toronto

Higher Education

75 ARGUMENTS: AN ANTHOLOGY
Published by McGraw-Hill, a business unit of The McGraw-Hill Companies,
Inc., 1221 Avenue of the Americas, New York, NY, 10020. Copyright © 2008 by
The McGraw-Hill Companies, Inc. All rights reserved. No part of this publica-
tion may be reproduced or distributed in any form or by any means, or stored
in a database or retrieval system, without the prior written consent of The
McGraw-Hill Companies, Inc., including, but not limited to, in any network or
other electronic storage or transmission, or broadcast for distance learning.
Some ancillaries, including electronic and print components, may not be available to customers outside the United States.

This book is printed on acid-free paper.

2 3 4 5 6 7 8 9 0 DOC/DOC 0 9 8

ISBN: 978-0-07-249664-2
MHID: 0-07-249664-9

Vice President and Editor in chief: *Emily Barrosse*
Publisher: *Lisa Moore*
Sponsoring editor: *Victoria Fullard*
Editorial assistant: *Jesse Hassenger*
Marketing manager: *Lori DeShazo*
Senior project manager: *Diane M. Folliard*
Designer: *Marianna Kinigakis*
Production supervisor: *Jason I. Huls*
Composition: *10/12 Palatino, by Techbooks*
Printing: *45# New Era Matte, R. R. Donnelley & Sons*

Library of Congress Cataloging–in–Publication Data

75 Arguments : An Anthology / [edited by] Alan Ainsworth.
   p. cm.
   ISBN-13: 978-0-07-249664-2 (softcover : alk. paper)
   ISBN-10: 0-07-249664-9 (softcover: alk. paper)
  1. College readers. 2. English language—Rhetoric. 3. Persuasion (Rhetoric)
4. Report writing. I. Ainsworth, Alan. II. Title: Seventy five arguments.
   PE1417.A128 2008
   808' .0427—dc22

                                                            2006012054

The Internet addresses listed in the text were accurate at the time of publication.
The inclusion of a Web site does not indicate an endorsement by the authors or
McGraw-Hill, and McGraw-Hill does not guarantee the accuracy of the informa-
tion presented at these sites.

www.mhhe.com

Table of Contents

Chapter 3
POP CULTURE AND THE MEDIA: DO WE COVER EVENTS OR INVENT THEM?   118

Chapter 4
GLOBALIZATION AND CULTURE: SHOULD SLOW INVASIONS BE STOPPED?   164

Chapter 7
MARRIAGE AND DIVORCE: HOW SHOULD YOU TAKE THIS PERSON TO BE YOUR SPOUSE?   318

Chapter 8
RESPONSIBILITY AND THE ECONOMY: SHOULD MONEY HAVE A MIND OF ITS OWN?   345

Chapter 9
ETHNICITY: IF RACE DOESN'T EXIST, WHY IS IT
SO IMPORTANT?   406

Chapter 10
NATURE AND ITS RESOURCES: TO SUSTAIN OR
TO EXPLOIT?   436

ALTERNATIVE TABLE OF CONTENTS

This Table of Contents classifies the essays in the anthology by several means of argument. It is by no means conclusive or definitive. Many essays have been placed in several categories.

Ethos

Pathos

Deductive

Inductive Causal Evidence

Inductive Analogy

Evaluation

Proposal

Classification

Comparison/Contrast

Narrative

Preface

APPROACH:

75 Arguments is a new anthology to complement the *75 Readings* family of anthologies priced with students in mind. It is designed for any number of courses where argumentative essays are studied and written. First, it can be used for students to practice the various methods of analysis of argument (including those covered briefly in an Introduction to Argument section). Second, the readings can be used as models for their own argument (students and instructors should take care here: most of the arguments include nonacademic prose and some include fallacies). Third, the readings can be used as sources to produce documented synthesis papers. They can also be used as springboards for further research and the writing of full research papers.

AUDIENCE:

Students and instructors will find argumentative essays written by a great diversity of authors from Plato to a contemporary blogger. The readings are intended to provide not only many viewpoints but various methods of argument, length and complexity, style, and organization. The readings in this anthology are purposefully not accompanied by apparatus other than a brief introduction to argument. *75 Arguments* can, because of this, be integrated into a variety of courses, approaches, and teaching methods. The readings stand on their own for analysis by the instructor and students.

CONTENT/ORGANIZATION:

The argumentative essays are organized loosely around twelve themes. Each of these thematic sections offers six or seven essays, one or several of which ask timeless questions. In addition, each section also offers very specific arguments, mostly on contemporary applications to the general issue. For instance, the first section Languages of Argument: Can Names Really Hurt You? includes two timeless ways of thinking about language: George Orwell's "Politics and the English Language" and a selection from George Lakoff and Mark Johnson's "Metaphors We Live By." The other essays in the section offer several contemporary arguments ranging from one about profanity by fans at athletic events to a very current argument about how to argue on the Internet.

A VALUE PRICE:

At less than half the price of argument readers currently popular among college instructors, *75 Arguments* is part of a McGraw-Hill franchise of value-priced titles put together to address the very real concerns about textbook costs for students. Other value-priced books available through McGraw-Hill include *75 Readings* (a rhetorically arranged reader), *75 Readings Plus* (that same rhetorically arranged reader with editorial apparatus), *75 Thematic Readings* (a thematic reader), and *75 Readings Across the Curriculum* (a thematic reader with an interdisciplinary focus). To keep the cost low, *75 Arguments* has been compiled as a reader only; it has only readings—no headnotes, no questions before or after the selections, no writing assignments—which we hope appeals particularly to professors who prefer to develop their own sequence of discussion questions to support particular goals of their courses. Equally important, we hope that both the selections and the price of this text will meet the needs of your classes.

SUPPLEMENTS:

Catalyst 2.0, which accompanies each new copy of *75 Arguments,* is a thorough online writing resource which includes peer review software, grammar exercises, and diagnostic tests; writing guides and sample student papers for common assignments; interactive tutorials on key topics; a guide to evaluating online sources; *Bibliomaker* software that automatically formats source information in a variety of documentation styles. Instructors can choose from a variety of classroom management tools including an online grade book.

ACKNOWLEDGMENTS:

Special thanks to the instructors who reviewed the readings in this anthology:

James Allen, *College of DuPage*

M.D. Allen, *University of Wisconsin, Fox Valley*

Daniel Bender, *Pace University*

Michael Cooley, *Berry College*

Litasha Dennis, *Winthrop University*

Anne Herbert, *Bradley University*

Amanda Lawrence, *Young Harris College*

Paul Mahaffey, *University of Montevallo*

Mark Scamahorn, *San Diego Miramar College*

Olga Skorapa, *University of New England*

Kimberleigh Stallings, *University of North Carolina, Charlotte*

Ryan Van Cleave, *Clemson University*

Kim Whitehead, *Mississippi University for Women*

I would like to thank the following at McGraw-Hill: Barbara Duhon, Ray Kelley, Chris Bennem, Melissa Hunt, and especially Lisa Moore and Victoria Fullard. I'd like to thank my students, colleagues, and friends at Houston Community College and the

University of Houston, especially George Trail. Finally, I'd like to thank Lee Harrison, Michael Ainsworth, Joan Ainsworth, Joe Ainsworth (in memory), and the rest of my family.

Finally, we want to hear what you think about this text. Please e-mail English@mcgraw-hill.com to make suggestions or comments about *75 Arguments* or to ask any questions about its use.

Alan Ainsworth
Alan.Ainsworth@hccs.edu

A Very Brief Introduction to Argument

Let's start by defining the term *argument*. There are two major definitions of the term, one of which has become more popular in everyday speech and writing:

> **Ar´gu•ment** (är-gyə-ment) *n*. **1.** A discussion in which disagreement is expressed; a debate. A quarrel; a dispute. **2.** A set of statements in which one follows as a conclusion from the others.

Both definitions are important in the college experience and beyond. There are many occasions in many classes where opposing views (or those that seem opposing) are discussed and debated. The arguments (definition 1, debate) are then supported by the other definition of argument as a set of assertions, one of which is said to follow from the others. We, of course, use this definition of argument every day of our lives. Any time you use the term "because" you are connecting a conclusion with the supporting reasons.

This book of *75 Arguments* is a collection of seventy-five writings which primarily demonstrate reasoned argument rather than debate. At the same time, some of the issues being argued can be paired with another writing to create debate. They can also be grouped to help us see that most issues are more complex than simple pro/con stances suggest.

SEVERAL METHODS OF ANALYZING ARGUMENT

There are many ways of analyzing argument. We will briefly consider some of them as follows:

Aristotle's Appeals Modernized

Three key terms have come to us from the Greek philosopher Aristotle that help us analyze and write arguments: *ethos, logos, pathos*. Each of these appeals is directed to the three elements of communication. Aristotle was primarily thinking of how these might apply to spoken messages. His insights, however, have been imposed onto written communication to some success. We can also impose them onto the other methods of communication in our media age of audio, video, Internet, etc.

	Ethos	*Logos*	*Pathos*
Speech	Speaker	Speech	Listener(s) or Audience
Writing	Writer	Text	Reader(s)
Media	Developer	Media	User(s)

In Greek "*ethos*" means "good man," but since we are all good people, we will translate it as "good person." The appeal *ethos* is related to the word "ethics," the study of good and evil. The *ethos* of an argument is the "character" of the speaker as in "character reference." In writing the *ethos* is what allows the reader to believe the writer's reasonableness or authority in her point of view.

Aristotle thought of the *logos* as the logic that is used to support the point of view of the writer. He was reacting to the Sophists, who were more interested in oratorical fireworks than argument as an attempt to determine truths. The Greek word "*logos*," however, is a word packed with meaning and could be used to include a great deal more than just logic. *Logos* has been translated as a variety of concepts including "word," "thought," "principle," or "speech." The power of words is included in this concept. Additionally, it can be thought of as a "sign," "symbol," or "icon." The contemporary English world "logo," meaning a clean pictorial design signifying a company or product, is directly related. In summary, in addition to the power of logic and reason, *logos* also includes all the power of symbols such as the American flag, the Christian cross, or the Nike Swoosh.

Pathos is the appeal to the listener, to the group of listeners as an audience. We listen to a speaker in different ways when we are alone than when we are in small groups than when we are in large audiences. The *pathos* of an argument is the emotion evoked by the information and presentation of the point of the view of the speaker. *Pathos* comes from the same root as "pathetic" in the meaning "full of pity." Aristotle's insight that a speaker can change a group's emotions is easily seen today in churches, comedy clubs, or classrooms. And we as speakers change our speech depending on the intended listener. Think about how you would tell a story to a police officer in a different way than you would your best friend. We then have to translate this idea that Aristotle had for speech to written communication. How a writer shapes her text for a particular reader or sets of readers is vitally important, but she does not have the luxury of immediate feedback from her reader in the same way that a speaker does with his listener. Consider these four possible target readers and argumentative contexts:

- Visitors to a national church Web site advocating the right to life movement
- Readers of a local underground paper promoting saving the wetlands of Florida
- Chat room participants interested in high performance race cars
- Your instructor reading your paper

As you can see, the writer should consider her reader(s) before beginning her argument. Speakers, on the other hand, are able to receive instant feedback from their listeners and can change their messages accordingly.

Deductive Reasoning

Aristotle sought not only to understand the three aspects of rhetoric with his appeals, he also wrote extensively on deductive reasoning. Deductive reasoning deals with statements that can be held to be necessary conclusions given earlier assertions. For instance, the general statement that "All English teachers are boring" is followed by the specific statement "Dr. Ainsworth is an English teacher." The only conclusion to be drawn from this reasoning is that "Dr. Ainsworth must be boring."

Inductive Reasoning

Inductive reasoning deals with probable inference rather than necessary inference. This simply means that inductive reasoning will lead you to a *likely* conclusion based on the premises, but not the only possible conclusion. Inductive reasoning incorporates many types of reasoning including causal arguments in courtrooms, arguments used by scientists to support theories, and analogies between like systems.

Causal Arguments:

In an everyday example, we see how we would use induction to hypothesize the causes of particular actions. John and Joe go out to breakfast one morning. John excuses himself for a minute and leaves his chocolate-iced donut on the table. When he returns, his donut is missing, Joe has chocolate icing on his fingers and donut crumbs on the table in front of him. Inductive reasoning tells us that Joe ate John's donut.

Argument Using Evidence in Science and the Social Sciences:

Scientific argument uses experimental methods codified in the 17th and 18th centuries. Here various experimental methods are combined with mathematical analysis to provide evidence for theorems. The social sciences have adapted these methods to their fields. A complex example from sociology is the proposition that adult survivors of child abuse are more likely to abuse their own children than those who were not abused themselves. The social scientist uses this data to arrive at arguments for root causes.

Argument by Analogy:

Argument by analogy is basically an argument using an extended comparison of two "like" systems. The question becomes whether the systems actually do compare in all of their aspects. Imagine a speaker at a high school graduation who compares life to a football game and says that one has to prepare for the game, play the game well, and live with the wins and the losses. We must question how far we can take this analogy for it to remain useful.

Toulmin's Approach

The contemporary philosopher Stephen Toulmin has taken Aristotle's original philosophy of deductive reasoning and tried to create a system that would take into account probabilities and other features of inductive reasoning into what he called "practical reasoning." The vocabulary associated with Stephen Toulmin sounds like something you'd expect to hear in a courtroom:

- Claim
- Data
- Warrant
- Qualifiers
- Rebuttal

First, we need to make the basic connections between Data and Claim and Warrant through a simple diagram:

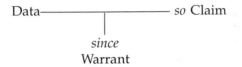

We then need to define the key terms below:

Claim: The claim of your argument is the central thesis or assertion.

Data: The claim is supported by data or facts. These facts can also be called "grounds" or "evidence."

Warrant: You've seen enough TV police shows to know what it means when a court approves a warrant for finding evidence. A warrant in legal terms is explicit permission from a court to do something, usually search a property or arrest someone. A warrant in Toulmin's argument is a justified assumption that evidence may be found to support a claim, and that your audience shares that assumption. In argument, the warrant is the link between your data and your claim.

The final two parts of this simplified version of Toulmin's approach to argument allow for probable claims rather than absolute ones.

Qualifiers: Most of the time, claims are not considered absolute. Most fields of argument allow for claims to be qualified or contingent on certain conditions.

Rebuttals: Rebuttals allow for exceptions to your argument without having to concede your claim completely. Rebuttals anticipate holes or weaknesses your opposition might find in your argument. For instance, you may argue that jogging is a *generally* healthy form of exercise and good for the body except to the extent that it's hard on the knees. By acknowledging that stress on the knees is the only significant downside to jogging, you're supporting your claim that jogging is *generally* healthy and good for the body.

The diagram showing Toulmin's argument form above becomes more complex with the insertion of Qualifiers and Rebuttals:

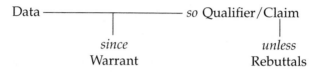

Toulmin tried to incorporate both reason and practicality into one method of analyzing arguments.

Rogerian Argument

Psychologist Carl Rogers offers an alternative method to the Aristotelian approach described above and the combative approach employed in debate and courtroom law. He encouraged the practice of "empathic listening," in which a listener puts aside his own biases and predispositions to see an issue sympathetically from the opposition's side. This strategy requires a listener to understand the opposition's values, ideas, and reasoning. The key to successfully employing Rogerian argument in written communication is to find common ground between the writer and resistant readers.

OTHER APPROACHES TO ARGUMENT:

Satire

Satire tries to use humor and irony in order to try to convince a reader of the folly of a particular argument. Sometimes the author creates a naïve "persona" through which a situation is seen from a new perspective. We should distinguish the term "persona" from "*ethos*" in that the "*persona*" means "character" as in a fictional "character" distinct from the actual person writing the satire. Satire, because it involves extended use of irony, can be more obvious in speech or through the media than in writing. For instance, Jon Stewart's satire on *The Daily Show with Jon Stewart* is easily seen as ironic and humorous because of his use of facial expressions and joking voices. Many written satires have been taken literally on first reading, including Jonathan Swift's "A Modest Proposal" and Judy Brady's "I Want a Wife," included in this anthology.

Parody

A related term, *parody*, involves using a very similar form of another work for comic or argumentative effect. *The Daily Show* in addition to being a satire, is also a parody of television newscasts. *America, A Users Guide,* written by Jon Stewart and others, is a parody of high school history textbooks. Parodies mock the original form. In addition to other arguments, *America* argues against the pose of sincerity and glib answers of textbook writers.

Homage

A term related to parody, "*homage*" is using the form that others use in order to praise the form or change the argument of the original. *The Declaration of Sentiments*, included in this anthology, argues against the tyranny of men using the form and power of *The Declaration of Independence*, which argued against the tyranny of George III.

Legal Arguments

Legal Arguments come in two major and differing forms. First, there are the arguments which a trial lawyer makes before a judge or jurors concerning the facts of a particular case. The second kind of argument is one a lawyer makes concerning the law of a particular case and its relationship to other laws within the legal system. This kind is usually made during the appeal process to a judge or a panel of judges who then render opinions based on settled law.

ARGUMENT IN ACADEMIC PAPERS

In academic papers, students encounter several different kinds of argumentative assignments in the various disciplines. Almost all of the assignments will require that you write a cogent, well-reasoned, organized, and researched argument. Sometimes the instructor will give very specific directions and resources to use. In this case, you should try to take these directions into an assignment that you can value and make your own. Sometimes, assignments are more open. When considering possible issues to write about, consider applying the aspects of your life that interest you in the particular discipline. What around you prompts a strong reaction? You should have a desire to learn more about an issue that may motivate you throughout the process.

Focusing your argument on a specific perspective will help you to give depth to a particular subject. Take the problem of homelessness, for example. By narrowing the focus from homelessness in general to the federal government's responsibility to provide aid to the homeless in your hometown, you move from an overwhelmingly large and indistinct topic to a specific issue about which you can take a stand.

Similarly, claiming that distance learning through online classes makes education accessible to previously disenfranchised students with extreme time limitations and personal obligations is far more debatable than the general topic of educational technology.

Another example is the broad topic of vegetarianism versus this debatable assertion: People should convert to vegetarianism because the energy required to sustain a meat-free diet is much less than that needed for a carnivorous diet; the surplus of food created by this less energy-intensive process could make strides toward ending hunger.

In all of these examples, you would need to support your thesis by using the terms, theories, and research from other scholars that are pertinent to the particular discipline you are studying. For instance, the vegetarian paper would be very different for a class in economics than for a class in biology; the paper on online classes would be different for a class in education, sociology, or instructional technology.

Academic arguments very commonly fall into four categories:

- *Definition* (What is it?): As you may have guessed, this type of argument focuses primarily on what things are, how we label them, and changes they have gone (or are going) through.
- *Causal* (How did it get that way?): Causal arguments look both to the past and to the future to hypothesize about how and why events took place and/or to predict what may happen down the road.
- *Evaluation* (Is it good or bad?): Evaluation arguments require commonly agreed upon criteria or standards of judgment. Only after both you and your audience agree that fuel efficiency, longevity, safety, and appearance are the considerations in rating automobiles can you argue whether or not Ford is the best car available. Evaluation arguments often require definition arguments to be interspersed throughout.
- *Proposals* (What should we do about it?): This type of argument is built around a call for action. It consists of two types of arguments: the claim that there is, in fact, a problem and a proposal of a solution.

When writing an argument, you may find your argument will cover some combination of these four areas of development or fall squarely into one of these types.

ARGUMENT IN THE MEDIA

Finally, a brief note about the analysis of arguments in media other than speech or writing. Images have made arguments long before the advent of writing. Painting and sculpture show images and can be powerful religious arguments. Before the majority of people were literate, artists and architects knew the power of images and incorporated them into the powerful religious argument embodied in cathedrals. There are countless didactic paintings. With the invention of photography and, later, film, images took on different meanings, different arguments. The integration of recorded sound into film, and the instant transmission over long distances that radio and television signals allowed changed meanings of messages. Individuals in political movements used these powerful tools to make arguments about their ideas, sometimes for ill. We need only think of the powerful propaganda machines of Adolph Hitler's Germany to see an example. Since the advent of the interactive Internet and all it allows, media has changed, and perhaps become more individual again. Today, we need to pay attention to the TV news we wake up to, to the billboards we see on the way to work or class, to the magazine we flip through at the gym, to the visuals in the games we play or the blogs we read. All of these are making an argument. With the powerful tools afforded us with word processors, easily accessible visuals, graphs, and videos, and the even more powerful instant publishing of the Web and blogs, we can become our own producers of multimedia. As such, we should be equally as adept at analyzing our use of speech, writing, the media we hear, read, and use. And equally so, we must be good speakers, writers, and producers.

A FINAL WORD ON THE USE OF *75 ARGUMENTS*

75 Arguments can be used in several ways. First, it can be used for students to practice the various methods of analysis of argument (some mentioned below, briefly). Second, the readings can be used as models for their own arguments. Third, the readings can be used as sources to produce documented synthesis papers. They can also be used as springboards for further research and the writing of full research papers.

Chapter

Languages of Argument: Can Names Really Hurt You?

Politics and the English Language

George Orwell

Most people who bother with the matter at all would admit that 1
the English language is in a bad way, but it is generally assumed
that we cannot by conscious action do anything about it. Our civilization is decadent, and our language—so the argument runs—
must inevitably share in the general collapse. It follows that any
struggle against the abuse of language is a sentimental archaism,
like preferring candles to electric light or hansom cabs to air-
planes. Underneath this lies the half-conscious belief that language is a natural growth and not an instrument which we shape
for our own purposes.

Now, it is clear that the decline of a language must ulti- 2
mately have political and economic causes: it is not due simply
to the bad influence of this or that individual writer. But an
effect can become a cause, reinforcing the original cause and
producing the same effect in an intensified form, and so on
indefinitely. A man may take to drink because he feels himself
to be a failure, and then fail all the more completely because
he drinks. It is rather the same thing that is happening to the
English language. It becomes ugly and inaccurate because our
thoughts are foolish, but the slovenliness of our language makes
it easier for us to have foolish thoughts. The point is that the

process is reversible. Modern English, especially written English, is full of bad habits which spread by imitation and which can be avoided if one is willing to take the necessary trouble. If one gets rid of these habits one can think more clearly, and to think clearly is a necessary first step towards political regeneration: so that the fight against bad English is not frivolous and is not the exclusive concern of professional writers. I will come back to this presently, and I hope that by that time the meaning of what I have said here will have become clearer. Meanwhile, here are five specimens of the English language as it is now habitually written.

3 These five passages have not been picked out because they are especially bad—I could have quoted far worse if I had chosen—but because they illustrate various of the mental vices from which we now suffer. They are a little below the average, but are fairly representative samples. I number them so that I can refer back to them when necessary:

(1) I am not, indeed, sure whether it is not true to say the Milton who once seemed not unlike a seventeenth-century Shelley had not become, out of an experience even more bitter in each year, more alien (sic) to the founder of that Jesuit sect which nothing could induce him to tolerate.

—Professor Harold Laski (essay in *Freedom of Expression*)

(2) Above all, we cannot play ducks and drakes with a native battery of idioms which prescribes such egregious collocations of vocables as the basic *put up with* for *tolerate* or *put at a loss* for *bewilder*.

—Professor Lancelot Hogben (*Interglossa*)

(3) On the one side we have the free personality: by definition it is not neurotic, for it has neither conflict nor dream. Its desires, such as they are, are transparent, for they are just what institutional approval keeps in the forefront of consciousness; another institutional pattern would alter their number and intensity; there is little in them that is natural, irreducible, or culturally dangerous. But on the other side, the social bond itself is nothing but the mutual reflection of these self-secure integrities. Recall the definition of love. Is not this the very picture of a small academic? Where is there

a place in this hall of mirrors for either personality or fraternity?

—Essay on psychology in *Politics* (New York)

(4) All the "best people" from the gentlemen's clubs, and all the frantic Fascist captains, united in common hatred of Socialism and bestial horror of the rising tide of the mass revolutionary movement, have turned to acts of provocation, to foul incendiarism, to medieval legends of poisoned wells, to legalize their own destruction to proletarian organizations, and rouse the agitated petty-bourgeoisie to chauvinistic fervor on behalf of the fight against the revolutionary way out of the crisis.

—Communist pamphlet

(5) If a new spirit is to be infused into this old country, there is one thorny and contentious reform which must be tackled, and that is the humanization and galvanization of the BBC. Timidity here will bespeak canker and atrophy for the soul. The heart of Britain may be sound and of strong beat, for instance, but the British lion's roar at present is like that of Bottom in Shakespeare's *Midsummer Night's Dream*—as gentle as any sucking dove. A virile new Britain cannot continue indefinitely to be traduced in the eyes, or rather ears, of the world by the effete languors of Langham Place, brazenly masquerading as "standard English." When the Voice of Britain is heard at nine o'clock, better far and infinitely less ludicrous to hear aitches honestly dropped than the present priggish, inflated, inhibited, schoolma' amish braying of blameless bashful mewing maidens!

—Letter in *Tribune*

Each of these passages has faults of its own, but, quite apart 4 from avoidable ugliness, two qualities are common to all of them. The first is staleness of imagery; the other is lack of precision. The writer either has a meaning and cannot express it, or he inadvertently says something else, or he is almost indifferent as to whether his words mean anything or not. This mixture of vagueness and sheer incompetence is the most marked characteristic of modern English prose, and especially of any kind of political writing. As soon as certain topics are raised, the concrete melts into the abstract and no one seems able to think of turns of speech that are not hackneyed: prose consists less and less of *words* chosen for the sake of their meaning, and more of *phrases* tacked together like the sections of a prefabricated henhouse. I list below, with notes and examples, various of the tricks by means of which the work of prose construction is habitually dodged:

DYING METAPHORS

5 A newly invented metaphor assists thought by evoking a visual image, while on the other hand a metaphor which is technically "dead" (e. g., *iron resolution*) has in effect reverted to being an ordinary word and can generally be used without loss of vividness. But in between these two classes there is a huge dump of wornout metaphors which have lost all evocative power and are merely used because they save people the trouble of inventing phrases for themselves. Examples are: *Ring the changes on, take up the cudgels for, toe the line, ride roughshod over, stand shoulder to shoulder with, play into the hands of, no axe to grind, grist to the mill, fishing in troubled waters, rift within the lute, on the order of the day, Achilles' heel, swan song, hotbed.* Many of these are used without knowledge of their meaning (what is a "rift," for instance?), and incompatible metaphors are frequently mixed, a sure sign that the writer is not interested in what he is saying. Some metaphors now current have been twisted out of their original meaning without those who use them even being aware of the fact. For example, *toe the line* is sometimes written *tow the line.* Another example is *the hammer and the anvil,* now always used with the implication that the anvil gets the worst of it. In real life it is always the anvil that breaks the hammer, never the other way about: a writer who stopped to think what he was saying would be aware of this, and would avoid perverting the original phrase.

OPERATORS, OR VERBAL FALSE LIMBS

6 These save the trouble of picking out appropriate verbs and nouns, and at the same time pad each sentence with extra syllables which give it an appearance of symmetry. Characteristic phrases are: *render inoperative, militate against, prove unacceptable,*

make contact with, be subjected to, give rise to, give grounds for, have the effect of, play a leading part (role) in, make itself felt, take effect, exhibit a tendency to, serve the purpose of, etc. etc. The keynote is the elimination of simple verbs. Instead of being a single word, such as *break, stop, spoil, mend, kill,* a verb becomes a *phrase,* made up of a noun or adjective tacked on to some general-purposes verb such as *prove, serve, form, play, render.* In addition, the passive voice is wherever possible used in preference to the active, and noun constructions are used instead of gerunds (*by examination of* instead of *by examining*). The range of verbs is further cut down by means of the *-ize* and *de-* formations, and banal statements are given an appearance of profundity by means of the *not un-* formation. Simple conjunctions and prepositions are replaced by such phrases as *with respect to, having regard to, the fact that, by dint of, in view of, in the interests of, on the hypothesis that;* and the ends of sentences are saved from anti-climax by such resounding commonplaces as *greatly to be desired, cannot be left out of account, a development to be expected in the near future, deserving of serious consideration, brought to a satisfactory conclusion,* and so on and so forth.

PRETENTIOUS DICTION

Words like *phenomenon, element, individual* (as noun), *objective,* 7 *categorical, effective, virtual, basic, primary, promote, constitute, exhibit, exploit, utilize, eliminate, liquidate,* are used to dress up simple statements and give an air of scientific impartiality to biased judgments. Adjectives like *epoch-making, epic, historic, unforgettable, triumphant, age-old, inevitable, inexorable, veritable,* are used to dignify the sordid processes of international politics, while writing that aims at glorifying war usually takes on an archaic color, its characteristic words being: *realm, throne, chariot, mailed fist, trident, sword, shield, buckler, banner, jackboot, clarion.* Foreign words and expressions such as *cul de sac, ancien régime, deus ex machina, mutatis mutandis, status quo, Gleichschaltung, Weltanschauung,* are used to give an air of culture and elegance. Except for the useful abbreviations *i.e., e.g.,* and *etc.,* there is no real need for any of the hundreds of foreign phrases now current in English. Bad writers, and especially scientific, political and sociological writers, are nearly always haunted by the notion that Latin or Greek words are grander than Saxon ones, and unnecessary words like *expedite, ameliorate, predict, extraneous, deracinated, clandestine, subaqueous* and hundreds of others constantly gain ground from their Anglo-Saxon opposite numbers.[1] The jargon peculiar to Marxist writing (*hyena, hangman, cannibal, petty bourgeois, these gentry, lacquey, flunkey, mad dog, White Guard,* etc.) consists largely of words and phrases translated from Russian, German or French; but the normal way of coining a new word is to use a Latin or Greek root with the appropriate affix and, where necessary, the *-ize* formation. It is often easier to make up words of this kind (*deregionalize, impermissible, extramarital, non-fragmentatory* and so forth) than to think up the English words that will cover one's meaning. The result, in general, is an increase in slovenliness and vagueness.

MEANINGLESS WORDS

8 In certain kinds of writing, particularly in art criticism and literary criticism, it is normal to come across long passages which are almost completely lacking in meaning.[2] Words like *romantic, plastic, values, human, dead, sentimental, natural, vitality,* as used in art criticism, are strictly meaningless, in the sense that they not only do not point to any discoverable object, but are hardly even expected to do so by the reader. When one critic writes, "The outstanding features of Mr. X's work is its living quality," while another writes, "The immediately striking thing about Mr. X's

---

[1]An interesting illustration of this is the way in which the English flower names which were in use till very recently are being ousted by Greek ones, *snapdragon* becoming *antirrhinum, forget-me-not* becoming *myosotis,* etc. It is hard to see any practical reason for this change of fashion: it is probably due to an instinctive turning-away from the more homely word and a vague feeling that the Greek word is scientific.

[2]*Example:* "Comfort's catholicity of perception and image, strangely Whitmanesque in range, almost the exact opposite in aesthetic compulsion, continues to evoke that trembling atmospheric accumulative hinting at a cruel, and inexorably serene timelessness. . . . Wrey Gardiner scores by aiming at simple bullseyes with precision. Only they are not so simple, and through this contented sadness runs more than the surface bittersweet of resignation." (*Poetry Quarterly*)

work is its peculiar deadness," the reader accepts this as a simple difference of opinion. If words like *black* and *white* were involved, instead of the jargon words *dead* and *living*, he would see at once that language was being used in an improper way. Many political words are similarly abused. The word *Fascism* has now no meaning except in so far as it signifies "something not desirable." The words *democracy, socialism, freedom, patriotic, realistic, justice,* have each of them several different meanings which cannot be reconciled with one another. In the case of a word like *democracy,* not only is there no agreed definition, but the attempt to make one is resisted from all sides. It is almost universally felt that when we call a country democratic we are praising it: consequently the defenders of every kind of régime claim that it is a democracy, and fear that they might have to stop using the word if it were tied down to any one meaning. Words of this kind are often used in a consciously dishonest way. That is, the person who uses them has his own private definition, but allows his hearer to think he means something quite different. Statements like *Marshal Pétain was a true patriot, The Soviet press is the freest in the world, The Catholic Church is opposed to persecution,* are almost always made with intent to deceive. Other words used in variable meanings, in most cases more or less dishonestly, are: *class, totalitarian, science, progressive, reactionary, bourgeois, equality.*

Now that I have made this catalogue of swindles and perversions, let me give another example of the kind of writing that they lead to. This time it must of its nature be an imaginary one. I am going to translate a passage of good English into modern English of the worst sort. Here is a well-known verse from *Ecclesiastes:*

> I returned, and saw under the sun, that the race is not to the swift, nor the battle to the strong, neither yet bread to the wise, nor yet riches to men of understanding, nor yet favor to men of skill; but time and chance happeneth to them all.

Here it is in modern English:

> Objective consideration of contemporary phenomena compels the conclusion that success or failure in competitive activities exhibits no tendency to be commensurate with innate capacity, but that a considerable element of the unpredictable must invariably be taken into account.

11   This is a parody, but not a very gross one. Exhibit (3) above, for instance, contains several patches of the same kind of English. It will be seen that I have not made a full translation. The beginning and ending of the sentence follow the original meaning fairly closely, but in the middle the concrete illustrations—race, battle, bread—dissolve into the vague phrase "success or failure in competitive activities." This had to be so, because no modern writer of the kind I am discussing—no one capable of using phrases like "objective consideration of contemporary phenomena"—would ever tabulate his thoughts in that precise and detailed way. The whole tendency of modern prose is away from concreteness. Now analyze these two sentences a little more closely. The first contains 49 words but only 60 syllables, and all its words are those of everyday life. The second contains 38 words of 90 syllables: 18 of its words are from Latin roots, and one from Greek. The first sentence contains six vivid images, and only one phrase ("time and chance") that could be called vague. The second contains not a single fresh, arresting phrase, and in spite of its 90 syllables it gives only a shortened version of the meaning contained in the first. Yet without a doubt it is the second kind of sentence that is gaining ground in modern English. I do not want to exaggerate. This kind of writing is not yet universal, and outcrops of simplicity will occur here and there in the worst-written page. Still, if you or I were told to write a few lines on the uncertainty of human fortunes, we should probably come much nearer to my imaginary sentence than to the one from *Ecclesiastes*.

12   As I have tried to show, modern writing at its worst does not consist in picking out words for the sake of their meaning and inventing images in order to make the meaning clearer. It consists in gumming together long strips of words which have already been set in order by someone else, and making the results presentable by sheer humbug. The attraction of this way of writing is that it is easy. It is easier—even quicker, once you have the habit—to say *In my opinion it is a not unjustifiable assumption that* than to say *I think.* If you use ready-made phrases, you not only don't have to hunt about for words; you also don't have to bother with the rhythms of your sentences, since these phrases are generally so arranged as to be more or less euphonious. When you are composing in a hurry—when you are dictating to a stenographer, for instance, or

making a public speech—it is natural to fall into a pretentious, latinized style. Tags like *a consideration which we should do well to bear in mind or a conclusion to which all of us would readily assent* will save many a sentence from coming down with a bump. By using stale metaphors, similes and idioms, you save much mental effort, at the cost of leaving your meaning vague, not only for your reader but for yourself. This is the significance of mixed metaphors. The sole aim of a metaphor is to call up a visual image. When these images clash—as in *The Fascist octopus has sung its swan song, the jackboot is thrown into the melting-pot*—can be taken as certain that the writer is not seeing a mental image of the objects he is naming; in other words he is not really thinking. Look again at the examples I gave at the beginning of this essay. Professor Laski (1) uses five negatives in 53 words. One of these is superfluous, making nonsense of the whole passage, and in addition there is the slip *alien* for akin, making further nonsense, and several avoidable pieces of clumsiness which increase the general vagueness. Professor Hogben (2) plays ducks and drakes with a battery which is able to write prescriptions, and, while disapproving of the everyday phrase *put up with,* is unwilling to look *egregious* up in the dictionary and see what it means. In (3), if one takes an uncharitable attitude towards it, [it] is simply meaningless: probably one could work out its intended meaning by reading the whole of the article in which it occurs. In (4) the writer knows more or less what he wants to say, but an accumulation of stale phrases chokes him like tealeaves blocking a sink. In (5) words and meaning have almost parted company. People who write in this manner usually have a general emotional meaning—they dislike one thing and want to express solidarity with another—but they are not interested in the detail of what they are saying. A scrupulous writer, in every sentence that he writes, will ask himself at least four questions, thus: What am I trying to say? What words will express it? What image or idiom will make it clearer? Is this image fresh enough to have an effect? And he will probably ask himself two more: Could I put it more shortly? Have I said anything that is avoidably ugly? But you are not obliged to go to all this trouble. You can shirk it by simply throwing your mind open and letting the ready-made phrases come crowding in. They will construct your sentences for you—even think your thoughts for you, to a certain extent—and at need they will perform the important service of partially concealing your meaning even from yourself. It is at this point that the special connection between politics and the debasement of language becomes clear.

13 In our time it is broadly true that political writing is bad writing. Where it is not true, it will generally be found that the writer is some kind of rebel, expressing his private opinions, and not a "party line." Orthodoxy, of whatever color, seems to demand a lifeless, imitative style. The political dialects to be found in pamphlets, leading articles, manifestos, White Papers and the speeches of Under-Secretaries do, of course, vary from party to party, but they are all alike in that one almost never finds in them a fresh, vivid, home-made turn of speech. When one watches some tired hack on the platform mechanically repeating the familiar phrases—*bestial atrocities, iron heel, blood-stained tyranny, free peoples of the world, stand shoulder to shoulder*—one often has a curious feeling that one is not watching a live human being but some kind of dummy: a feeling which suddenly becomes stronger at moments when the light catches the speaker's spectacles and turns them into blank discs which seem to have no eyes behind them. And this is not altogether fanciful. A speaker who uses that kind of phraseology has gone some distance towards turning himself into a machine. The appropriate noises are coming out of his larynx, but his brain is not involved as it would be if he were choosing his words for himself. If the speech he is making is one that he is accustomed to make over and over again, he may be almost unconscious of what he is saying, as one is when one utters the responses in church. And this reduced state of consciousness, if not indispensable, is at any rate favorable to political conformity.

14 In our time, political speech and writing are largely the defense of the indefensible. Things like the continuance of British rule in India, the Russian purges and deportations, the dropping of the atom bombs on Japan, can indeed be defended, but only by arguments which are too brutal for most people to face, and which do not square with the professed aims of political parties. Thus political language has to consist largely of euphemism, question-begging and sheer cloudy vagueness. Defenseless villages are bombarded from the air, the inhabitants driven out into the countryside, the cattle machine-gunned, the huts set on fire with incendiary bullets: this is called *pacification*. Millions of peasants are robbed of their

farms and sent trudging along the roads with no more than they can carry: this is called *transfer of population* or *rectification of frontiers*. People are imprisoned for years without trial, or shot in the back of the neck or sent to die of scurvy in Arctic lumber camps: this is called *elimination of unreliable elements*. Such phraseology is needed if one wants to name things without calling up mental pictures of them. Consider for instance some comfortable English professor defending Russian totalitarianism. He cannot say outright, "I believe in killing off your opponents when you can get good results by doing so." Probably, therefore, he will say something like this:

> While freely conceding that the Soviet régime exhibits certain features which the humanitarian may be inclined to deplore, we must, I think, agree that a certain curtailment of the right to political opposition is an unavoidable concomitant of transitional periods, and that the rigors which the Russian people have been called upon to undergo have been amply justified in the sphere of concrete achievement.

The inflated style is itself a kind of euphemism. A mass of Latin words falls upon the facts like soft snow, blurring the outlines and covering up all the details. The great enemy of clear language is insincerity. When there is a gap between one's real and one's declared aims, one turns as it were instinctively to long words and exhausted idioms, like a cuttlefish squirting out ink. In our age there is no such thing as "keeping out of politics." All issues are political issues, and politics itself is a mass of lies, evasions, folly, hatred and schizophrenia. When the general atmosphere is bad, language must suffer. I should expect to find—this is a guess which I have not sufficient knowledge to verify—that the German, Russian and Italian languages have all deteriorated in the last ten or fifteen years, as a result of dictatorship.

But if thought corrupts language, language can also corrupt thought. A bad usage can spread by tradition and imitation, even among people who should and do know better. The debased language that I have been discussing is in some ways very convenient. Phrases like *a not unjustifiable assumption, leaves much to be desired, would serve no good purpose, a consideration which we should do well to bear in mind,* are a continuous temptation, a packet of aspirins always at one's elbow. Look back through this essay, and for certain you will find that I have again and again committed the very faults I am protesting against. By this morning's post I have received a pamphlet dealing with conditions in Germany. The author tells me that he "felt impelled" to write it. I open it at random, and here is almost the first sentence that I see: "[The Allies] have an opportunity not only of achieving a radical transformation of Germany's social and political structure in such a way as to avoid a nationalistic reaction in Germany itself, but at the same time of laying the foundations of a cooperative and unified Europe." You see, he "feels impelled" to write—feels, presumably, that he has something new to say—and yet his words, like cavalry horses answering the bugle, group themselves automatically into the familiar dreary pattern. This invasion of one's mind by ready-made phrases (*lay the foundations, achieve a radical transformation*) can only be prevented if one is constantly on guard against them, and every such phrase anaesthetizes a portion of one's brain.

17   I said earlier that the decadence of our language is probably curable. Those who deny this would argue, if they produced an argument at all, that language merely reflects existing social conditions, and that we cannot influence its development by any direct tinkering with words and constructions. So far as the general tone or spirit of a language goes, this may be true, but it is not true in detail. Silly words and expressions have often disappeared, not through any evolutionary process but owing to the conscious action of a minority. Two recent examples were *explore every avenue* and *leave no stone unturned*, which were killed by the jeers of a few journalists. There is a long list of fly-blown metaphors which could similarly be got rid of if enough people would interest themselves in the job; and it should also be possible to laugh the *not un-* formation out of existence,[3] to reduce the amount of Latin and Greek in the average sentence, to drive out foreign phrases and strayed scientific words, and, in general, to make pretentiousness unfashionable. But all these are minor points. The defense of the English language implies more than this, and perhaps it is best to start by saying what it does *not* imply.

18   To begin with, it has nothing to do with archaism, with the salvaging of obsolete words and turns of speech, or with the setting

[3]One can cure oneself of the *not un-* formation by memorizing this sentence: *A not unblack dog was chasing a not unsmall rabbit across a not ungreen field.*

up of a "standard English" which must never be departed from. On the contrary, it is especially concerned with the scrapping of every word or idiom which has outworn its usefulness. It has nothing to do with correct grammar and syntax, which are of no importance so long as one makes one's meaning clear, or with the avoidance of Americanisms, or with having what is called a "good prose style." On the other hand it is not concerned with fake simplicity and the attempt to make written English colloquial. Nor does it even imply in every case preferring the Saxon word to the Latin one, though it does imply using the fewest and shortest words that will cover one's meaning. What is above all needed is to let the meaning choose the word, and not the other way about. In prose, the worst thing one can do with words is to surrender to them. When you think of a concrete object, you think wordlessly, and then, if you want to describe the thing you have been visualizing, you probably hunt about till you find the exact words that seem to fit it. When you think of something abstract you are more inclined to use words from the start, and unless you make a conscious effort to prevent it, the existing dialect will come rushing in and do the job for you, at the expense of blurring or even changing your meaning. Probably it is better to put off using words as long as possible and get one's meaning as clear as one can through pictures or sensations. Afterwards one can choose—not simply *accept*—the phrases that will best cover the meaning, and then switch around and decide what impression one's words are likely to make on another person. This last effort of the mind cuts out all stale or mixed images, all prefabricated phrases, needless repetitions, and humbug and vagueness generally. But one can often be in doubt about the effect of a word or a phrase, and one needs rules that one can rely on when instinct fails. I think the following rules will cover most cases:

  i. Never use a metaphor, simile of other figure of speech which you are used to seeing in print.

  ii. Never use a long word where a short one will do.

  iii. If it is possible to cut a word out, always cut it out.

  iv. Never use the passive where you can use the active.

  v. Never use a foreign phrase, a scientific word or a jargon word if you can think of an everyday English equivalent.

  vi. Break any of these rules sooner than say anything outright barbarous.

19   These rules sound elementary, and so they are, but they demand a deep change of attitude in anyone who has grown used to writing in the style now fashionable. One could keep all of them and still write bad English, but one could not write the kind of stuff that I quoted in those five specimens at the beginning of this article.

20   I have not here been considering the literary use of language, but merely language as an instrument for expressing and not for concealing or preventing thought. Stuart Chase and others have come near to claiming that all abstract words are meaningless, and have used this as a pretext for advocating a kind of political quietism. Since you don't know what Fascism is, how can you struggle against Fascism? One need not swallow such absurdities as this, but one ought to recognize that the present political chaos is connected with the decay of language, and that one can probably bring about some improvement by starting at the verbal end. If you simplify your English, you are freed from the worst follies of orthodoxy. You cannot speak any of the necessary dialects, and when you make a stupid remark its stupidity will be obvious, even to yourself. Political language—and with variations this is true of all political parties, from Conservatives to Anarchists—is designed to make lies sound truthful and murder respectable, and to give an appearance of solidity to pure wind. One cannot change this all in a moment, but one can at least change one's own habits, and from time to time one can even, if one jeers loudly enough, send some worn-out and useless phrase—some *jackboot, Achilles' heel, hotbed, melting pot, acid test, veritable inferno* or other lump of verbal refuse—into the dustbin where it belongs.

From "Metaphors We Live By"

George Lakoff and Mark Johnson

CONCEPTS WE LIVE BY

1 Metaphor is for most people a device of the poetic imagination and the rhetorical flourish—a matter of extraordinary rather than ordinary language. Moreover, metaphor is typically viewed as

characteristic of language alone, a matter of words rather than thought or action. For this reason, most people think they can get along perfectly well without metaphor. We have found, on the contrary, that metaphor is pervasive in everyday life, not just in language but in thought and action. Our ordinary conceptual system, in terms of which we both think and act, is fundamentally metaphorical in nature.

The concepts that govern our thought are not just matters of 2 the intellect. They also govern our everyday functioning, down to the most mundane details. Our concepts structure what we perceive, how we get around in the world, and how we relate to other people. Our conceptual system thus plays a central role in defining our everyday realities. If we are right in suggesting that our conceptual system is largely metaphorical, then the way we think, what we experience, and what we do every day is very much a matter of metaphor.

But our conceptual system is not something we are normally 3 aware of. In most of the little things we do every day, we simply think and act more or less automatically along certain lines. Just what these lines are is by no means obvious. One way to find out is by looking at language. Since communication is based on the same conceptual system that we use in thinking and acting, language is an important source of evidence for what that system is like.

Primarily on the basis of linguistic evidence, we have found 4 that most of our ordinary conceptual system is metaphorical in nature. And we have found a way to begin to identify in detail just what the metaphors are that structure how we perceive, how we think, and what we do.

To give some idea of what it could mean for a concept to be 5 metaphorical and for such a concept to structure an everyday activity, let us start with the concept ARGUMENT and the conceptual metaphor ARGUMENT IS WAR. This metaphor is reflected in our everyday language by a wide variety of expressions:

Argument is War

Your claims are *indefensible*.

He *attacked* every weak point in my argument.

His criticisms were right on *target*.

I *demolished* his argument.

I've never *won* an argument with him.

You disagree? Okay, *shoot!*

If you use that *strategy,* he'll *wipe you out.*

He *shot down* all of my arguments.

6   It is important to see that we don't just *talk* about arguments in terms of war. We can actually win or lose arguments. We see the person we are arguing with as an opponent. We attack his positions and we defend our own. We gain and lose ground. We plan and use strategies. If we find a position indefensible, we can abandon it and take a new line of attack. Many of the things we *do* in arguing are partially structured by the concept of war. Though there is no physical battle, there is a verbal battle, and the structure of an argument—attack, defense, counter-attack, etc.— reflects this. It is in this sense that the ARGUMENT IS WAR metaphor is one that we live by in this culture; it structures the actions we perform in arguing.

7   Try to imagine a culture where arguments are not viewed in terms of war, where no one wins or loses, where there is no sense of attacking or defending, gaining or losing ground. Imagine a culture where an argument is viewed as a dance, the participants are seen as performers, and the goal is to perform in a balanced and aesthetically pleasing way. In such a culture, people would view arguments differently, experience them differently, carry them out differently, and talk about them differently. But *we* would probably not view them as arguing at all: they would simply be doing something different. It would seem strange even to call what they were doing "arguing." Perhaps the most neutral way of describing this difference between their culture and ours would be to say that we have a discourse form structured in terms of battle and they have one structured in terms of dance.

8   This is an example of what it means for a metaphorical concept, namely, ARGUMENT IS WAR, to structure (at least in part) what we do and how we understand what we are doing when we argue. *The essence of metaphor is understanding and experiencing one kind of thing in terms of another.* It is not that arguments are a subspecies of war. Arguments and wars are different kinds of

things—verbal discourse and armed conflict—and the actions performed are different kinds of actions. But ARGUMENT is partially structured, understood, performed, and talked about in terms of WAR. The concept is metaphorically structured, the activity is metaphorically structured, and, consequently, the language is metaphorically structured.

Moreover, this is the *ordinary* way of having an argument and talking about one. The normal way for us to talk about attacking a position is to use the words "attack a position." Our conventional ways of talking about arguments presuppose a metaphor we are hardly ever conscious of. The metaphors not merely in the words we use—it is in our very concept of an argument. The language of argument is not poetic, fanciful, or rhetorical; it is literal. We talk about arguments that way because we conceive of them that way—and we act according to the way we conceive of things.

The most important claim we have made so far is that metaphor is not just a matter of language, that is, of mere words. We shall argue that, on the contrary, human *thought processes* are largely metaphorical. This is what we mean when we say that the human conceptual system is metaphorically structured and defined. Metaphors as linguistic expressions are possible precisely because there are metaphors in a person's conceptual system. Therefore, whenever in this book we speak of metaphors, such as ARGUMENT IS WAR, it should be understood that *metaphor* means *metaphorical concept*.

THE SYSTEMATICITY OF METAPHORICAL CONCEPTS

Arguments usually follow patterns; that is, there are certain things we typically do and do not do in arguing. The fact that we in part conceptualize arguments in terms of battle systematically influences the shape arguments take and the way we talk about what we do in arguing. Because the metaphorical concept is systematic, the language we use to talk about that aspect of the concept is systematic.

We saw in the ARGUMENT IS WAR metaphor that expressions from the vocabulary of war, e.g., *attack a position, indefensible, strategy, new line of attack, win, gain ground,* etc., form a systematic way of talking about the battling aspects of arguing. It is no accident that these expressions mean what they mean when we use them to talk about arguments. A portion of the conceptual network of battle partially characterizes the concept of an argument, and the language follows suit. Since metaphorical expressions in our language are tied to metaphorical concepts in a systematic way, we can use metaphorical linguistic expressions to study the nature of metaphorical concepts and to gain an understanding of the metaphorical nature of our activities.

13 To get an idea of how metaphorical expressions in everyday language can give us insight into the metaphorical nature of the concepts that structure our everyday activities, let us consider the metaphorical concept TIME IS MONEY as it is reflected in contemporary English.

Time is Money

You're *wasting* my time.

This gadget will *save* you hours.

I don't have the time to *give* you.

How do you *spend* your time these days?

That flat tire *cost* me an hour.

I've *invested* a lot of time in her.

I don't *have enough* time to *spare* for that.

You're *running out* of time.

You need to *budget* your time.

Put aside some time for ping pong.

Is that *worth your while?*

Do you *have* much time *left?*

He's living on *borrowed* time.

You don't *use* your time *profitably.*

I *lost* a lot of time when I got sick.

Thank you for your time.

14 Time in our culture is a valuable commodity. It is a limited resource that we use to accomplish our goals. Because of the way that the concept of work has developed in modern Western culture,

where work is typically associated with the time it takes and time is precisely quantified, it has become customary to pay people by the hour, week, or year. In our culture TIME IS MONEY in many ways: telephone message units, hourly wages, hotel room rates, yearly budgets, interest on loans, and paying your debt to society by "serving time." These practices are relatively new in the history of the human race, and by no means do they exist in all cultures. They have arisen in modern industrialized societies and structure our basic everyday activities in a very profound way. Corresponding to the fact that we *act* as if time is a valuable commodity—a limited resource, even money—we *conceive* of time that way. Thus we understand and experience time as the kind of thing that can be spent, wasted, budgeted, invested wisely or poorly, saved, or squandered.

TIME IS MONEY, TIME IS A LIMITED RESOURCE, and TIME IS A VALUABLE COMMODITY are all metaphorical concepts. They are metaphorical since we are using our everyday experiences with money, limited resources, and valuable commodities to conceptualize time. This isn't a necessary way for human beings to conceptualize time; it is tied to our culture. There are cultures where time is none of these things. 15

The metaphorical concepts TIME IS MONEY, TIME IS A RESOURCE, and TIME IS A VALUABLE COMMODITY form a single system based on sub-categorization, since in our society money is a limited resource and limited resources are valuable commodities. These sub categorization relationships characterize entailment relationships between the metaphors. TIME IS MONEY entails that TIME IS A LIMITED RESOURCE, which entails that TIME IS A VALUABLE COMMODITY. 16

We are adopting the practice of using the most specific metaphorical concept, in this case TIME IS MONEY, to characterize the entire system. Of the expressions listed under the TIME IS MONEY metaphor, some refer specifically to money (*spend*, *invest*, *budget*, *profitably*, *cost*), others to limited resources (*use*, *use up*, *have enough of*, *run out of*), and still others to valuable commodities (*have*, *give*, *lose*, *thank you for*). This is an example of the way in which metaphorical entailments can characterize a coherent system of metaphorical concepts and a corresponding coherent system of metaphorical expressions for those concepts. 17

METAPHORICAL SYSTEMATICITY: HIGHLIGHTING AND HIDING

18   The very systematicity that allows us to comprehend one aspect of a concept in terms of another (e.g., comprehending an aspect of arguing in terms of battle) will necessarily hide other aspects of the concept. In allowing us to focus on one aspect of a concept (e.g., the battling aspects of arguing), a metaphorical concept can keep us from focusing on other aspects of the concept that are inconsistent with that metaphor. For example, in the midst of a heated argument, when we are intent on attacking our opponent's position and defending our own, we may lose sight of the cooperative aspects of arguing. Someone who is arguing with you can be viewed as giving you his time, a valuable commodity, in an effort at mutual understanding. But when we are preoccupied with the battle aspects, we often lose sight of the cooperative aspects.

19   A far more subtle case of how a metaphorical concept can hide an aspect of our experience can be seen in what Michael Reddy has called the "conduit metaphor." Reddy observes that our language about language is structured roughly by the following complex metaphor:

IDEAS (or MEANINGS) ARE OBJECTS.

LINGUISTIC EXPRESSIONS ARE CONTAINERS.

COMMUNICATION IS SENDING.

20   The speaker puts ideas (objects) into words (containers) and sends them (along a conduit) to a bearer who takes the idea/objects out of the word/containers. Reddy documents this with more than a hundred types of expressions in English, which he estimates account for at least 70 percent of the expressions we use for talking about language. Here are some examples:

The CONDUIT *Metaphor*

It's hard to *get* that idea *across to* him.

I *gave* you that idea.

Your reasons *came through* to us.

It's difficult to *put* my ideas *into* words.

When you *have* a good idea, try to *capture* it immediately *in* words.

Try to *pack* more thought *into* fewer words.

You can't simply *stuff* ideas *into* a sentence any old way.

The meaning is right there *in* the words.

Don't *force* your meanings *into* the wrong words.

His words *carry* little meaning.

The introduction *has* a great deal of thought *content*.

Your words seem *hollow*.

The sentence is *without* meaning.

The idea is *buried in* terribly dense paragraphs.

In examples like these it is far more difficult to see that there [21] is anything hidden by the metaphor or even to see that there is a metaphor here at all. This is so much the conventional way of thinking about language that it is sometimes hard to imagine that it might not fit reality. But if we look at what the CONDUIT metaphor entails, we can see some of the ways in which it masks aspects of the communicative process.

First, the LINGUISTIC EXPRESSIONS ARE CONTAINERS [22] FOR MEANINGS aspect of the CONDUIT metaphor entails that words and sentences have meanings in themselves, independent of any context or speaker. The MEANINGS ARE OBJECTS part of the metaphor, for example, entails that meanings have an existence independent of people and contexts. The part of the metaphor that says LINGUISTICS EXPRESSIONS ARE CONTAINERS FOR MEANING entails that words (and sentences) have meanings, again independent of contexts and speakers. These metaphors are appropriate in many situations—those where context differences don't matter and where all the participants in the conversation understand the sentences in the same way. These two entailments are exemplified by sentences like

The meaning is *right there in* the words,

which, according to the CONDUIT metaphor, can correctly be said of any sentence. But there are many cases where context does matter. Here is a celebrated one recorded in actual conversation by Pamela Downing:

Please sit in the apple-juice seat.

23   In isolation this sentence has no meaning at all, since the expression "apple-juice seat" is not a conventional way of referring to any kind of object. But the sentence makes perfect sense in the context in which it was uttered. An overnight guest came down to breakfast. There were four place settings, three with orange juice and one with apple juice. It was clear what the apple-juice seat was. And even the next morning, when there was no apple juice, it was still clear which seat was the apple-juice seat.

24   In addition to sentences that have no meaning without context, there are cases where a single sentence will mean different things to different people. Consider:

> We need new alternative sources of energy.

This means something very different to the president of Mobil Oil from what it means to the president of Friends of the Earth. The meaning is not right there in the sentence—it matters a lot who is saying or listening to the sentence and what his social and political attitudes are. The CONDUIT metaphor does not fit cases where context is required to determine whether the sentence has any meaning at all and, if so, what meaning it has.

25   These examples show that the metaphorical concepts we have looked at provide us with a partial understanding of what communication, argument, and time are and that, in doing this, they hide other aspects of these concepts. It is important to see that the metaphorical structuring involved here is partial, not total. If it were total, one concept would actually *be* the other, not merely be understood in terms of it. For example, time isn't really money. If you *spend your time* trying to do something and it doesn't work, you can't get your time back. There are no time banks. I can *give you a lot of time*, but you can't give me back the same time, though you can *give me back the same amount of time*. And so on. Thus, part of a metaphorical concept does not and cannot fit.

26   On the other hand, metaphorical concepts can be extended beyond the range of ordinary literal ways of thinking and talking into the range of what is called figurative, poetic, colorful, or fanciful thought and language. Thus, if ideas are objects, we can *dress them up in fancy clothes, juggle them, line them up nice and neat*, etc. So when we say that a concept is structured by a metaphor, we mean that it is partially structured and that it can be extended in some ways but not others.

Sexism in English: Embodiment and Language

Alleen Pace Nilsen

> If a woman is swept off a ship into the water, the cry is "Man overboard!" If she is killed by a hit-and-run driver, the charge is "manslaughter." If she is injured on the job, the coverage is "workmen's compensation." But if she arrives at a threshold marked "Men Only," she knows the admonition is not intended to bar animals or plants or inanimate objects. It is meant for her.
>
> *Alma Graham*

During the late 1960s, I lived with my husband and three young children in Kabul, Afghanistan. This was before the Russian invasion, the Afghan civil war, and the eventual taking over of the country by the Taleban Islamic movement and its resolve to return the country to a strict Islamic dynasty, in which females are not allowed to attend school or work outside their homes.

But even when we were there and the country was considered moderate rather than extremist, I was shocked to observe how different were the roles assigned to males and females. The Afghan version of the *chaderi* prescribed for Moslem women was particularly confining. Women in religious families were required to wear it whenever they were outside their family home, with the result being that most of them didn't venture outside.

The household help we hired were made up of men, because women could not be employed by foreigners. Afghan folk stories and jokes were blatantly sexist, as in this proverb: "If you see an old man, sit down and take a lesson; if you see an old woman, throw a stone."

But it wasn't only the native culture that made me question women's roles, it was also the American community within Afghanistan.

Most of the American women were like myself—wives and mothers whose husbands were either career diplomats, employees of USAID, or college professors who had been recruited to work on various contract teams. We were suddenly bereft of our traditional roles. The local economy provided few jobs for women and certainly none for foreigners; we were isolated from former friends and the social goals we had grown up with. Some of us became alcoholics, others got very good at bridge, while still others searched desperately for ways to contribute either to our families or to the Afghans.

6   When we returned in the fall of 1969 to the University of Michigan in Ann Arbor, I was surprised to find that many other women were also questioning the expectations they had grown up with. Since I had been an English major when I was in college, I decided that for my part in the feminist movement I would study the English language and see what it could tell me about sexism. I started reading a desk dictionary and making note cards on every entry that seemed to tell something different about male and female. I soon had a dog-eared dictionary, along with a collection of note cards filling two shoe boxes.

7   The first thing I learned was that I couldn't study the language without getting involved in social issues. Language and society are as intertwined as a chicken and an egg. The language a culture uses is telltale evidence of the values and beliefs of that culture. And because there is a lag in how fast a language changes—new words can easily be introduced, but it takes a long time for old words and usages to disappear—a careful look at English will reveal the attitudes that our ancestors held and that we as a culture are therefore predisposed to hold. My note cards revealed three main points. While friends have offered the opinion that I didn't need to read a dictionary to learn such obvious facts, the linguistic evidence lends credibility to the sociologic observations.

WOMEN ARE SEXY; MEN ARE SUCCESSFUL

8   First, in American culture a woman is valued for the attractiveness and sexiness of her body, while a man is valued for his physical strength and accomplishments. A woman is sexy. A man is successful.

9   A persuasive piece of evidence supporting this view are the eponyms—words that have come from someone's name—found in English. I had a two-and-a-half-inch stack of cards taken from men's names but less than a half-inch stack from women's names, and most of those came from Greek mythology. In the words that

came into American English since we separated from Britain, there are many eponyms based on the names of famous American men: Bartlett pear, boysenberry, Franklin stove, Ferris wheel, Gatling gun, mason jar, sideburns, sousaphone, Schick test, and Winchester rifle. The only common eponyms that I found taken from American women's names are Alice blue (after Alice Roosevelt Longworth), bloomers (after Amelia Jenks Bloomer), and Mae West jacket (after the buxom actress). Two out of the three feminine eponyms relate closely to a woman's physical anatomy, while the masculine eponyms (except for "sideburns" after General Burnsides) have nothing to do with the namesake's body, but, instead, honor the man for an accomplishment of some kind.

In Greek mythology women played a bigger role than they did   10 in the biblical stories of the Judeo-Christian cultures, and so the names of goddesses are accepted parts of the language in such place names as Pomona, from the goddess of fruit, and Athens, from Athena, and in such common words as *cerea* from Ceres, *psychology* from Psyche, and *arachnoid* from Arachne. However there is the same tendency to think of women in relation to sexuality as shown through the eponyms "aphrodisiac" from Aphrodite, the Greek name for the goddess of love and beauty, and "venereal disease" from Venus, the Roman name for Aphrodite.

Another interesting word from Greek mythology is *Amazon*.   11 According to Greek folk etymology, the *a-* means "without," as in *atypical* or *amoral*, while *-mazon* comes from "mazos," meaning "breast," as still seen in *mastectomy*. In the Greek legend, Amazon women cut off their right breasts so they could better shoot their bows. Apparently, the storytellers had a feeling that for women to play the active, "masculine" role the Amazons adopted for themselves, they had to trade in part of their femininity.

This preoccupation with women's breasts is not limited to the   12 Greeks; it's what inspired the definition and the name for "mammals" (from Indo-European "mammae" for "breasts"). As a volunteer for the University of Wisconsin's *Dictionary of American Regional English (DARE)*, I read a western trapper's diary from the 1830s. I was to make notes of any unusual usages or language patterns. My most interesting finding was that the trapper referred to a range of mountains as "The Teats," a metaphor based on the similarity between the shapes of the mountains and women's breasts. Because today we use the French wording "The Grand Tetons," the metaphor isn't as obvious, but I wrote to mapmakers and found the following listings: Nipple Top and Little Nipple Top near Mount Marcy in the Adirondacks; Nipple Mountain in Archuleta County, Colorado; Nipple Peak in Coke County, Texas; Nipple Butte in Pennington, South Dakota; Squaw Peak in Placer County, California (and many other locations); Maiden's Peak and Squaw Tit (they're the same mountain) in the Cascade Range in Oregon; Mary's Nipple near Salt Lake City, Utah; and Jane Russell Peaks near Stark, New Hampshire.

13   Except for the movie star Jane Russell, the women being referred to are anonymous—it's only a sexual part of their body that is mentioned. When topographical features are named after men, it's probably not going to be to draw attention to a sexual part of their bodies but instead to honor individuals for an accomplishment.

14   Going back to what I learned from my dictionary cards, I was surprised to realize how many pairs of words we have in which the feminine word has acquired sexual connotations while the masculine word retains a serious businesslike aura. For example, a *callboy* is the person who calls actors when it is time for them to go on stage, but a *callgirl* is a prostitute. Compare *sir* and *madam*. *Sir* is a term of respect, while *madam* has acquired the specialized meaning of a brothel manager. Something similar has happened to *master* and *mistress*. Would you rather have a painting "by an old master" or "by an old mistress"?

15   It's because the word *woman* had sexual connotations, as in "She's his woman," that people began avoiding its use, hence such terminology as ladies' room, lady of the house, and girl's school or school for young ladies. Those of us who in the 1970s began asking that speakers use the term *woman* rather than *girl* or *lady* were rejecting the idea that *woman* is primarily a sexual term.

16   I found two-hundred pairs of words with masculine and feminine forms; for example, *heir-heiress, hero-heroine, steward/stewardess, usher/usherette*. In nearly all such pairs, the masculine word is considered the base, with some kind of a feminine suffix being added. The masculine form is the one from which compounds are made; for example, from king/queen comes kingdom but not queendom, from sportsman/sportslady comes sportsmanship but not sportsladyship. There is one—and only one—semantic area in

which the masculine word is not the base or more powerful word. This is in the area dealing with sex, marriage, and motherhood. When someone refers to a *virgin,* a listener will probably think of a female unless the speaker specifies male or uses a masculine pronoun. The same is true for *prostitute.*

In relation to marriage, linguistic evidence shows that wed- 17 dings are more important to women than to men. A woman cherishes the wedding and is considered a bride for a whole year, but a man is referred to as a groom only on the day of the wedding. The word *bride* appears in *bridal attendant, bridal gown, bridesmaid, bridal shower,* and even *bridegroom. Groom* comes from Old Middle English *grom,* meaning "man," and in that sense is seldom used outside of the wedding. With most pairs of male/female words, people habitually put the masculine word first: *Mr. and Mrs., his and hers, boys and girls, men and women, kings and queens, brothers and sisters, guys and dolls,* and *host and hostess.* But it is the *bride and groom* who are talked about, not the *bride and groom.*

The importance of marriage to a woman is also shown by the 18 fact that when a marriage ends in death, the woman gets the title of widow. A man gets the derived title of widower. This term is not used in other phrases or contexts, but widow is seen in *widowhood, widow's peak,* and *widow's walk.* A widow in a card game is an extra hand of cards, while in typesetting it is a leftover line of type.

Changing cultural ideas bring changes to language, and since 19 I did my dictionary study three decades ago the word *singles* has largely replaced such gender-specific and value-laden terms as *bachelor, old maid, spinster, divorcée, widow,* and *widower.* In 1970 I wrote that when people hear a man called "a professional," they usually think of him as a doctor or a lawyer, but when people hear a woman referred to as "a professional," they are likely to think of her as a prostitute. That's not as true today because so many women have become doctors and lawyers, it's no longer incongruous to think of women in those professional roles.

Another change that has taken place is in wedding announce- 20 ments. They used to be sent out from the bride's parents and did not even give the names of the groom's parents. Today, most couples choose to list either all or none of the parents' names. Also it is now much more likely that both the bride and groom's picture will be in the newspaper, while twenty years ago only the bride's picture was published on the "Women's" or the "Society" page. In the weddings I have recently attended, the official has pronounced the couple "husband and wife" instead of the traditional "man and wife," and the bride has been asked if she promises to "love, honor, and cherish," instead of to "love, honor, and obey."

WOMEN ARE PASSIVE; MEN ARE ACTIVE

21   However, other wording in the wedding ceremony relates to a second point that my cards showed, which is that women are expected to play a passive or weak role while men plan an active or strong role. In the traditional ceremony the official asks, "Who gives the bride away?" and the father answers, "I do." Some fathers answer, "Her mother and I do," but that doesn't solve the problem inherent in the question. The idea that a bride is something to be handed over from one man to another bothers people because it goes back to the days when a man's servants, his children, and his wife were all considered to be his property. They were known by his name because they belonged to him, and he was responsible for their actions and their debts.

22   The grammar used in talking or writing about weddings as well as other sexual relationships shows the expectation of men playing the active role. Men *wed* women while women *become* brides of men. A man *possesses* a woman; he *deflowers* her; he *performs;* he *scores;* he *takes away* her virginity. Although a woman can *seduce* a man, she cannot offer him her virginity. When talking about virginity, the only way to make the woman the actor in the sentence is to say that "she lost her virginity," but people lose things by accident rather than by purposeful actions, and so she's only the grammatical, not the real-life, actor.

23   The reason that women brought the term *Ms.* into the language to replace *Miss* and *Mrs.* relates to this point. Many married women resent being identified in the "Mrs. Husband" form. The dictionary cards showed what appeared to be an attitude on the part of the editors that it was almost indecent to let a respectable woman's name march unaccompanied across the pages of a

dictionary. Women were listed with male names whether or not the male contributed to the woman's reason for being in the dictionary or whether or not in his own right he was as famous as the woman. For example:

> Charlotte Brontë = Mrs. Arthur B. Nicholls
>
> Amelia Earhart = Mrs. George Palmer Putnam
>
> Helen Hayes = Mrs. Charles MacArthur
>
> Jenny Lind = Mme. Otto Goldschmit
>
> Cornelia Otis Skinner = daughter of Otis
>
> Harriet Beecher Stowe = sister of Henry Ward Beecher
>
> Dame Edith Sitwell = sister of Osbert and Sacheverell

Only a small number of rebels and crusaders got into the dictionary without the benefit of a masculine escort: temperance leaders Frances Elizabeth Caroline Willard and Carry Nation, women's rights leaders Carrie Chapman Catt and Elizabeth Cady Stanton, birth control educator Margaret Sanger, religious leader Mary Baker Eddy, and slaves Harriet Tubman and Phillis Wheatley.   24

Etiquette books used to teach that if a woman had Mrs. in front of her name, then the husband's name should follow because Mrs. is an abbreviated form of Mistress and a woman couldn't be a mistress of herself. As with many arguments about "correct" language usage, this isn't very logical because Miss is also an abbreviation of Mistress. Feminists hoped to simplify matters by introducing Ms. as an alternative to both Mrs. and Miss, but what happened is that Ms. largely replaced Miss to become a catch-all business title for women. Many married women still prefer the title Mrs., and some even resent being addressed with the term Ms. As one frustrated newspaper reporter complained, "Before I can write about a woman I have to know not only her marital status but also her political philosophy." The result of such complications may contribute to the demise of titles, which are already being ignored by many writers who find it more efficient to simply use names; for example, in a business letter: "Dear Joan Garcia," instead of "Dear Mrs. Joan Garcia," "Dear Ms. Garcia," or "Dear Mrs. Louis Garcia."   25

26   Titles given to royalty show how males can be disadvantaged by the assumption that they always play the more powerful role. In British royalty when a male holds a title, his wife is automatically given the feminine equivalent. But the reverse is not true. For example, a count is a high political officer with a countess being his wife. The same pattern holds true for a duke and a duchess and a king and a queen. But when a female holds the royal title, the man she marries does not automatically acquire the matching title. For example, Queen Elizabeth's husband has the title of prince rather than king, but when Prince Charles married Diana, she became Princess Diana. If they had stayed married and he had ascended to the throne, then she would have become Queen Diana. The reasoning appears to be that since masculine words are stronger, they are reserved for true heirs and withheld from males coming into the royal family by marriage. If Prince Phillip were called "King Phillip," British subjects might forget who had inherited the right to rule.

27   The names that people give their children show the hopes and dreams they have for them, and when we look at the differences between male and female names in a culture, we can see the cumulative expectations of that culture. In our culture girls often have names taken from small, aesthetically pleasing items; for example, Ruby, Jewel, and Pearl. Esther and Stella mean "star," and Ada means "ornament." One of the few women's names that refers to strength is Mildred, and it means "mild strength." Boys often have names with meanings of power and strength; for example, Neil means "champion"; Martin is from Mars, the God of war; Raymond means "wise protection"; Harold means "chief of the army"; Ira means "vigilant"; Rex means "king"; and Richard means "strong king."

28   We see similar differences in food metaphors. Food is a passive substance just sitting there waiting to be eaten. Many people have recognized this and so no longer feel comfortable describing women as "delectable morsels." However, when I was a teenager, it was considered a compliment to refer to "a girl" (we didn't call anyone a "woman" until she was middle-aged) as "a cute tomato," "a peach," "a dish," "a cookie," "honey," "sugar," or "sweetie-pie." When being affectionate, women will occasionally

call a man "honey" or "sweetie," but in general, food metaphors are used much less often with men than with women. If a man is called "a fruit," his masculinity is being questioned. But it's perfectly acceptable to use a food metaphor if the food is heavier and more substantive than that used for women. For example, pin-up pictures of women have long been known as "cheesecake," but when Burt Reynolds posed for a nude centerfold the picture was immediately dubbed "beefcake," that is, a hunk of meat. That such sexual references to men have come into the language is another reflection of how society is beginning to lessen the differences between their attitudes toward men and women.

Something similar to the fruit metaphor happens with refer- 29 ences to plants. We insult a man by calling him a "pansy," but it wasn't considered particularly insulting to talk about a girl being "a wallflower," "a clinging vine," or a "shrinking violet," or to give girls such names as Ivy, Rose, Lily, Iris, Daisy, Camelia, Heather, and Flora. A positive plant metaphor can be used with a man only if the plant is big and strong; for example, Andrew Jackson's nickname of *Old Hickory*. Also, the phrases *blooming idiots* and *budding geniuses* can be used with either sex, but notice how they are based on the most active thing a plant can do, which is to bloom or bud.

Animal metaphors also illustrate the different expectations for 30 males and females. Men are referred to as "studs," "bucks," and "wolves," while women are referred to with such metaphors as "kitten," "bunny," "beaver," "bird," "chick," and "lamb." In the 1950s we said that boys went "tom catting," but today it's just "catting around," and both boys and girls do it. When the term "foxy," meaning that someone was sexy, first became popular it was used only for females, but now someone of either sex can be described as a "fox." Some animal metaphors that are used predominantly with men have negative connotations based on the size and/or strength of the animals; for example, "beast," "bullheaded," "jackass," "rat," "loanshark," and "vulture." Negative metaphors used with women are based on smaller animals; for example, "social butterfly," "mousey," "catty," and "vixen." The feminine terms connote action, but not the same kind of large scale action as with the masculine terms.

WOMEN ARE CONNECTED WITH NEGATIVE CONNOTATIONS; MEN WITH POSITIVE CONNOTATIONS

31 The final point that my note cards illustrated was how many positive connotations are associated with the concept of masculinity, while there are either trivial or negative connotations connected with the corresponding feminine concept. An example from the animal metaphors makes a good illustration. The word *shrew* taken from the name of a small but especially vicious animal was defined in my dictionary as "an ill-tempered scolding woman," but the word *shrewd* taken from the same root was defined as "marked by clever, discerning awareness" and was illustrated with the phrase "a shrewd businessman."

32 Early in life, children are conditioned to the superiority of the masculine role. As child psychologists point out, little girls have much more freedom to experiment with sex roles than do little boys. If a little girl acts like a tomboy, most parents have mixed feelings, being at least partially proud. But if their little boy acts like a sissy (derived from *sister*), they call a psychologist. It's perfectly acceptable for a little girl to sleep in the crib that was purchased for her brother, to wear his hand-me-down jeans and shirts, and to ride the bicycle that he has outgrown. But few parents would put a boy baby in a white-and-gold crib decorated with frills and lace, and virtually no parents would have their little boy wear his sister's hand-me-down dresses, nor would they have their son ride a girl's pink bicycle with a flower-bedecked basket. The proper names given to girls and boys show this same attitude. Girls can have "boy" names—Cris, Craig, Jo, Kelly, Shawn, Teri, Toni, and Sam—but it doesn't work the other way around. A couple of generations ago, Beverly, Frances, Hazel, Marion, and Shirley were common boys' names. As parents gave these names to more and more girls, they fell into disuse for males, and some older men who have these names prefer to go by their initials or by such abbreviated forms as Haze or Shirl.

33 When a little girl is told to be a lady, she is being told to sit with her knees together and to be quiet and dainty. But when a little boy is told to be a man, he is being told to be noble, strong, and virtuous—to have all the qualities that the speaker looks on

as desirable. The concept of manliness has such positive connotations that it used to be a compliment to call someone a *he-man*, to say that he was doubly a man. Today many people are more ambivalent about this term and respond to it much as they do to the word *macho*. But calling someone a manly man or a virile man is nearly always meant as a compliment. Virile comes from the Indo-European *vir*, meaning "man," which is also the basis of *virtuous*. Consider the positive connotations of both virile and virtuous with the negative connotations of *hysterical*. The Greeks took this latter word from their name for uterus (as still seen in *hysterectomy*). They thought that women were the only ones who experienced uncontrolled emotional outbursts, and so the condition must have something to do with a part of the body that only women have. But how word meanings change is regularly shown at athletic events where thousands of *virtuous* women sit quietly beside their *hysterical* husbands.

Differences in the connotations between positive male and negative female connotations can be seen in several pairs of words that differ denotatively only in the matter of sex. *Bachelor* as compared to *spinster* or *old maid* has such positive connotations that women try to adopt it by using the term *bachelor-girl* or *bachelorette*. *Old maid* is so negative that it's the basis for metaphors: pretentious and fussy old men are called "old maids," as are the leftover kernels of unpopped popcorn and the last card in a popular children's card game. 34

Patron and *matron* (Middle English for "father" and "mother") have such different levels of prestige that women try to borrow the more positive masculine connotations with the word *patroness*, literally "female father." Such a peculiar term came about because of the high prestige attached to *patron* in such phrases as *a patron of the arts* or *a patron saint*. *Matron* is more apt to be used in talking about a woman in charge of a jail or a public restroom. 35

When men are doing jobs that women often do, we apparently try to pay the men extra by giving them fancy titles. For example, a male cook is more likely to be called a "chef," while a male seamstress will get the title of "tailor." The armed forces have a special problem in that they recruit under such slogans as "The Marine Corps builds men!" and "Join the Army! Become a Man." Once the recruits are enlisted, they find themselves doing 36 much of the work that has been traditionally thought of as "women's work." The solution to getting the work done and not insulting anyone's masculinity was to change the titles as shown below:

waitress = orderly

nurse = medic or corpsman

secretary = clerk-typist

assistant = adjutant

dishwasher = KP (kitchen police) or kitchen helper

37   Compare *brave* and *squaw*. Early settlers in America truly admired Indian men and hence named them with a word that carried connotations of youth, vigor, and courage. But for Indian women they used an Algonquin slang term with negative sexual connotations that are almost opposite to those of brave. *Wizard* and *witch* contrast almost as much. The masculine *wizard* implies skill and wisdom combined with magic, while the feminine *witch* implies evil intentions combined with magic. When *witch* is used for men, as in *witch-doctor,* many mainstream speakers feel some carry-over of the negative connotations.

38   Part of the unattractiveness of both *witch* and *squaw* is that they have been used so often to refer to old women, something with which our culture is particularly uncomfortable, just as the Afghans were. Imagine my surprise when I ran across the phrases *grandfatherly advice* and *old wives' tales* and realized that the underlying implication is the same as the Afghan proverb about old men being worth listening to while old women talk only foolishness.

39   Other terms that show how negatively we view old women as compared to young women are *old nag* as compared to *filly,* *old crow* or *old bat* as compared to *bird,* and being *catty* as compared to being *kittenish.* There is no matching set of metaphors for men. The chicken metaphor tells the whole story of a woman's life. In her youth she is a "chick." Then she marries and begins "feathering her nest." Soon she begins feeling "cooped up," so she goes to "hen parties" where she "cackles" with her friends. Then she has her "brood," begins to "henpeck" her husband, and finally turns into an old "biddy."

I embarked on my study of the dictionary not with the intentions of prescribing language change but simply to see what the language would tell me about sexism. Nevertheless, I have been both surprised and pleased as I've watched the changes that have occurred over the past three decades. I'm one of those linguists who believes that new language customs will cause a new generation of speakers to grow up with different expectations. This is why I'm happy about people's efforts to use inclusive languages, to say "he or she" or "they" when speaking about individuals whose names they do not know. I'm glad that leading publishers have developed guidelines to help writers use language that is fair to both sexes. I'm glad that most newspapers and magazines list women by their own names instead of only by their husbands' names. And I'm so glad that educated and thoughtful people no longer begin their business letters with "Dear Sir" or "Gentlemen," but instead use a memo form or begin with such salutations as "Dear Colleagues," "Dear Reader," or "Dear Committee Members." I'm also glad that such words as *poetess, authoress, conductress,* and *aviatrix* now sound quaint and old-fashioned and that *chairman* is giving way to *chair* or *head, mailman* to *mail carrier, clergyman* to *clergy,* and *stewardess* to *flight attendant.* I was also pleased when the National Oceanic and Atmospheric Administration bowed to feminist complaints and in the late 1970s began to alternate men's and women's names for hurricanes. However, I wasn't so pleased to discover that the change did not immediately erase sexist thoughts from everyone's mind, as shown by a headline about Hurricane David in a 1979 New York tabloid, "David Rapes Virgin Islands." More recently a similar metaphor appeared in a headline in the *Arizona Republic* about Hurricane Charlie, "Charlie Quits Carolinas, Flirts with Virginia."

What these incidents show is that sexism is not something existing independently in American English or in the particular dictionary that I happened to read. Rather, it exists in people's minds. Language is like an X-ray in providing visible evidence of invisible thoughts. The best thing about people being interested in and discussing sexist language is that as they make conscious decisions about what pronouns they will use, what jokes they will tell or laugh at, how they will write their names, or how they will begin their letters, they are forced to think about the underlying issue of sexism. This is good because as a problem that begins in people's assumptions and expectations, it's a problem that will be solved only when a great many people have given it a great deal of thought.

For Argument's Sake: Why Do We Feel Compelled to Fight About Everything?

Deborah Tannen

1　I was waiting to go on a television talk show a few years ago for a discussion about how men and women communicate, when a man walked in wearing a shirt and tie and a floor-length skirt, the top of which was brushed by his waist-length red hair. He politely introduced himself and told me that he'd read and liked my book *You Just Don't Understand,* which had just been published. Then he added, "When I get out there, I'm going to attack you. But don't take it personally. That's why they invite me on, so that's what I'm going to do."

2　We went on the set and the show began. I had hardly managed to finish a sentence or two before the man threw his arms out in gestures of anger, and began shrieking—briefly hurling accusations at me, and then railing at length against women. The strangest thing about his hysterical outburst was how the studio audience reacted: They turned vicious—not attacking me (I hadn't said anything substantive yet) or him (who wants to tangle with someone who screams at you?) but the other guests: women who had come to talk about problems they had communicating with their spouses.

3　My antagonist was nothing more than a dependable provocateur, brought on to ensure a lively show. The incident has stayed with me not because it was typical of the talk shows I have appeared on—it wasn't, I'm happy to say—but because it exemplifies the ritual nature of much of the opposition that pervades our public dialogue.

Everywhere we turn, there is evidence that, in public discourse, we prize contentiousness and aggression more than cooperation and conciliation. Headlines blare about the Starr Wars, the Mommy Wars, the Baby Wars, the Mammography Wars; everything is posed in terms of battles and duels, winners and losers, conflicts and disputes. Biographies have metamorphosed into demonographies whose authors don't just portray their subjects warts and all, but set out to dig up as much dirt as possible, as if the story of a person's life is contained in the warts, only the warts, and nothing but the warts.

It's all part of what I call the argument culture, which rests on the assumption that opposition is the best way to get anything done: The best way to discuss an idea is to set up a debate. The best way to cover news is to find people who express the most extreme views and present them as "both sides." The best way to begin an essay is to attack someone. The best way to show you're really thoughtful is to criticize. The best way to settle disputes is to litigate them.

It is the automatic nature of this response that I am calling into question. This is not to say that passionate opposition and strong verbal attacks are never appropriate. In the words of the Yugoslavian-born poet Charles Simic, "There are moments in life when true invective is called for, when it becomes an absolute necessity, out of a deep sense of justice, to denounce, mock, vituperate, lash out, in the strongest possible language." What I'm questioning is the ubiquity, the knee-jerk nature of approaching almost any issue, problem or public person in an adversarial way.

Smashing heads does not open minds. In this as in so many things, results are also causes, looping back and entrapping us. The pervasiveness of warlike formats and language grows out of, but also gives rise to, an ethic of aggression: We come to value aggressive tactics for their own sake—for the sake of argument. Compromise becomes a dirty word, and we often feel guilty if we are conciliatory rather than confrontational—even if we achieve the result we're seeking.

Here's one example. A woman called another talk show on which I was a guest. She told the following story: "I was in a place where a man was smoking, and there was a no-smoking sign. Instead of saying 'You aren't allowed to smoke in here. Put that out!' I said, 'I'm awfully sorry, but I have asthma, so your smoking makes it hard for me to breathe. Would you mind terribly not smoking?' When I said this, the man was extremely polite and solicitous, and he put his cigarette out, and I said, 'Oh, thank you, thank you!' as if he'd done a wonderful thing for me. Why did I do that?"

9   I think this woman expected me—the communications expert—to say she needs assertiveness training to confront smokers in a more aggressive manner. Instead, I told her that her approach was just fine. If she had tried to alter his behavior by reminding him of the rules, he might well have rebelled: "Who made you the enforcer? Mind your own business!" She had given the smoker a face-saving way of doing what she wanted, one that allowed him to feel chivalrous rather than chastised. This was kinder to him, but it was also kinder to herself, since it was more likely to lead to the result she desired.

10   Another caller disagreed with me, saying the first caller's style was "self-abasing." I persisted: There was nothing necessarily destructive about the way the woman handled the smoker. The mistake the second caller was making—a mistake many of us make—was to confuse ritual self-effacement with the literal kind. All human relations require us to find ways to get what we want from others without seeming to dominate them.

11   The opinions expressed by the two callers encapsulate the ethic of aggression that has us by our throats, particularly in public arenas such as politics and law. Issues are routinely approached by having two sides stake out opposing positions and do battle. This sometimes drives people to take positions that are more adversarial than they feel—and can get in the way of reaching a possible resolution. I have experienced this firsthand.

12   For my book about the workplace, *Talking from 9 to 5,* I spent time in companies, shadowing people, interviewing them and having individuals tape conversations when I wasn't there. Most companies were happy to proceed on a verbal agreement setting forth certain ground rules: Individuals would control the taping, identifying names would be changed, I would show them what I wrote about their company and change or delete

anything they did not approve. I also signed confidentiality agreements promising not to reveal anything I learned about the company's business.

Some companies, however, referred the matter to their attor- 13 neys so a contract could be written. In no case where attorneys became involved—mine as well as theirs—could we reach an agreement on working together.

Negotiations with one company stand out. Having agreed on 14 the procedures and safeguards, we expected to have a contract signed in a matter of weeks. But six months later, after thousands of dollars in legal fees and untold hours of everyone's time, the negotiations reached a dead end. The company's lawyer was demanding veto power over my entire book; it meant the company could (if it chose) prevent me from publishing the book even if I used no more than a handful of examples from this one company. I could not agree to that. Meanwhile, my lawyer was demanding for me rights to use the videotapes of conversations any way I wanted. The company could not agree to that; it meant I could (if I chose) put videotapes of their company on national television, make them look bad, reveal company secrets and open them up to being sued by their own employees.

The people I was working with at the company had no desire 15 to pass judgment on any part of my book that did not involve them, and I had no intention of using the videotapes except for analysis. These extreme demands could have been easily dismissed by the principals—except they had come after months of wrangling with the language of drafts passed back and forth. Everybody's patience and good will had worn out. The adversarial nature of the legal process had polarized us beyond repair.

Requiring people to behave like enemies can stir up mutual 16 enmity that remains long after a case has been settled or tried, and the lawyers have moved on. Because our legal system is based on the model of ritual battle, the object—like the object of all fights—is to win, and that can interfere with the goal of resolving disputes.

The same spirit drives the public discourse of politics and the 17 press, which are increasingly being given over to ritual attacks. On Jan. 18, 1994, retired admiral Bobby Ray Inman withdrew as nominee for secretary of defense after several news stories raised questions about his business dealings and his finances. Inman, who had held high public office in both Democratic and Republican administrations, explained that he did not wish to serve again because of changes in the political climate—changes that resulted in public figures being subjected to relentless attack. Inman said he was told by one editor, "Bobby, you've just got to get thicker skin. We have to write a bad story about you every day. That's our job."

18   Everyone seemed to agree that Inman would have been confirmed. The news accounts about his withdrawal used words such as "bizarre," "mystified" and "extraordinary." A New York Times editorial reflected the news media's befuddlement: "In fact, with the exception of a few columns, . . . a few editorials and one or two news stories, the selection of Mr. Inman had been unusually well received in Washington." This evaluation dramatizes just how run-of-the-mill systematic attacks have become. With a wave of a subordinate clause ("a few editorials . . . "), attacking someone personally and (from his point of view) distorting his record are dismissed as so insignificant as to be unworthy of notice.

19   The idea that all public figures should expect to be criticized ruthlessly testifies to the ritualized nature of such attack: It is not sparked by specific wrongdoing but is triggered automatically.

20   I once asked a reporter about the common journalistic practice of challenging interviewees by repeating criticism to them. She told me it was the hardest part of her job. "It makes me uncomfortable," she said. "I tell myself I'm someone else and force myself to do it." But, she said she had no trouble being combative if she felt someone was guilty of behavior she considered wrong. And that is the crucial difference between ritual fighting and literal fighting: opposition of the heart.

21   It is easy to find examples throughout history of journalistic attacks that make today's rhetoric seem tame. But in the past, such vituperation was motivated by true political passion, in contrast with today's automatic, ritualized attacks—which seem to grow out of a belief that conflict is high-minded and good, a required and superior form of discourse.

22   The roots of our love for ritualized opposition lie in the educational system that we all pass through. Here's a typical scene: The teacher sits at the head of the classroom, pleased with herself and her class. The students are engaged in a heated debate. The

very noise level reassures the teacher that the students are participating. Learning is going on. The class is a success.

But look again, cautions Patricia Rosof, a high school history 23
teacher who admits to having experienced just such a wave of satisfaction. On closer inspection, you notice that only a few students are participating in the debate; the majority of the class is sitting silently. And the students who are arguing are not addressing subtleties, nuances or complexities of the points they are making or disputing. They don't have that luxury because they want to win the argument—so they must go for the most dramatic statements they can muster. They will not concede an opponent's point—even if they see its validity—because that would weaken their position.

This aggressive intellectual style is cultivated and rewarded 24
in our colleges and universities. The standard way to write an academic paper is to position your work in opposition to someone else's. This creates a need to prove others wrong, which is quite different from reading something with an open mind and discovering that you disagree with it. Graduate students learn that they must disprove others' arguments in order to be original, make a contribution and demonstrate intellectual ability. The temptation is great to oversimplify at best, and at worst to distort or even misrepresent other positions, the better to refute them.

I caught a glimpse of this when I put the question to someone 25
who I felt had misrepresented my own work: "Why do you need to make others wrong for you to be right?" Her response: "It's an argument!" Aha, I thought, that explains it. If you're having an argument, you use every tactic you can think of—including distorting what your opponent just said—in order to win.

Staging everything in terms of polarized opposition limits the 26
information we get rather than broadening it. For one thing, when a certain kind of interaction is the norm, those who feel comfortable with that type of interaction are drawn to participate, and those who do not feel comfortable with it recoil and go elsewhere. If public discourse included a broad range of types, we would be making room for individuals with different temperaments. But when opposition and fights overwhelmingly predominate, only those who enjoy verbal sparring are likely to take part. Those who cannot comfortably take part in oppositional discourse—or choose not to—are likely to opt out.

27   But perhaps the most dangerous harvest of the ethic of aggression and ritual fighting is—as with the audience response to the screaming man on the television talk show—an atmosphere of animosity that spreads like a fever. In extreme forms, it rears its head in road rage and workplace shooting sprees. In more common forms, it leads to what is being decried everywhere as a lack of civility. It erodes our sense of human connection to those in public life—and to the strangers who cross our paths and people our private lives.

Fan Profanity

Howard M. Wasserman

1   Many free-speech controversies, especially on college campuses, are grounded in concerns for civility, politeness, and good taste. They also tend to follow the same path and end the same way. A government entity regulates speech in an effort to elevate discourse, limit the profane and protect public and personal sensitivities; courts strike down the regulations as violating the First Amendment freedom of speech; and we end up right where we started.

2   Colleges may be pursuing a similar course in trying to deal with objectionable cheering by students at sporting events. University of Maryland officials expressed anger and embarrassment following a men's basketball game against conference rival Duke University in January 2004, when fans chanted and sported T-shirts with the slogan "F--- Duke" and directed epithets at Duke players. This was one of many incidents of offensive or obnoxious cheering by students throughout the country during the 2004 college basketball season.

3   John K. Anderson, chief of the Educational Affairs Division of the Maryland Attorney General's Office, advised the university that a written code of fan conduct applicable at a university-owned and -operated athletic facility, if "carefully drafted," would be constitutionally permissible. University of Maryland Associate Athletics Director Michael Lipitz began working with a committee of

students to consider rules of conduct. The committee ultimately recommended that the university promote voluntary compliance, although rules and formal punishment remain a "last resort" if a proposed standing monitoring committee determines that voluntary compliance is ineffective. Other schools, such as Western Michigan University, currently have, or are studying the need for, similar codes to restrict profanity and other abusive language. And the approach of a new academic year may bring new incidents and new university attempts at regulating fan expression.

One can envision guidelines restricting profanity and epithets 4 in signs and chants, as well as imposing a general requirement that students keep things stylish, clever, clean, and classy. Presumably, the sanction would be removal from the arena. The ostensible purpose behind such guidelines is to enable the majority of fans to enjoy the game unburdened by objectionable or offensive signs, messages, and chants. But any such policy enacted and enforced at a public university such as Maryland should not and perhaps will not survive First Amendment scrutiny. On the other hand, a private college, not bound by the strictures of the First Amendment, obviously remains free to impose such restrictions.

The speech at issue is expression by fans related to a sporting 5 event, to all aspects of the game and all the participants in the game—what we can call "cheering speech." Cheering speech can be directed at players, coaches, officials, executives, administrators, or other fans. It can be in support of one's own players and team, against the opposing players and team or even critical of one's own players and team. It can be about events on the field or it can target broader social and political issues surrounding the game, the players on sport in general.

In advising the university that it could regulate cheering 6 speech, Anderson insisted that fans at sporting events, particularly children, are "captive auditors." They are captives in the arena or stadium; the only way to avoid being offended by the chants or signs is to leave the arena or stop coming to games. This captive status, Anderson argued, alters the ordinary First Amendment burden. Rather than requiring objecting listeners to "avert their eyes" (or ears) to avoid objectionable speech, the university can force speakers, especially students, to alter their manner of communicating to protect the sensibilities of these captive fans.

7   In reality, the captive-audience doctrine is far more limited than Anderson suggests. Courts have found listeners to be captives in only four places: their own homes, the workplace, public elementary and secondary schools, and inside and around abortion clinics. And even in those places, captive-audience status permits government to limit oral expression but not the same message in written form on pickets, signs, or clothing. One certainly could avert one's eyes to avoid viewing the message written on a sign or on the body of a student at a basketball game.

8   Of course, one problem with cheering speech is that much of it is oral. Fans have complained not only about signs and T-shirts, but also about chants and taunts targeting players, coaches and officials, which other fans may be unable to avoid no matter where in the arena they sit. Objectors must perform the more difficult task to averting their ears to avoid offensive cheers, something that children may be even less able to do. It is true that courts have upheld content-neutral regulations on sound and noise levels to protect captive audiences, beginning with the Supreme Court case *Kovacs v. Cooper* in 1949. But government never has been permitted to protect captive auditors by singling out particular profane or offensive oral messages for selective restriction while leaving related messages on the same subject, uttered at the same volume, undisturbed.

9   More important, the captive-audience doctrine never has been applied to listeners in public places of recreation and entertainment, places to which people voluntarily go for the particular purpose of engaging in expressive activity, in this case cheering on their favorite college team. Fans who pay to attend a college basketball game at an on-campus arena are not captive auditors there, any more than an individual walking on a city street who stumbles across an objectionable political rally or an individual whose office sits above the route of an objectionable parade.

10   The Hobson's Choice that Anderson believes this creates for fans—leave the arena and stop attending games or tolerate offensive cheers—is precisely the choice people make in any public place at which expression occurs. It is the same choice that people in the California courthouse had to make when confronted with a jacket emblazoned with the message "F--- the Draft," a message and manner of expression that the Supreme Court found

to be protected from prosecution under a disturbing-the-peace statute in the 1971 landmark case *Cohen v. California*. In fact, leaving was even less of an option there for an objecting auditor whose job required her to remain in the courthouse or an objector conducting business before the court and likely required to be there on pain of contempt or default. It is difficult to reconcile that "F--- the Draft" is a protected message in a courthouse, but "F--- Duke" is unprotected amid the cacophony of 20,000 screaming basketball fans. It is even less comprehensible that Paul Cohen's intellectual heir could be prohibited from wearing his jacket (for example, to protest the so-called "backdoor draft"[1] created by extending reservists' service) at a university sports arena governed by a fan speech code.

The real import of *Cohen* is the principle that a speaker's 11 choice of words and manner of communication are essential elements of the overall message expressed and government cannot prohibit certain words or manner without also suppressing certain messages in the process. A cheering fan's point of view is bound up in the decision to formulate a particular message by telling an opponent that he "sucks" or by targeting more personal issues. Fans have created controversy by targeting a player whose girlfriend had posed in *Playboy*, chanting "rapist" at a player who had pled guilty to sexual assault and waving fake joints at a player with a history of use. "Fear the Turtle," "We Hate Duke" and "Duke Sucks" are three ways of cheering for the Maryland Terrapins, as well as cheering against Duke. But each conveys a distinct message and point of view and each has ample grounds for constitutional protection within the expressive milieu of a college sports stadium.

Because word choice and communicative manner are essen- 12 tial components of free-speech protection, it becomes impossible to enforce any fan-conduct policy in a uniform, non-arbitrary way. The state cannot neutrally define what words or manner are offensive or establish any meaningful standard to measure offensiveness. Justice John Marshall Harlan's memorable phrase in *Cohen* was that "one man's vulgarity is another's lyric," and government's

---

[1]Some say that extending the hours of duty of National Guard and reservist troops beyond their expected length of time amounts to a form of conscription.

inability to make principled distinctions means "the Constitution leaves matters of taste and style so largely to the individual."

13   Under current doctrine, offensiveness cannot be measured from the standpoint of the most sensitive person in the crowd; the level of permissible expression cannot be reduced to what the least-tolerant listener will accept. Nor should it be measured from the standpoint of children in the crowd, because, as the Court long has insisted, the level of discourse for an adult audience cannot be reduced to what is fit or proper for children. The university sports arena exemplifies the problem of the mixed audience—how can government regulate speech in the interest of protecting children when the speech occurs before a mixed audience of children and adults? The pithy answer may be that it simply cannot do so. There is no, and can be no, baseline for oral speech before a mixed audience; either children unavoidably hear some "adult" expression or we reduce the level of speech to what is suitable for a sandbox.

14   In seeking to control abusive cheering speech, universities apparently do not distinguish among expressive forms. On one hand is blatant use of profanity; on the other hand are epithets or chants that do not employ any of the seven dirty words, but that target opposing teams, players, coaches or officials, perhaps with references to personal life or criminal difficulties. The presumption apparent in Anderson's recommendation to the University of Maryland was that a public university could serve the same interest in protecting children through a single conduct policy that banned both "F--- Duke" chants and signs and chants and signs targeting a player accused of sexual assault. One can imagine attempts to require students to keep things "polite" or "positive"—cheer for your team and your players, but do not jeer or criticize the opponent (or, for that matter, your own team). Even conceding a government interest in protecting sensitive and juvenile ears from the seven dirty words in public spaces, government goes a step beyond when it begins to restrict particular nonprofane messages that bear on the game played on the field or on the participants in that game.

15   Moreover, the sexual-assault example presents on additional wrinkle. Taunting a player who has been accused of sexual assault may be, at least in part, a social or political statement, protesting or drawing attention to the problem of athlete misbehavior or to

the fact that this player continues to be allowed to play for the school despite his off-court misconduct.

Perhaps the level of protection turns on the subtlety of the 16 chants. Students are obvious in their attempts to offend when they use profanity, chant "rapist," or wave fake joints. But what if Maryland students chant or wear T-shirts bearing the slogan "Duck Fuke"? This is an obvious play on the profanity that created controversy at Maryland, but it does not use (as opposed to hinting at) dirty words. Should hinting at profanity be enough to justify a restriction on protected manner of expression?

Or what if the offensiveness is lost on those who might oth- 17 erwise be offended? Students at Allen Field House at the University of Kansas were praised for their cleverness during the 2004 season when they chanted "salad tosser" at Texas Tech Basketball Coach Bob Knight. On the surface, the taunt was a reference to Knight's infamous verbal altercation several days earlier with the Texas Tech chancellor at a salad bar in Lubbock. But the phrase also is a slang reference to a particular sexual act, a double entendre the students surely knew when they began the chant, but many listeners likely did not.

Dissenting in *Cohen,* justice Harry Blackmun derided Paul 18 Cohen's jacket as "an absurd and immature antic." By contrast, Justice Harlan insisted that the expression at issue was, in fact, of "no small constitutional consequence." Free-speech scholars laud *Cohen* for recognizing that government must leave matters of expressive taste and style to the individual. One could dismiss offensive signs, T-shirts and taunts at college basketball games as similarly absurd and immature antics. However, as in *Cohen,* skirmishes over what fan expression will be permitted at public university sporting events are of no small constitutional consequence.

College sport has become, for better or for worse, a central 19 part of college life and culture. The prevailing belief among university administrators and most commentators is that successful athletic teams, particularly in high-profile football and men's basketball, can be a source of university pride, publicity, media attention, revenue and increased donations. The non-athlete students who pack the stadium provide an essential ingredient of that overall culture. Students are encouraged to attend games and make noise, to be excited and passionate about their school, to cheer for their team and players (and against the opposing team and players), and to create a playing environment that will be intimidating or distracting to the opponent and will give their team a homecourt advantage. Indeed, it is somewhat ironic that Duke players were at the receiving end of the taunts that prompted Maryland to consider an arena speech code. Duke students have attained wide notoriety for their sometimes-clever, sometimes-offensive cheering speech and the headaches they cause opposing teams and players.

20   The grandstand at the arena or stadium has become the central public forum for cheering speech. Fans are invited to the arena and encouraged to speak, loudly and in however vivid or stark terms, to support, oppose, cheer, jeer, criticize and even taunt teams, players, coaches, and officials in that game. Having created this forum for students to express themselves, a public university has ceded control over the manner in which students do so, at least within the parameters of protected speech. Fans must remain free to jeer as well as cheer players and teams and in as blatant or profane a manner as they wish.

21   Perhaps one may not particularly enjoy sitting, or having one's children sit, in an arena where students are shouting expletives throughout the game. But commitment to a neutral free-speech principle means tolerating a great deal of speech that one personally does not like or does not wish to hear. And there is nothing wrong with hortatory efforts by the university, coaches and, most important, other students to encourage fans, especially student fans, to keep their cheering stylish, clean, classy, and creative. The "voluntary compliance" policies recommended in June by the student committee at university of Maryland included a program under which students could exchange profane T-shirts for noncontroversial ones, contests that would encourage appropriate signs and banners, having coaches address students about the need for good sportsmanship and fan behavior and distributing newspapers at games with "creative witty cheers" for students to use.

22   The point is that a state university may not formally punish— even via non-criminal sanction such as removal from the arena— those students who depart generally accepted norms by loudly

wielding a particular loaded word to inform officials or opposing players that they are not very good at what they do.

How to Tame a Wild Tongue
Gloria Anzaldúa

We're going to have to control your tongue," the dentist says, 1 pulling out all the metal from my mouth. Silver bits plop and tinkle into the basin. My mouth is a motherlode. The dentist is cleaning out my roots. I get a whiff of the stench when I gasp. "I can't cap that tooth yet, you're still draining," he says.

"We're going to have to do something about your tongue," I 2 hear the anger rising in his voice. My tongue keeps pushing out the wads of cotton, pushing back the drills, the long thin needles. "I've never seen anything as strong or as stubborn," he says. And I think, how do you tame a wild tongue, train it to be quiet, how do you bridle and saddle it? How do you make it lie down?

> Who is to say that robbing a people of its language is less violent than war?
>
> *Ray Gwyn Smith*[1]

I remember being caught speaking Spanish at recess—that was 3 good for three licks on the knuckles with a sharp ruler. I remember being sent to the corner of the classroom for "talking back" to the Anglo teacher when all I was trying to do was tell her how to pronounce my name. "If you want to be American, speak 'American.' If you don't like it, go back to Mexico where you belong."

"I want you to speak English. *Pa' hallar buen trabajo tienes que* 4 *saber hablar el inglés bien. Qué vale toda tu educatión si todavía hablas inglés con un* 'accent,'" my mother would say, mortified that I spoke English like a Mexican. At Pan American University, I and all Chicano students were required to take two speech classes. Their purpose: to get rid of our accents.

Attacks on one's form of expression with the intent to censor 5 are a violation of the First Amendment. *El Anglo con care de inocente nos arrancó la lengua.* Wild tongues can't be tamed, they can only be cut out.

OVERCOMING THE TRADITION OF SILENCE

*Ahogadas, escupimos el oscuro. Peleando con
nuestra propia sombra el silencio nos sepulta.*

6 *En boca cerrada no entran moscas.* "Flies don't enter a closed mouth"
is a saying I kept hearing when I was a child. *Ser habladora* was to
be a gossip and a liar, to talk too much. *Muchachitas bien criadas,* well-
bred girls don't answer back. *Es una falta de respeto* to talk back to
one's mother or father. I remember one of the sins I'd recite to the
priest in the confession box the few times I went to confession: talking back to my mother, *hablar pa' 'tras, repelar. Hocicona, repelona,
chismosa,* having a big mouth, questioning, carrying tales are all signs
of being *mal criada.* In my culture they are all words that are deroga-
tory if applied to women—I've never heard them applied to men.

7   The first time I heard two women, a Puerto Rican and a
Cuban, say the word *"nosotras,"* I was shocked. I had not known
the word existed. Chicanas use *nosotros* whether we're male or
female. We are robbed of our female being by the masculine plu-
ral. Language is a male discourse.

> And our tongues have become dry the wilderness has dried out
> our tongues and we have forgotten speech.
>
> *Irena Klepfisz*[2]

8   Even our own people, other Spanish speakers *nos quieren poner
candados en la boca.* They would hold us back with their bag of
reglas de academia.

OYÉ COMO LADRA: EL LENGUAJE DE LA FRONTERA

Quien tiene boca se equivoca.
    Mexican saying

9 *"Pocho,* cultural traitor, you're speaking the oppressor's language
by speaking English, you're ruining the Spanish language," I have
been accused by various Latinos and Latinas. Chicano Spanish is
considered by the purist and by most Latinos deficient, a mutilation of Spanish.

But Chicano Spanish is a border tongue which developed nat- 10
urally. Change, *evolución, enriquecimiento de palabras nuevas por
invención o adopción* have created variants of Chicano Spanish,
un nuevo lenguaje. Un lenguaje que corresponde a un modo de vivir.
Chicano Spanish is not incorrect, it is a living language.

For a people who are neither Spanish nor live in a country in 11
which Spanish is the first language; for a people who live in a
country in which English is the reigning tongue but who are not
Anglo; for a people who cannot entirely identify with either standard (formal, Castilian) Spanish nor standard English, what
recourse is left to them but to create their own language? A language which they can connect their identity to, one capable of
communicating the realities and values true to themselves—a language with terms that are neither *español ni inglés,* but both. We
speak a patois, a forked tongue, a variation of two languages.

Chicano Spanish sprang out of the Chicanos' need to identify 12
ourselves as a distinct people. We need a language with which we
could communicate with ourselves, a secret language. For some
of us, language is a homeland closer than the Southwest—for
many Chicanos today live in the Midwest and the East. And
because we are a complex, heterogeneous people, we speak many
languages. Some of the languages we speak are

1. Standard English
2. Working-class and slang English
3. Standard Spanish
4. Standard Mexican Spanish
5. North Mexican Spanish dialect
6. Chicano Spanish (Texas, New Mexico, Arizona, and California
   have regional variations)
7. Tex-Mex
8. *Pachuco* (called *caló*)

My "home" tongues are the languages I speak with my sister 13
and brothers, with my friends. They are the last five listed, with
6 and 7 being closest to my heart. From school, the media, and job
situations, I've picked up standard and working class English.
From Mama-grande Locha and from reading Spanish and Mexican literature, I've picked up Standard Spanish and Standard Mexican Spanish. From *los recién llegados,* Mexican immigrants, and

braceros, I learned the North Mexican dialect. With Mexicans I'll try to speak either Standard Mexican Spanish or the North Mexican dialect. From my parents and Chicanos living in the Valley, I picked up Chicano Texas Spanish, and I speak it with my mom, younger brother (who married a Mexican and who rarely mixes Spanish with English), aunts, and older relatives.

14   With Chicanas from *Nuevo México* or *Arizona* I will speak Chicano Spanish a little, but often they don't understand what I'm saying. With most California Chicanas I speak entirely in English (unless I forget). When I first moved to San Francisco, I'd rattle off something in Spanish, unintentionally embarrassing them. Often it is only with another Chicana *tejano* that I can talk freely.

15   Words distorted by English are known as anglicisms or *pochismos.* The *pocho* is an anglicized Mexican or American of Mexican origin who speaks Spanish with an accent characteristic of North Americans and who distorts and reconstructs the language according to the influence of English.[3] Tex-Mex, or Spanglish, comes most naturally to me. I may switch back and forth from English to Spanish in the same sentence or in the same word. With my sister and my brother Nune and with Chicano *tejano* contemporaries I speak in Tex-Mex.

16   From kids and people my own age I picked up *Pachuco.* *Pachuco* (the language of the zoot suiters) is a language of rebellion, both against Standard Spanish and Standard English. It is a secret language. Adults of the culture and outsiders cannot understand it. It is made up of slang words from both English and Spanish. *Ruca* means girl or woman, *vato* means guy or dude, *chale* means no, *simón* means yes, *churro* is sure, talk is *periquiar,* *pigionear* means petting, *que gacho* means how nerdy, *ponte águila* means watch out, death is called *la pelona.* Through lack of practice and not having others who can speak it, I've lost most of the *Pachuco* tongue.

CHICANO SPANISH

17   Chicanos, after 250 years of Spanish/Anglo colonization, have developed significant differences in the Spanish we speak. We collapse two adjacent vowels into a single syllable and sometimes

shift the stress in certain words such as *maíz/maiz, cohete/cuete*. We leave out certain consonants when they appear between vowels: *lado/lao, mojado/mojao*. Chicanos from South Texas pronounce *f* as *j* as in *jue* (*fue*). Chicanos use "archaisms," words that are no longer in the Spanish language, words that have been evolved out. We say *semos, truje, haiga, ansina,* and *naiden*. we retain the "archaic" *j*, as in *jalar*, that derives from an earlier *h* (the French *halar* or the Germanic *halon* which was lost to standard Spanish in the sixteenth century), but which is still found in several regional dialects such as the one spoken in South Texas. (Due to geography, Chicanos from the Valley of South Texas were cut off linguistically from other Spanish speakers. We tend to use words that the Spaniards brought over from Medieval Spain. The majority of the Spanish colonizers in Mexico and the Southwest came from Extremadura—Hernán Cortés was one of them—and Andalucía. Andalucians pronounce *ll* like a *y*, and their *d*'s tend to be absorbed by adjacent vowels: *tirado* becomes *tirao*. They brought *el lenguaje popular, dialectos y regionalismos*.)[4]

    Chicanos and other Spanish speakers also shift *ll* to *y* and *z* to *s*.[5] We leave out initial syllables, saying *tar* for *estar, toy* for *estoy, hora* for *ahora* (*cubanos* and *puertorriqueños* also leave out initial letters of some words). We also leave out the final syllable such as *pa* for *para*. The intervocalic *y*, the *ll* as in *tortilla, ella, botella*, gets replaced by *tortia* or *tortiya, ea, botea*. We add an additional syllable at the beginning of certain words: *atocar* for *tocar, agastar* for *gastar*. Sometimes we'll say *lavaste las vacijas*, other times *lavates* (substituting the *ates* verb endings for the *aste*). 18

    We used anglicisms, words borrowed from English: *bola* from ball, *carpeta* from carpet, *máchina de lavar* (instead of *lavadora*) from washing machine. Tex-Mex argot, created by adding a Spanish sound at the beginning or end of an English word such as *cookiar* for cook, *watchar* for watch, *parkiar* for park, and *rapiar* for rape, is the result of the pressures on Spanish speakers to adapt to English. 19

    We don't use the word *vosotros/as* or its accompanying verb form. We don't say *claro* (to mean yes), *imagínate*, or *me emociona*, unless we picked up Spanish from Latinas, out of a book, or in a classroom. Other Spanish-speaking groups are going through the same, or similar, development in their Spanish. 20

LINGUISTIC TERRORISM

> *Deslenguadas. Somos los del español deficiente.* We are your lin-
> guistic nightmare, your linguistic aberration, your linguistic
> *mestisaje,* the subject of your *burla.* Because we speak with
> tongues of fire we are culturally crucified. Racially, culturally,
> and linguistically *somos huérfanos*—we speak an orphan
> tongue.

21   Chicanas who grew up speaking Chicano Spanish have internalized the belief that we speak poor Spanish. It is illegitimate, a bastard language. And because we internalize how our language has
been used against us by the dominant culture, we use our language differences against each other.

22   Chicana feminists often skirt around each other with suspicion and hesitation. For the longest time I couldn't figure it out.
Then it dawned on me. To be close to another Chicana is like
looking into the mirror. We are afraid of what we'll see there.
Pena. Shame. Low estimation of self. In childhood we are told
that our language is wrong. Repeated attacks on our native
tongue diminish our sense of self. The attacks continue throughout our lives.

23   Chicanas feel uncomfortable talking in Spanish to Latinas,
afraid of their censure. Their language was not outlawed in their
countries. They had a whole lifetime of being immersed in their
native tongue; generations, centuries in which Spanish was a first
language, taught in school, heard on radio and TV, and read in
the newspaper.

24   If a person, Chicana or Latina, has a low estimation of my
native tongue, she also has a low estimation of me. Often with
mexicanas y latinas we'll speak English as a neutral language. Even
among Chicanas we tend to speak English at parties or conferences. Yet, at the same time, we're afraid the other will think we're
agringadas because we don't speak Chicano Spanish. We oppress
each other trying to out-Chicano each other, vying to be the "real"
Chicanas, to speak like Chicanos. There is no one Chicano language just as there is no one Chicano experience. A monolingual
Chicana whose first language is English or Spanish is just as much
a Chicana as one who speaks several variants of Spanish. A

Chicana from Michigan or Chicago or Detroit is just as much a Chicana as one from the Southwest. Chicano Spanish is as diverse linguistically as it is regionally.

By the end of this century, Spanish speakers will comprise the biggest minority group in the United States, a country where students in high schools and colleges are encouraged to take French classes because French in considered more "cultured." But for a language to remain alive it must be used.[6] By the end of this century English, and not Spanish, will be the mother tongue of most Chicanos and Latinos.

So, if you want to really hurt me, talk badly about my language. Ethnic identity is twin skin to linguistic identity—I am my language. Until I can take pride in my language, I cannot take pride in myself. Until I can accept as legitimate Chicano Texas Spanish, Tex-Mex, and all the other languages I speak, I cannot accept the legitimacy of myself. Until I am free to write bilingually and to switch codes without having always to translate, while I still have to speak English or Spanish when I would rather speak Spanglish, and as long as I have to accommodate the English speakers rather than having them accommodate me, my tongue will be illegitimate.

I will no longer be made to feel ashamed of existing. I will have my voice: Indian, Spanish, white. I will have my serpent's tongue—my woman's voice, my sexual voice, my poet's voice. I will overcome the tradition of silence.

> My fingers
> move sly against your palm
> Like women everywhere, we speak in code . . .
> *Melanie Kaye/Kantrowitz*[7]

NOTES

1. Ray Gwyn Smith, *Moorland Is Cold Country,* unpublished book.
2. Irena Klepfisz, *"Di rayze aheym/*The Journey Home," in *The Tribe of Dina: A Jewish Women's Anthology,* Melanie Kaye/Kantrowitz and Irena Klepfisz, eds. (Montpelier, VT: Sinister Wisdom Books, 1986), 49.

3. R. C. Ortega, *Dialectologia Del Barrio*, trans. Hortencia S. Alwan (Los Angeles, CA: R. C. Ortega Publisher & Bookseller, 1977), 132.

4. Eduardo Hernandéz-Chávez, Andrew D. Cohen, and Anthony F. Beltramo, *El Lenguaje de los Chicanos: Regional and Social Characteristics of Language Used by Mexican Americans* (Arlington, VA: Center for Applied Linguistics, 1975), 39.

5. Hernandéz-Chávez, xvii.

6. Irena Klepfisz, "Secular Jewish Identity: Yidishkayt in America," in *The Tribe of Dina*, Kaye/Kantrowitz and Klepfisz, eds., 43.

7. Melanie Kaye/Kantrowitz, "Sign," in *We Speak in Code: Poems and Other Writings* (Pittsburgh, PA: Motheroot Publications, Inc., 1980), 85.

Arguing on the Internet

Luis Poza

1   I remember my first experience in public debate on a computer network. I forget if it was Usenet access I enjoyed as a student at San Francisco State University, or if it was on the discussion forums at GEnie, one of those "Online Services" like Prodigy before general dial-up Internet access became available for $20 a month.

2   I had wandered into a discussion area on gun control, and read a couple of posts. Nothing really representative, just what had been posted recently. I then quite naively decided to post my own beliefs on the issue. Now, such discussion groups were relatively new (it was in the very early 1990's, when web pages were just being invented), and I had no idea what was waiting for me. Worse, I had not before engaged in public debate, nor had I carefully studied the topic in detail. I just had some uninformed personal opinions, untested by opposing listeners—in other words, weak views, not founded in fact, just casual opinions. And I publicly posted them in the gun control forum.

3   I might as well have just walked into a maximum security prison stark naked and shouted, "fresh meat!"

Needless to say, the pro-gun advocates went into a feeding 4
frenzy. When you're on an Internet discussion group in a disputed
topic populated by extremists on both sides, anyone showing
naiveté immediately draws out even those who don't usually participate in debate, taking the golden opportunity to "win" an
argument, demonstrating how right they are against an opponent
who presents very little risk of making a skilled riposte. Within
hours, my post had drawn about a dozen replies by the pro-gun
element, all of them gleefully tearing my statement to shreds.

It was a very sudden and powerful education. 5

I could have simply been repelled by the reaction, ashamed 6
of how foolish I must have appeared, and avoided visiting such
places ever again in hopes of forgetting it had ever happened. If
I had done so, things would have developed so that I probably
would never have started this blog. Instead, I hung on, took the
electronic beating, and decided to rough out my inglorious debut
on the discussion groups, maintaining my arguments while putting a great deal of effort into finding out the facts, hopefully
never to post so naively again. I felt my opinions were essentially
correct, I just didn't have the facts at my disposal to prove it.

· And so began my career debating social and political issues over 7
the Internet, an experience which has not been a waste of time. While
I doubt I have converted too many souls, the experience has nonetheless provided a strong incentive to study, to research the subjects I am
commenting on. It has vastly sharpened my debating skills, teaching
me through painful experience how to engage in public debate. And
more than just a few times it has proven me wrong (more often on
small points than on broad ones) and taught me things I probably
would not have learned elsewhere or otherwise. The main problem,
and what keeps me from engaging in such forum debates for too
many months is the fact that I tend to be wordy (you haven't
noticed?), and if I am present long enough on a forum, researching
my points and writing new posts begin to eat up too many hours of
my day, leaving me little free time—even more frustrating when my
debate opponents never do their research but demand I do mine to
a tee. This blog took over as an alternative once I figured out the Movable Type system; nevertheless, I am sure I will find a new discussion
group somewhere and jump in again, for another several months at
least, before it gets to be too much work again.

8   But that's not what I wanted to write about.

9   More specifically, that history is just background to the main point I intended for this post: how to argue and debate on the Internet. Like any other endeavor, there are tricks and strategies and techniques and pitfalls. I felt like going over a few, to share a bit of what I've learned. That's part of what a blog is for, right? Showing off and acting all superior. So here goes.

10   As I've mentioned, the first thing you should do is to research your topic. Relying on what you think you know without checking can be perilous. Your opponents have search engines ready and waiting, not to mention their collective experience—you will be writing in opposition to dozens, if not hundreds of people; though few will come out and reply, it will more often be those who know more about the particular facts of the case that you have brought up. If you get your facts wrong, there will be several people ready to jump down your throat, point out all your errors, and proclaim you to be their bitch.

11   You also have to be honest in how you present your information; you cannot ignore contradictory evidence. You cannot only quote the facts that support your case. True, that is easier on a blog, but a blog is more about exposition and less about debate. I hope that in this blog, I never commit the former offense, and not very often the latter. But in a forum debate, where vociferous antagonists wait readily to prove you wrong, you can't get away with that kind of stuff. So save yourself the embarrassment and attacks and check yourself. Say what you know you can support with facts from a credible source. Quote your cited material in the correct context. And don't omit contradictory evidence, because someone else will bring it up anyway and make you look like your were hiding it. Instead, quote it and refute it right away.

12   Next, remember to explain yourself sufficiently. This can be hard. We all think within our own minds, and we fully understand our own context. We often mistakenly assume others will as well. That's a common error that my college writing students commit, making it hard sometimes for me to understand what they are writing about. For example, let's say that I want to explain a political point to my students, who are all Japanese. If I explained to them, for example, Bush's Social Security plan, in the same way I write about it here on this blog, they would not

understand. They do not have the social or political context, nor an understanding of the nature of the American pension system or its history, the kind of stuff Americans will absorb through experience.

That's an extreme example, though; usually the kind of con- 13 text differential you experience will be much more subtle. An example of that would be one time in a college linguistics course when the topic of "English as the official language" came up. A lot of students in the class got angry with me because I suggested that English was a logical base language for universal communication within the U.S. They were angry not at my concept of a common linguistic experience serving as a communications bridge, but at what they assumed to be the underlying context of making English into the only respected or required language, disenfranchising other languages and cultures—meanings I had not spoken and did not intend to relay. The meaning of a word or a set of ideas can be very tricky when each individual presumes different definitions and connotations.

In short, you must explain your argument in detail, not 14 depending on people to make the same assumptions you do—they most often will not, especially if they have a different ideology than you have.

Next, do "opposition research." After forming your argument, 15 look at it from the other side. If you were to argue against your own writing, how would you go about it? What holes would you poke in it? What research would you do to try to get ammunition to knock it down? Then apply those findings to your argument, shoring up weaknesses, tearing out easily assailed segments, and adding fortifications in the form of added evidence or further argumentation.

Finally, edit. Cut. Whittle. It is a common failing for a writer to 16 say everything they want to say, to make every point they think of. Especially for gabby writers like me. One of the first things an opponent will do is pick out your weakest argument and focus on that. If you give three different points in your argument, one strong, one moderate, and one weak, guess which one will get attacked? So cut the weak one, and if possible, the moderate one as well.

That leads me to how you should deal with your debate 17 opponent. As I said, they will attack your weakest point—but they will also use that as an excuse to fully avoid your strongest point. This can wholly decimate even the strongest argument. A case in point: Bush's National Guard disgrace. Public debate was fierce about that one, and Bush's argument was weak in the face of many unexplained facts, or facts that could not be challenged. I collected and detailed those facts in a blog post. There was a lot of damning stuff, and the arguments showing Bush had gotten special preference and dodged the draft, and then later deserted the Guard and was never punished for it; these arguments were pretty strong, and Bush's denials sounded pretty weak.

18   Then the *60 Minutes* story on Bush came out, and the Killian memos, though described by those who served at the time to be more or less accurate, were shown to be fakes. And at that, the debate was over. Sure, the fakes did not weaken any of the other evidence by one iota, nor did they exonerate Bush, proving he did nothing wrong. But in a debate, if one side sets forth a weak point that can be just obliterated by the other side, all the stronger facts and arguments seem to vanish, and the other side will proclaim righteous victory—and the audience will accept it. Try it out: read my blog post <http://www.blogd.com/archives/000458.html.>, and go to even a moderate citizen and state the facts. Their reply will almost certainly center on the faked memos, even though they are irrelevant to the other facts of the case. I am certain that Bush would have loved to give Dan Rather a big wet one right on the lips, as Rather had handed him a huge victory.

19   The same goes for your own arguments: get something wrong, forward a weak point, and your opponents will find it easy to attack the weak point and completely ignore all of your iron-clad arguments. So don't give them the chance. Get rid of the weak stuff yourself, before you present your argument to others. Force your opponents to face only your strongest arguments and nothing else. Sure, they may use straw men anyway, but don't give them the opportunity to gain the same advantage without resorting to trickery.

20   Even still, opponents will focus on even the smallest details to nitpick, avoiding the main thrust of your argument. That happens a lot when conservatives come to comment on my blogging. After the Killian memos were shown up, I posted on the outstanding weight of evidence against Bush in his National Guard

misdeeds. In my list of evidence, I included a document that was not fake—but one conservative visitor jumped on that one document and tried to tie it in with the discredited memos. That was his response to a long, well-evidenced writing demonstrating how Bush dodged the draft by using his family's influence, and then went AWOL without being punished—99% of my argument was just ignored and a single detail was attacked, as if to discredit the whole argument. That will happen to you, so be prepared.

If a debate opponent does any of this, and you want them to   21 answer the strong points or the main thrust of your argument, then press them. Word your main point and prime evidence as succinctly as possible, then demand that they respond to it before anything else. Usually they'll shut up at that point. Which makes the case for being as succinct as possible in the first place— something I'm not good at.

Aside from avoiding the strong points and focusing on the   22 weak ones, your opponents will try other tricks. The next most common one will be the undocumented source. After all, if you can't see where they got their "facts," how can you respond to them? One of the most common examples of that technique on this blog is in the discussions about the ratings for the Air America Radio network. When I post about Air America Radio doing well, conservative readers often respond with attacks about how AAR's ratings are in the toilet, how Limbaugh and Dr. Laura and others are doing well and AAR is showing poorly, etc. etc. But few ever cite specifics, nor do they usually cite sources. The reason becomes apparent when I demand they do and the results show up: their sources are usually right-wing rags which ignore vital data (e.g., they quote overalls and ignore demographics), cherry-pick their data (pointing to the least successful AAR stations or shows while touting conservative strongholds), and intentionally mislead with vague and inaccurate representations (for example, one conservative journalist blasted AAR because of ratings one member radio station got before AAR even went on their air).

So when your opponent cites any information and you don't   23 know where to find the original, press them for it, demand they produce it, and refuse to accept their argument until they do. Naturally, you're going to have to be prepared to do the same— but that was my first point of advice in any case, and it only serves to strengthen your argument. So certify your data, and don't let your opponent get away with passing off shoddy merchandise.

24   Certifying the data can be tricky in itself. Take the AAR ratings. Media ratings are tricky. The original *Star Trek* was cancelled on the weight of its bad ratings, but when it had finally been killed off, a network analyst told the network executives that they'd just killed their most popular show. How could that be? Demographics. If the audience for a show is made up more of people with disposable income, then low overall numbers don't mean much. Many of Rush Limbaugh's listeners, on the other hand, are older people who do not spend as much. Air America performs poorly in overall ratings, but does very well in demographics, which is why they're still on the air, picking up more sponsors and expanding into new markets.

25   But the main argument conservative journalists make about AAR failing is in its ratings—and even though they have access to the expensive demographic data for radio, they only refer to the overall ratings—because those look the worst.

26   Furthermore, don't let them get away with grabbing "facts" from biased sites. If their source was Michelle Malkin, Ann Coulter or Bill O'Reilly, call them out on it. If you cited Al Franken, Jesse Jackson, and Janeane Garofalo as your sources, chances are your opponent would call you out for it. Point that out to them if they try to pawn off Rush Limbaugh or Joe Scarborough as credible sources for data. And, of course, keep to the same standards in your own writing.

27   If they do come up with apparently credible sources, then investigate. Never take it for granted. When I first started debating gun control, I was overwhelmed by the number of facts and figures that the pro-gun advocates peppered their arguments with. I almost was ready to throw in the towel when I started getting the feeling that I was being lied to—some of the "facts" they produced sounded fishy. That's when I discovered that SFSU had started an account with Lexis Nexis, and started doing searches—and immediately discovered that my opponents' source of "facts" had been NRA literature; seemingly credible sources either turned out to be biased or simply were reporting the biased data. Lexis also provided me with powerful

supplies of ammunition to shoot back with, in addition to cutting down my opponents' arguments as being full of half-truths, shoddy and biased studies, and NRA propaganda. I went from almost losing the argument to actually winning it; I recall that in the end, only one opponent survived the arguments I posed, and he was a professional writer. And in the end, he was reduced to admitting that the law stood behind my statements, adding that he felt the Supreme Court justices would burn in hell for their judgments interpreting the 2nd Amendment to apply only to organized militias like the National Guard. But then, he was a professional writer, which meant he was less willing to ignore facts.

And that'll be another roadblock to winning arguments: 28 obstinacy. Pigheadedness. The stubborn refusal of an opponent to admit a point, no matter how clearly you have presented your evidence, no matter how desperately weak and unsupported their own argument may be. You'll always come up against people who will never admit they're wrong, even when faced with overwhelming evidence to the contrary. With the Bush National Guard case, it did not matter in the least to Bush supporters that there was ironclad proof that Bush had used his family influence to get into the guard and was catapulted to officer rank and the much-sought piloting slot after just a few days, after scoring the absolute minimum (25%) on his aptitude test. These facts are not in question, they are firmly established. But try to approach a conservative on a debate forum and get them to admit that Bush used undue influence to get into the Guard and avoid Vietnam. It'll be like pulling teeth, except that teeth at one point or another finally come out.

So the above points should be a guide to surviving (or at least 29 tolerating) public debate on the Internet—or, in reverse, a guide to obfuscating and winning arguments by cheating. If you want to win the quick and dirty way, just pick at the weakest point in your opponents' writing, make up fake facts and refuse to cite your sources, mine the ultra-biased talking heads for ammo (again, don't cite), avoid making any arguments yourself except for the most vague and insinuating kinds, and never, ever admit to being wrong no matter how badly you get thrashed—just keep insisting that you're right.

2

Dissent and Censorship: Should Law Abridge the Freedom of Speech?

The Zenger Case Revisited:

Satire, Sedition and Political Debate in Eighteenth Century America

Alison Olson

1 On 4 August 1734 Governor William Cosby of New York, stung by a series of satirical attacks that had appeared in John Peter Zenger's *New York Weekly Journal*, brought the printer to trial for publishing a seditious libel. Zenger's attorney conceded at the outset that his client had done the printing; by most existing legal precedent the fact of publication was all that the jury was to consider, and the judges, who could be expected to side with the governor, were to determine the libelousness of the content. But in this case the attorney for the printer went on to argue that the precedent was in fact not binding; the jury, not the judge, should consider the content of the attacks as well as the act of publication and should acquit his client if the articles were based on truth. The jury agreed: after a brief recess they returned with a verdict of "not guilty." As a result of the trial, a rapacious governor was momentarily humbled and a powerful defense lawyer turned into a popular hero; the story of the trial came to be written up by the defense in a way that has made it grist for popular history ever since.

But does it provide anything more than a good story? Recent 2 writers have said a regretful "No." Preoccupied with the search for a binding legal precedent, they have found in the case nothing more than an inconclusive partisan confrontation. It did not produce across-the-board freedom of the press (nor did any of Zenger's advocates argue that this was a good thing). It did not change the English definition of a free press or of libel. It did not even affect the outcome of the upcoming election. Stephen Botein called its "celebrity as a landmark case" no longer justified, and thought the case "nothing more than a matter of historical accident" (11). Leonard Levy thought that "Zenger's acquital had little if any appreciable effect upon the freedom of the press in New York or elsewhere in the colonies" (Levy 1985, 37, 45; see also Levy 1960), and Stanley Katz agreed: the trial "did not directly further the development either of political liberty or of freedom of the press in America" (34). James Morton Smith, studying the press for a later period, found the issues addressed in the Zenger case still unsettled by the last decade of the eighteenth century. A gloomy set of verdicts to be sure.

But are these nay-sayers really correct? If they are, how do we 3 explain the explosive growth of satirical attacks on various colonial governments in the decades immediately after the case was settled? Before the trial the only political satires that could be safely printed were those written by imperial officials themselves, governors and proprietary representatives, in particular.[1] In the years between the trial and the Stamp Act, by contrast, over two dozen political satires appeared in print, virtually all of them in opposition to established governments and imperial officials. Fables, parodied speeches and proclamations, mock addresses, lethal thrusts masquerading as praise appeared in pamphlets, broadsides, poets' corners, advertisements, news items, and the like; of all the printers of these items only one was prosecuted (even his charges were dropped).[2] Our futile search for binding precedents, it would seem, has made us miss what the Zenger trial really did accomplish: it made possible the dynamic growth of political expression in the colonies by making it relatively safe for American writers to publish political humor—particularly satire—critical of men in office.

Before the Zenger case there was no agreed upon procedure 4 for trying a political satirist for seditious libel in either England or America. Americans had never tried such a case; English precedents were inconsistent though of late they had been tending to go against printers. In two English trials less than a decade before Zenger's, the guilt or innocence of accused printers had been left to judges who labeled virtually all humorous attacks on the government threats to political stability and hence seditious libels. After Zenger's acquittal, by contrast, American courts generally left determination of guilt or innocence to juries likely to see such satire as a useful correction to political transgressions and hence to excuse the printers: public officials, be they royal governors or locally elected legislators, were loath to prosecute cases they could not win.

5   But there was more to it even than that. After the trial, any politician was a fool to take a satirist to court. The Zenger case lay at the crossroads of literature and law. It revealed that the press and the courts together could produce a kind of double trial, not only for the satirist, but also for the public official he satirized. Satire isolated, tried, condemned and pilloried the objects of its attack by showing that they had violated community norms. If the targeted official then decided to charge the satirist with libel, the satirist would defend himself by arguing that he had portrayed community values as everyone understood them, and the official's behavior exactly as everyone saw him, so the official's reputation itself would be on trial again. And if, like the Zenger jury, the jurors believed the truth of the charges, the governor, not the printer, would be convicted in the court of public opinion. Zenger's *Journal* used satire to mock the Governor and his supporters; Zenger's lawyers used it to mock the prosecuting attorney.[3] Since satire tried people by laughter, Zenger's case was in effect a trial of a trial in which the defense attorney used satire to defend satirists. A "style" of courtroom performance intersected with a style of journalism; a vision of the newspaper world where humorists ridiculed men in power before a public audience intersected with a vision of the courtroom functioning the same way. Above all, the *Journal* and the trial revealed that satire could focus the values of an American provincial community, make clear that a politician had not respected them, and show that laughter was the gentlest way of belittling and isolating him and even of turning him out. The trial was, therefore, an essential step in legitimizing the emerging opposition in a fledgling

political democracy. It could, indeed, be a landmark without its verdict determining the legal outcome of any further trials.

The outline of the trial is clear. . . .   6

The *Journal*, which had first appeared in November 1733, was 7 essentially the mouthpiece of two of the Governor's leading political opponents, James Alexander and Lewis Morris, bent on revenge for Cosby's dismissal of Morris from his position as Chief Justice for the colony. The idea of an opposition paper in the colonies was not entirely new when the *Journal* began production. A decade earlier James Franklin's *New England Courant* had jibed satirically at Massachusetts officialdom until Franklin himself had been jailed and forced to apologize. But the *Courant* had been as much a literary journal as newspaper, its direct concerns were far more with the smallpox inoculation than with politics, and it had lost its punch when Franklin was jailed (Clark 136, 127, 137, 177; Tourtellot 256–57). The *Journal* took up where the *Courant* had left off. It attacked Cosby in a veriety of ways, mixing long solemn passages and shorter quotes from a leading London opposition journal, the *Independent Reflector,* with partisan reports of domestic affairs, articles purporting to be about neighboring colonies but in fact raising questions, about New York, songs and satirical poems about the fickleness of government support and even more satirical mock advertisements containing thinly disguised descriptions of the Governor or his supporters. The serious tracts took up the bulk of the columns but the satirical pieces were funnier and far harder for the Governor to respond to; significantly, the four issues ordered by the Governor to be burnt all contained particularly witty satirical ads or poems.

The humorous contributions that worried the government so 8 much emerged in the colonies from a satirical style of political attack that had been developing in the Anglo-American world, particularly on the English side, over the first quarter of the eighteenth century. The earlier works of Dryden and Shaftesbury fueled an explosion of English satirical literature which was at its greatest from the late 1720s to the late 1750s, peaking in the years when Zenger's *Journal* appeared. The extraordinary group of English satirists writing then included Pope, Gay, Swift, Bolingbroke, Pulteney, and enough other interested authors to raise the number of pamphlets about satire from twelve in the 1720s to sixty-one in the 1730s.

9   The appearance of a generation of great satirists, all of whom opposed Walpole's administration, was hardly fortuitous: it correlated exactly with a change in English law about censorship of the press. In the seventeenth century satirical attacks on the government were likely to be headed off before they were printed, by licensing acts in England and the colonies which required government approval before writings could be published. In 1695, however, Parliament refused to renew the English Licensing Act and similar acts were subsequently relaxed in the various colonies; publications were no longer censored before they were published but were subject ot prosecution—generally for libel— once they had appeared. This meant two things: first, rather than attempting to decide the subversiveness of material before it was printed the government now waited to assess its effect on the public. Second, if the criticisms of the government were to be effective and at the same time avoid prosecution, they must be carefully disguised, packaged as innocent humor whose intent to attack the government could not be proven in court.

10   How did one banter against the government and get away with it? The satirists developed a bag of techniques which made it extremely difficult to prove beyond legal doubt just who or what they were talking about. They got at their subjects by suggestion rather than direct identification, using methods suggested by Jonathan Swift. "First, never to print a man's name out at length; but as I do that of Mr. Stggesle. . . Secondly, by putting cases; thirdly by insinuation; fourthly by celebrating the actions of others, who acted directly contrary to the persons we would reflect on; fifthly, by nicknames . . . which everybody can tell how to apply" (see Spector 6–7).[4] They wrote histories of past events or societies or governments which could pass for generalized commentaries on humanity but in fact were thinly disguised descriptions of current parallels. They created fictionalized accounts or travels abroad to countries that strikingly resembled their own, or fictionalized commentaries of travelers from abroad. They described animal behavior when they were really referring to people or, following the guidelines Swift had drawn up to help writers avoid legal prosecution, they identified people with only the first and last letters of their names. The *Journal* picked up on these disguises: one of defense attorney Andrew Hamilton's earliest points

in Zenger's defense was "I own, when I read the Information I had not the art to find out that the Governour was the Person meant in every Period of that Newspaper" (*Case and Tryal* 19).

Free to publish political attacks without censorship, but 11 constrained to disguise those attacks in order to avoid prosecution once their works had appeared in print, writers made the most of satirical techniques to attack political figures, especially unpopular ministers like Sir Robert Walpole and his associates. They came to regard satire as a substitute for law, as a way to reveal the public crimes of men they could not reach through the courts. "Where law cannot extend its awe and authority, satire wields the scourge of disgrace" (Stevens 100), they wrote; it "shake[s] the writer beyond the reach of law" (Harte 1). Through ridicule satirists tried public figures in a court of public opinion, assured their conviction by laughter and sentenced them to the pillory of public scorn: getting people to laugh at a public official could disgrace him almost as badly as condemnation by a court of law.

It is the publicness of the laughter that is important here, its 12 effectiveness in what Michael Warner calls the "public sphere of print discourse" (57; see also Burke 270 and Gilreath). Satire's object was to hold its victim up to public scorn by poking fun at him: it "intentionally humiliated" (Ingram 51), and in so doing it flattered the intelligence of readers who were able to recognize both the person targeted and the behavior that provoked the attack. The community of citizens judged for themselves whether a writing was "valid" (and therefore, in the case of satire, funny) or not. Satire temporarily bonded its readers in laughter, thereby isolating its victim further. Since it shrank people through mockery it was particularly useful in reducing "great men" to disposable size.

For both public officials and their opposition, satire offered a 13 gamble. For a critic of the government to print satire was risky, but for the government to take the satirist to court for libel was even more so. The printer/author took the chance that his publication might be shut down or his voice silenced during or after a libel trial if the publisher could find no one to pay his costs or take his place while he was in jail. The defendants/satirists were further handicapped at the trial by the fact that judges, appointed by the same royal authority as the targeted officials, and in some cases dependent on those officials for influence at court, generally decided the libellousness of works in question and juries generally representing readers were left only to decide if the publications originated in the shop of the accused printer.

14   So the political satirist faced possible prosecution in a trial where he might not be whole heartedly supported even by those who shared his political views. On the other hand, publications marked for government prosecution sold especially well (printers actually made extra copies of pamphlets or journal issues they expected to be the object of government attack); being prosecuted was itself a measure of success (the government would not go after something beneath its notice), and the printer's conviction in court was not likely to reduce the damage already done to the public official satirized. Printing satire was a risk, but probably one worth taking.

15   The satirist had to gamble on publication; his victim had to gamble on taking the author to court, and for the politician who found himself the butt of satire, the risks involved in bringing his critic to trial were even greater. At the onset he ran into the skillful satirists' obfuscation of his subject. It was very hard to prove in a court of law that a satirist intended more than simple fun or at most a general lament for the vices of the times. More serious, his charge would probably be seditious libel but the courts had never determined exactly what seditious libel really was. At Zenger's trial the Attorney General explained the standard definition: "scandal as is expressed in a scoffing and ironical manner . . . a taunting manner . . . in a strain of ridicule . . . [tending] to a Breach of Public Peace" (*Case and Tryal* 26). (Zenger had been charged with publishing a "false, malicious, seditious, and scandalous libel.") In *DeLibellis Famosas*, a Star Chamber Case of 1606, "libel" was defined simply as "defamation, tending to expose another to public hatred, contempt or ridicule" and at the time of Zenger's case, the definition was still in effect.

16   The main difficulty in this definition besides its vagueness is that it contained virtually nothing to distinguish it from legitimate satire. Contemporaries recognized this, and used the terms interchangeably. A number of contemporaries tried to develop their own distinctions. In particular, they argued that libel was based on falsehood whereas satire could not be effective unless it was

perceived as being largely based on truth. Readers do not laugh very hard at a description whose real subject they cannot recognize and they do not laugh at all at a description so distorted it is grotesque. Truth, argued Shaftesbury, was the innocent man's best defense against satirical attack (61). But the courts had been very erratic in approaching the question of truth. In *DeLibellis Famosas* in 1606 the court had reversed previous rulings which had based conviction on the falseness of the argument, and the 1606 definition was still in effect when Zenger was tried. But even this interpretation was not always observed. Libel was a Star Chamber doctrine, which had been very incompletely adapted to Common Law when the Star Chamber was abolished early in the English Civil Wars. At the end of the seventeenth century and the beginning of the eighteenth, truth was increasingly allowed as a defense. In Fuller's Case, early in the eighteenth century, for example, the Chief Justice had actually instructed the defendant to prove the truth of his case. But in 1729 and 1731 the pendulum swung back, first in the trial of the publisher of *Mist's Journal,* then in the trial of the *Craftsman's* printer (Holdsworth 10: 674; Cooper 61–62, 73–74; Siebert 380–82). In both cases the jury was not allowed to consider the truth behind the cited writings; indeed, it was argued, if there was truth behind the satirical exposures the satire could be all the more dangerous. Where, anyway, did one draw the line between the satirist's lesser distortions and exaggerations, and actual falsehood?

Besides this, the suer would not find making the distinction [17] between truth and falsehood to his own advantage because by claiming that a writer had defamed his character he was implicitly admitting that he found his own character recognizable in the writer's description and admitting, too, that general readers found his character in need of reform. By suing, the targeted public official implicitly gave substance to an author's defense of truth, and to Cato's defense of satires that "Guilty men alone fear them" (*Cato's Letters* 4: 298). The distinction between truth and falsehood was hardly one he would want to emphasize.

Since, then, contemporaries were unclear about the distinction [18] between libel and legitimate satire, legal decisions ended up being made on an *ad hoc* basis. But who made the definition each time? Was it the victim (the judge, speaking for the targeted official) healing his wounds, the author knowing his original intent, or the reader/hearer (the jury) responding to the humor? The answer was not obvious.

19   By the time of Lewis Morris' quarrel with Governor Cosby, then, English satirists were already realizing the immense damage their writings could inflict on public figures in and out of government. In Cosby, who became New York's chief executive in 1732, Morris and Alexander soon perceived an inept but nevertheless dangerous imitation of the English satirists' favorite target, Sir Robert Walpole. Cosby lacked both Walpole's resources and his political savvy, but soon after he fell out with the two New Yorkers he sought to use what powers he had to undermine them and their political circle. He counted on the colony's one newspaper, the *New York Gazette,* publishing only hostile accounts of them because its publisher was indebted to Cosby for government contracts. He arbitrarily dismissed Morris from his post as Chief Justice of the colony's Supreme Court because as governor, Cosby had authority to appoint judges "on good behavior." He refused to call a new election for the New York legislature and thus kept in session an assembly at least marginally compliant, and when Morris himself ran in a by-election Cosby prevailed on the local sheriff to disqualify some of his supporters. When significant issues came before the council he failed to notify Morris' councillors of the meetings (Bonomi). As Morris and Alexander saw it, in Cosby's administration, like Walpole's, "the persecuting spirit" was certainly in a fair way to ". . . raise the bantering one."

20   The techniques of the satirical attack were familiar to Morris, a frequent traveler to England, a reader of English literature, and a "fringe" member of one of the circles of London satirists. Well before the dispute with Cosby erupted in New York, Morris and his associates had already read *The Craftsman,* a contemporary English journal full of satirical attacks on Sir Robert Walpole; they had followed the editor's two trials for libel (at one of which "an honest jury" had refused to convict) and they were almost certainly aware of the voluminous pamphlet arguments, 1728–30, over the libellousness of particular articles in the journal, and again in 1732–33 against Walpole's proposed excise on wine and tobacco. They had had a chance to see *The Beggar's Opera,* which was being performed in the colonies, and to read Pope's *Dunciad,* which was already published there.

Morris's group had also written some satire of their own. 21
Morris's early patron and mentor in New York politics had been
Robert Hunter, governor of the province from 1709 to 1720 and
friend of Swift, Addison, Steele, and Defoe. Hunter was a satirist
himself; his play *Androboros* had satirized the imbecility of the
New York legislators the Governor had to deal with in the Assembly. Another protégé of Hunter's. William Livingston, had written
"A Satyr on the Times" and Morris himself had composed "The
Mock Monarch, or Kingdom of the Apes" satirizing another governor and his cronies (the same ones who ended up supporting
Cosby) as a group of apes (see Shields 1990, 138–41; 155–59). To
the New York writers, as to their English contemporaries, "the talent of satyr [should] be made use of to restrain men, by the fear
of shame, from immoral actions which do or do not fall under the
cognizance of the law."[5] "If an overgrown criminal . . . cannot
immediately be come at by ordinary Justice," argued Zenger's
writers, "let him yet receive the lash of satire."[6]

Morris, Alexander, and their group were clearly familiar also 22
with the contemporary English debate about the relation of satire to
libel. Virtually from the *Journal's* first appearance they appear to have
been daring the government to call their satires libelous and bring
them to trial on the charges. As early as 28 January 1733, under
"Domestic Affairs" they argued in the *Journal* that "Laws against
Libeling . . . may soon be shown to you and all men to be weak, and
have neither Law nor Reason for their Foundation."[7] In issue after
issue the *Journal* discussed what libel was and was not and argued
that only a jury (representing the reading public) was capable of
determining the libelousness of a given publication (Warner 33, 55).

Zenger's supporters argued that the paper simply was a vehi- 23
cle for satire; Cosby called it "full of false and scandalous libels"
(Smith 2: 19; Cosby 1734, 6: 5). When did a satire become a libel?
The authors hooked right into the English debate. The only clear
instance, according to the *Journal*, was when it contained (a) demon-
strably false statements against (b) a little known private individual who had no public reputation to protect him. A libel was
defined in the courts simply as a "malicious defamation", malicious
defaming itself being "falsely to take away from a man his good
name" (Katz 150). But to be a libel, a writing ". . . must descend to
particulars, and individuals."[8]

24   Like their English contemporaries the Governor's opponents argued that a successful satire could not be libelous almost by definition. For a satire to succeed, it had to be directed at a public figure whose shortcomings were well enough known that readers could recognize some truth in the charges.[9] No one would be interested in a satirical attack on a person he had never heard of. If a false statement was directed against a virtuous and respected public servant, no one would believe it, so the satire would fail.[10] At the same time if a satirical attack on "the vices of the age" was so general that readers could not identify the particular target, the satire would be useless, and not very funny anyway.[11] The master satirist concealed any direct identification of his subject that would convict him of libel in a court of law but developed indirect thrusts that were accurate enough to identify his target to the reading public.

25   If the very success of a satire demonstrated that readers accepted its general truthfulness, then a jury representing the public readership of a community would never find it false. Again and again the *Journal* reiterated this: "Every man may judge for himself whether [the] facts are true or not."[12] This meant of course, that the libellousness of a satirical writing must be determined not by a judge but by a jury "twelve good men and true," men returned from "the vicinage."[13] Cosby initially responded to the *Journal*'s attacks by trying to build up the *New York Gazette* as a counterweight on the Government's side. The *Gazette* called attention to "several things in Zenger's *Journal* which he has published as Matters of Fact though they were notorious falsehoods"[14] and particularly attacked the *Journal*'s assumption that readers were capable of judging the accuracy of what they read: "Why should the darling press be thus allowed / To midwife scandal to the brainless crowd."[15] When the *Gazette* failed to win away *Journal* readership Cosby, like his contemporaries in the English government, found himself in the uneasy position of having to decide whether to bring the publisher to trial. Despite Cosby's attempts to argue that "writers of seditious libels (like Morris) tell the world they speak the sentiments of the people" when they don't, the success of the *Journal* showed that its attacks on the Governor were largely perceived as being based on truth

and that he himself therefore was seen by the public to have faults of character in need of reform. Like Walpole and his colleagues, he realized that if he prosecuted the publisher for libeling him, he came close to admitting that he recognized himself in the writings; if he did not prosecute, Morris and Alexander would bait him more and more outrageously.[16]

In the end, Cosby prosecuted. The trial itself now shifted the   26 political audience from the reader to the jury and the spectators, and showed how telling a device satire could be in the courtroom. The satirical victim—in this case, the Governor—found himself on trial again, along with the printer Zenger.

At Zenger's trial the Attorney General himself served as pros-   27 ecutor; the defense employed Andrew Hamilton, prominent Philadelphia lawyer and political leader. There is considerable evidence that the leading figures were aware of the trial's potential to publicize the attack on the Governor beyond the *Journal's* readership. As the Governor's representative, Attorney General Bradley was clearly trying to minimize the trial's potential.

Bradley was trying to dispose of the case as quietly as possi-   28 ble. Second, Bradley seems almost deliberately to have avoided developing several rather powerful arguments he could have made had satire not been the principal issue of the trial. He could not develop at length the argument that satiric criticism undermined the popular respect and voluntary cooperation that were essential for a fledging government almost totally devoid of police power. Chief Justice Holt had given Bradley an opening in his instructions to an English jury of 1707, which Bradley quoted and then dropped: "If people should not be called to account for possessing the people with an ill opinion of the government, no government can exist" (Swift, *Examiner* #39, qtd. in Bell 179). Had Bradley developed this he would have walked right into the satirist's defense: far from undercutting the ties of a young community, satire reinforces them by highlighting the shared values and pouring ridicule on public officials whose behavior defies them.

Bradley cited a standard government argument that aggrieved   29 people should seek redress through legal action, not public appeals, and in the courts, not the press. But the satirists had already made clear their response to this, and Hamilton took it up:

most colonists did not have access to such legal redress, and one of the very purposes of satire was to censure "great abuses . . . which cannot be legally punished" (Swift again; Kernan 152). So Bradley could not do much with this either.

30   Nor could Bradley do more than mention the respect owed a governor as representative of the King. Hamilton was ready with the satirist's rejoinder here: one of the values New Yorkers shared was love of the King. If the misbehavior of a King's representative—in this case the Governor—undermined that love, the miscreant should be turned out of the community. The satirist encouraged this in the gentlest way, not by violence but by laughter. In sort, while Bradley was personally capable of replying to Hamilton with an emotive speech of his own, there were few appeals he could safely make in this particular trial.

31   On the defense side the star character, the satiric voice, was not the defendant, Zenger, but the defense attorney, Hamilton. (Zenger never testified in his own defense, a silence which was unusual at the time, though it became increasingly common later in the century.) Once on the floor Hamilton admitted Zenger's responsibility for the *Journal's* actual printing, hoping to rob the Attorney General of a cut-and-dried case. He then made clear his intention to approach the trial as a forum for public debate and an occasion to further isolate the Governor from the community:

32   Then having tried unsuccessfully to lure the Attorney General into a debate on the truth behind the *Journal* attacks, Hamilton deftly argued that the truthfulness of a writing—and indeed, whether its authors *meant* to tell the truth—was a matter of interpretation. Its "meaning" could be best assessed by the readers for whom it was written, and in this case the twelve jurors could stand for the reading public, the "rhetorical community" the author had in mind (Kern 21; Burns 14; Booth 49–50). They were representatives of their neighbors, he said again and again, "persons summoned out of the neighborhood" to "put their neighbors upon their guard against the craft . . . of men in authority" to "defend the liberty or property of . . . neighbors", to lay "a noble foundation for securing . . . liberty . . . to ourselves, our posterity, and our neighbors" (*Case and Tryal* 20, 21, 25, 28, 29, 39).

33   Why did he use the term "neighbors" so often? Because neighbors may have witnessed particular events the satirist was

talking about, but more importantly, because they could tell whether the behaviors of the public figures the satirist ridiculed actually did violate the norms of the community. Protection of liberty and property, safety of fellow subjects, the right to protest, the love of the King, honesty, respect for justice: all these are communal values Hamilton expressly mentioned (*Case and Tryal* 20, 23, 25, 28, 34). "Community" is a little vague here: in Hamilton's language it could stand for New York, the empire, all right-thinking people. It stands for a world view, which Hamilton managed to identify with the neighborhood as the satirist does with his readers. It is entirely rational to assume that a community must share some values in order to hang together, but once accepted the values become matters defended emotionally as "natural," taken for granted (Booth 33). Hamilton argued this point repeatedly: when the Governor violated norms of "common sense" it was "surprising," "monstrous," "astonishing," "strange," "a sad case," and any honest man had the right to complain about it (*Case and Tryal* 19, 20, 22, 28, 29).

The establishment of the author's rhetorical community was 34 absolutely key to Hamilton's point that the jury, not the judge, should decide whether a writing was better described as satire or libel. The Attorney General had left Hamilton an opening to argue that "breach of the peace" should be determined only by the readers of satire, not by its alledged victims, when he himself used two different meanings of the term. On the one hand, libel threatened to disturb the peace "by provoking the Parties injured, their Friends and Families, to Acts of Revenge," but on the other hand the *Journal* articles also were libelous because they "tend [ed.] . . . to disquiet the Minds of the People of this Province" (*Case and Tryal* 14, 18, 26). Who was provoked, the victim or the reader? This ambiguity let Hamilton point out that it was the arbitrary acts of the Governor that set people upon examining and enquiring into power"; the writings simply made the people (hence the jurors) sensible of the "sufferings of their fellow subjects" (*Case and Tryal* 28). The people of England had been similarly aroused by writings against Charles I's arbitrary government; it was the people, not the King's advisers, who were inspired to break the peace in a noble cause.

The reasoning here was pretty circular, but it worked. Only 35 members of a community—the rhetorical public—could decide whether a satirical writing could inspire their fellow members to acts of revenge which disturbed the peace. But this community had already been defined by the satirist himself to leave the accused public figures out.

36   Hamilton now clarified further the difficulty of calling satire "seditious libel." "If a libel is understood in the large and unlimited sense urged by Mr. Attorney, there is scarce a writing I know that may not be called a libel or scarce any person safe from being called to account as a libeller . . . when must [a man] laugh, so as to be secure from being taken up as a libeller?" (*Case and Tryal* 20, 37, 40).

37   What was more memorable and more imitable than his central argument, however, was his peroration. He began this with a masterful portrayal of himself as (again) a "neighbor," a fellow colonist with whom jurors could either sympathize or identify and whose arguments and political values they could therefore accept. Turning what might have been a handicap (the fact that he was an outsider, from Philadelphia) into an asset, Hamilton explained that he had come as a matter of duty, because "his neighbor's house [was] on fire": "a bad Precedent in one Government is soon set up for an authority in another." He moved on to adopt the satirist's mask, the persona of the venerable advocate for the people, used (sometimes almost verbatim) in later state trials: "I am truly unequal to such an undertaking on many accounts. And you see I labor under the weight of many years [in his fifties, at the prime of his career, able to make a sudden trip up from a town forty miles away] and I am borne down with great infirmities of body; yet old and weak as I am, I should think it my duty, if required, to go to the utmost part of the land."[17]

38   His style, moreover, relied on satiric humor as well as sympathy . . . "there may be a good Reason why Men should take the same care, to make an honest and upright Conduct a Fence and Security against the Injury of unruly Tongues." (Hamilton was explaining why the Governor's lack of such upright conduct merited Zenger's "unruly" attack.) "Were some Persons to go thro' the Streets of New York now-a-days, and read a Part of the Bible, if it was not known to be such, Mr. Attorney, with the help of his Innuendos, would easily turn it into a libel." (Hamilton was attacking the Attorney General's loose definition of libel in the

charge against Zenger.) Hamilton then went through selected verses of Isaiah, mocking so successfully the way the Attorney General would turn them into libel by using innuendo that Bradley had to concede that Hamilton "had made himself and the People very merry" (*Case and Tryal* 20, 37, 40). In the end, the jury took very little time in acquitting the printer.

So, how do we view the trial? There can be little doubt that 39 the verdict did deter future colonial office holders from charging unfriendly satirists with libel. Men in political authority were loath to face the public humiliation that a verdict of acquittal would bring. No longer could they rely on the determination of judges beholden to themselves. After Zenger's trial they were likely to face a jury which accepted full responsibility for deciding the guilt or innocence of a printer, on the assumption that if libels threatened the peace they did so by inspiring new readers (jurors) to protest, not their targets (office holders, including judges) to seek revenge. Reports of the trial and outcome were immediately sent "Abroad through the World" ("Remarks on Zenger's Trial"). "Remarks on the trial" were collected first in Barbados, London, and Philadelphia, then "plentifully dispersed through out the colonies," prompting at least a three way debate in the presses of New York, Philadelphia, and Barbados.[18] Accounts of Zenger's case reappeared in New York again in the late 1730s, in both New York and London in the 1760s, and in the English press in 1784.

No governor successfully undertook such a public trial again, 40 and most of them did not even try. The proprietary governor of Pennsylvania suffered in silence when Ben Franklin lampooned him for not putting down the Paxton Boys in 1764 (Franklin 55–76). Governor Fauquier of Virginia instructed a grand jury to "punish the Licentiousness of the Press" by indicting Robert Boling for a libel against the colony's General Court in the summer of 1766; the jury refused, and less than six months later when Boling published *A Satire on the Times* against Fauquier and his advisers, there was nothing the governor could do about it (Lemay). Jonathan Belcher, governor of Massachusetts and a Mason, had to put up with Joseph Greene's satirical attack on his own participation in Masonic rituals (Shields 1987, 109–26, esp. 112–15). Governor Dinwiddie of Virginia suffered the viciously satiric

"Dinwiddiance" which circulated in manuscript during his administration (see Brock) and Governor Hutchinson was utterly unable to bring his critics to trial in Massachusetts (Levy 65).

41   But note: "office holders" included legislators as well as governors, and though assemblies were growing increasingly aggressive in going after printers who challenged their legislative authority, even assemblymen became skittish about accusing a satirist of libel after the Zenger trial. The only publisher of satire so charged was Daniel Fowle of Boston for printing *Monster of Monsters*, an attack on the proposed Massachusetts excise in 1754. The legislature did not pursue Fowle's punishment ("public sympathy being with Fowle," it was argued, "the House dropped its charges"; Levy 34) and later gave back the examination cost it had initially charged him. Significantly, other publishers who offended legislators were charged with contempt, not libel, and even in the tense decades before the Revolution the political satirists on both sides remained unscathed (Granger, esp. 1–8; Nelson 10–12).

42   As important as the arguments that Zenger's trial introduced was the style of political satire that both the *Journal* writers and attorneys took up initially from contemporary English writers opposed to the government of Sir Robert Walpole. Colonial writers had certainly been aware of the marvelous adaptability of Augustan satire before the trial, but the Zenger case highlighted its usefulness for colonial America. After Zenger, the rhetoric and imagery the English satirists had directed against government corruption in general and Walpole's Excise Proposal in particular were to appear again and again as models for American writers throughout the century. *Monster of Monsters*, the Massachusetts anti-excise pamphlet we have just noted, drew from four anti-excise pamphlets in 1732 (Boyer 340–44); Pope, a consistent critic of Walpole, was at least in part behind the laughter at Governors Belcher, Dinwiddie, and even Fauquier (see, for example, Davis 21–22). Later on Charles Churchill's venomous stings of George III and Lord Bute featured in the Paxton Boys' (Olson; see Dunbar) attacks on Quaker legislators, Goldsmith's writings were an early model for Federalist attacks on Jefferson (Dowling, chap. 2). From the *Journal* at least through Joseph Dennie's *The Port Folio*, when American political writers laughed at their government they were thinking of the way the English laughed at theirs.

Through ridicule and laughter the trial showed satire could 43
create its own public (Ziff 46), communities of listeners or readers brought together by the literary indictment of any figure the
successful satirist targeted. Since satire tried people by laughter,
Zenger's case was in effect a trial of a trial in which the defense
attorney used satire to defend satirists. A "style" of courtroom
performance intersected with a style of journalism; a vision of the
newspaper world where adversaries debated before a public audience intersected with a vision of the courtroom functioning the
same way. The Zenger trial could, indeed, be a landmark without
its verdict determining the legal outcome of any further trials.

Neither the use of the press or the use of the courts as adver- 44
sarial forums was entirely new in the 1730s, nor was the use of a
bitingly effective satirical style by both journalists and jurists. But
the Zenger trial did mark one of the earliest occasions on which
all three coalesced, mutually enhancing each other. The combination was potent. It made the colonial world a little safer for
satirists and political opposition, a little less safe for unpopular
imperial officials. It added dynamic potential to the political trial
and helped constitute the "public" as part of political debate, and
the intersection it marked remained for the rest of the century.

NOTES

1. See Robert Hunter's *Androboros* (New York, 1714) in Walter
   Meserve and William Reardon, *Satiric Comedies* 1–40 and the
   four satirical pamphlets published by James Logan and Gov.
   William Keith in their 1724–5 controversy in Pennsylvania
   (Alison Olson, "Pennsylvania Satire Before the Stamp Act."
   Pennsylvania History).
2. The charges were against *Monster of Monsters*, published in
   1754 in Massachusetts.
3. For a discussion of juries as representative of colonial society
   see J. R. Pole, "Reflections on American Law and the American Revolution" and the responses to it by Peter Charles
   Hoffer, Bruce Mann, and James Henretta and James Rice in
   The William and Mary Quarterly (1993). William Smith wrote
   that Zenger's lawyers defended the truth behind the *Journal's*

allegations by the press, at clubs and other meetings for private conversation, "and considering the inflamed state of a small country, consisting at that time of less than a thousand freeholders qualified for jurors, it was easy to let every man perfectly into the full merits of the defence" (Kammen 2: 19).

4. Swift's advice is from "The Importance of the Guardian Considered" in *The Prose Works of Jonathan Swift, D.B.* V 297. For a general discussion of satirists and the law see Lawrence Hanson, *Government and the Press*, 1695–1763, 7–35.

5. *New York Weekly Journal*, 19 November 1733.

6. *New York Weekly Journal*, 12 November 1733.

7. *New York Weekly Journal*, 28 January 1733.

8. The argument that a satire can be truthful and still be a libel "only holds true as to private and personal failings; and it is quite otherwise when the crimes of men come to affect the publick." (*New York Weekly Journal*, 25 February 1733.)

9. ". . . the entertainment rises in proportion to the familiarity of the known haters" (Ramsay 81). But see also: "For general Satire will all Vices fit and ev'ry fool or knave will think he's hit" (*The Satirist: In Imitation of the Fourth Satire of The First Book of Horace* 11).

10. ". . . if Comedy and Satire Poems are:
. . . as some say that they to Libels tend
I'll only see if justly they offend" (*The Satirist* 11)
". . . if the actions clamoured at be thought just, then those who transacted them will never be afraid of submitting them to the judgment of the whole world by the Press." (*New York Weekly Journal*, 4 February 1733.)

11. "The essence of the satiric procedure is attack, and the attack launched impartially against everyone is no attack at all" (Rosenheim 29).

12. *New York Weekly Journal*, 12 November 1733.

13. *New York Weekly Journal*, 18 February 1733, 28 July 1735. (Copied from *The Craftsman* of Jan. 1, 1731–2.)

14. *New York Gazette*, 3–10 June 1734.

15. *New York Gazette*, 14 April 1735.

16. "The best way to prevent libels, is not to deserve them . . . the more notice is taken of them, the more they are published. Guilty men alone fear them . . ." (Cato 3: 298).

"The Facts exposed are not to be believed, because said or published; but it draws People's Attention . . . that everyone may judge for himself whether those facts are true or not" (*New York Weekly Journal*, 12 November 1733).

17. Compare this with Thomas Erskine's peroration in the trial of Thomas Hardy. "I am sinking under fatigue and weakness. I am at this moment scarcely able to stand up whilst I am speaking to you, deprived as I have been, for nights together, of everything that deserves the name of rest, repose, or comfort" (Wharam 170).

18. *Barbados Gazette*, 10 August 1737, in *Caribbeana*.

WORKS CITED

Baer, Marc. *Theatre and Disorder in Late Georgian London*. Oxford: Clarendon, 1992.

Bell, Ian. *Literature and Crime in Augustan England*. London: Routledge, 1991.

Bender, John. *Imagining the Penitentiary: Fiction and the Architecture of Mind in Eighteenth Century England*. Chicago: University of Chicago Press, 1987.

Bonomi, Patricia. *A Factious People: Politics and Society in Colonial New York*. New York, Columbia, 1971.

Booth, Wayne C. *Modern Dogma and the Rhetoric of Assent*. Notre Dame, Ind.: University of Notre Dame Press, 1974.

———. *A Rhetoric of Irony*. Chicago: University of Chicago Press, 1975.

Bolingbroke Lord Henry St. John. Aug. 28, 1727, *The Craftsman*, #60. *Lord Bolingbroke's Contributions to the Craftsman*. Ed. Simon Varey. Oxford: Oxford, 1982. 23.

Botein, Stephen. *Mr. Zenger's Malice and Falsehood*. Worcester, Mass.: American Antiquarian Society Facsimilies, 1985.

Boyer, Paul S. "Borrowed Rhetoric: The Massachusetts Excise Controversy of 1754." *William and Mary Quarterly* 3rd. ser. 21 (July 1964): 340–44.

Brock, R. A., ed. *Collections of the Virginia Historical Society I*. Richmond, Va.: Virginia Historical Society, 1971. #481.

Buranelli, Vincent, ed. *The Trial of Peter Zenger*. New York: New York, 1957.

Burke, Peter. *Popular Culture in Early Modern Europe*. Rev. imprint. Hants, England: Scolar Press, 1994.

Burns, Elizabeth. *Theatricality, A Study in Convention, the Theatre, and Social Life*. New York: Harper and Row, 1973.

A Brief Narrative of the Case and Tryal of John Peter Zenger. New York, 1736. 19.

Clark, Charles. *The Public Prints*. New York: Oxford, 1994.

Cohen, Daniel. *Pillars of Salt, Monuments of Grace*. New York: Oxford, 1993.

"The Colonial Virginia Satirist." Ed. Richard Beale Davis. *Transactions of the American Philosophical Society* N.S. 57, 11. Philadelphia, 1967.

Cooper, Thomas. *A Treatise on the Law of Libel and the Liberty of the Press*. 1830. New York: DaCapo Press, 1970.

Cosby, William. "Cosby to Lords of Trade, June 19, 1734." *Docs. re. Col. Hist. N.Y.* VI, 5. Rutherford Papers, New York Historical Society.

———. "Cosby to the Lords of Trade, Dec. 6, 1734." *Documents Relative to the Colonial History of the State of New York*. Vol. 6. Ed. E.B. O'Callaghan. Albany: Weed, Parson & Co., 1853–7.

Dowling, William C. *Literary Federalism in the Age of Jefferson Joseph Dennie and the Port Folio, 1801–1812*. Columbia: University of South Carolina Press, 1999.

Davis, Richard Beale. "The Colonial Virginia Satirist." *Transactions of the American Philosophical Society* N.S. 57, 11 (Philadelphia, 1967), 21–22.

Dunbar, John R., ed. *The Paxton Papers*. The Hague: Martinus Nijhoff, 1957.

Dunway, Clyde Augustus. *The Development of Freedom of the Press in Massachusetts*. Cambridge, Mass.: Harvard, 1906.

Finkelman, Paul. "Politics, The Press, and the Law: The Trial of John Peter Zenger." *American Political Trials*. Ed. Michael Belknap. Westport, Conn.: Greenwood, 1994.

Franklin, Benjamin. "Narrative of the Late Massacres in Lancaster County." *The Paxton Papers*. Ed. John R. Dunbar. The Hague: Martinus Nijhoff, 1957. 55–76.

Gilreath, James. "Government, Law, Public Opinion, and the Printed Word in Eighteenth Century America." *Publishing and Readership in Revolutionary France and America*. Ed. Carol Armbrustor. Westport, Conn.: Greenwood, 1993. 79–94.

Goebel, Julius and Raymond Naughton. *Law Enforcement in Colonial New York*. Montclair. N.J.: Patterson Smith, 1970.

Granger, Bruce Ingham. *Political Satire in the American Revolution, 1763–83*. Ithaca, N.Y.: Cornell, 1960.

Hanson, Lawrence. *Government and the Press, 1695–1763*. Oxford: Clarendon, 1967.

Hariman, Richard, ed. *Popular Trials: Rhetoric, Mass Media, and the Law*. Tuscaloosa, Al.: University of Alabama Press, 1990.

Harte, Walter. *An Essay on Satire, Particularly on the Dunciad*. 1730. Los Angeles: Clark Memorial Library, 1968.

Hoffer, Peter. *Law and People in Colonia, America*. Baltimore: Johns Hopkins, 1992.

Holdsworth, Sir William. *A History of English Law*. Vol. 10. London: Methuen, 1938.

Hunter, Robert. *Androboros*. New York, 1714. Reprinted in *Satiric Comedies*. Ed. Walter Meserve and William Reardon. Bloomington, Ind.: Indiana University Press, 1969. 1–40.

Ingram, Allan. *Intricate Laughter in the Satire of Swift and Pope*. Basingstoke: MacMillan, 1986.

James, Ellen Mosen. "Decoding the Zenger Trial: Andrew Hamilton's Fraudful Dexterity." *The Law in America*. Ed. William Penca and Wythe W. Holt, Jr. New York: New York Historical Society, 1989. 1–27.

Kammen, Michael, ed. *The History of the Province of New York*. Vol. 2. Cambridge, Mass.: Harvard, 1972.

Katz, Stanley N. *Brief Narrative of the Case and Trial of John Peter Zenger*. Cambridge, Mass.: Harvard, 1963.

Kern, Jean. *Dramatic Satire in the Age of Walpole, 1720–1750*. Ames, Iowa: University of Iowa Press, 1976.

Kernan, Alvin. *The Cankered Muse; Satire of the English Renaissance.* New Haven: Yale, 1959.

Landau, Norma. *The Justices of the Peace, 1679–1760.* Berkeley: University of California Press, 1984.

Lemay, J. A. Leo. "Robert Bolling and the Bailment of Colonel Chiswell." *Early American Literature* 6 (1971): 99–142.

Levy, Leonard W. *Emergence of a Free Press.* New York: Oxford, 1985.

———. "Did the Zenger Case Really Matter? Freedom of the Press in Colonial New York." *William & Mary Quarterly* 3rd ser. 18 (January 1960): 35–50.

Nelson, Harold. "Seditious Libel in Colonial America." *American Journal of Legal History* 60 (December 1973): 10–12.

Olson, Alison G. "The Pamphlet War over the Paxton Boys." *Pennsylvania Magazine of History and Biography* 123 (Fall 1999): 31–55.

———. "Pennsylvania Satire Before the Stamp Act." *Pennsylvania History* 68 (October 2001): 507–532.

Pole, J. R. "Reflections on American Law and the American Revolution." *The William and Mary Quarterly* 3rd ser. (Jan. 1993): 123–80.

Ramsay, Allan. *An Essay on Ridicule.* London, n.p. 1753.

"Remarks on Zenger's Tryal." *Barbados Gazette* 25 June 1737. ("The Tryal fell into many hands"). *Caribbeana, Containing Letters and Dissertations together with Political Essays on Various Subjects and Occasions.* London, n.p., 1741.

Roeber, A. G. *Faithful Magistrates and Republican: Lawyers: Creators of Virginia's Legal Culture, 1680–1810.* Chapel Hill, N. C.: University of North Carolina Press, 1980.

Rosenheim, Edward R. *Swift and the Satirist's Art.* Chicago: University of Chicago Press, 1963.

The Satirist: In Iimitation of the Fourth Satire of The First Book of Horace, London, n.p. 1933.

Shaftesbury, Lord Anthony *Characteristics of Men, Manners, Opinions, Times, etc.* London, Grant Richards, 1900.

Shields, David S. "Cleo Mocks the Masons: Joseph Greene's Masonic Satires." Ed. J. A. Leo Lemay. *Deism, Masonry, and* the Enlightenment. *Essays Honoring Alfred Owen Aldridge.* Newark, Del., University of Delaware, Press, 1987.

_____. *Oracles of Empire.* Chicago: University of Chicago Press, 1990.

Siebert, Frederick. *Freedom of the Press in England, 1476–1776.* Urbana, Ill.: University of Illinois Press, 1952.

Smith, James Morton. *Freedom's Fetters, The Alien and Sedition Laws and American Civil Liberties.* Ithaca, N.Y.: Cornell, 1956.

Smith, William. *The History of the Late Province of New York from its Discovery to the Appointment of Governor Colden in 1762.* Vol. 2. New York: New York Historical Society, 1830.

Spector, Robert D. *Political Controversy: A Study in Eighteenth-Century Propaganda.* New York: Greenwood, 1992.

Stevens, George Alexander. *An Essay on Satire.* London: G. Kearsley, 1785.

Swift, Jonathan. "The Importance of the Guardian Considered." *The Prose Works of Jonathan Swift*, D.D. Ed. Temple Scott. 12 vols. London: Bell, 1900–1914.

Thomas, Isaiah. *The History of Printing in America.* Vol. 1. Albany, 1874. New York: Weathervane Books, 1970.

Thumb, Thomas. *The Monster of Monsters: A True and Faithful Narrative of a Most Remarkable Phenomenon Lately Seen in this Metropolis.*

Trenchard, John, and Thomas Gordan. *Cato's Letters: Essays on Liberty, Civil and Religious, and Other Important Subjects. 1720–23.* Boston, 1754.

Tourtellot, Arthur Bernon. *Benjamin Franklin, the Shaping of Genius; the Boston Years,* New York: Doubleday, 1977.

Tyler, Moses Coit. *A History of American Literature, 1607–1783.* Ed. Archie Jones. Abr. ed. Chicago: University of Chicago Press, 1967.

Warner, Michael. *The Letters of the Republic: Publication and the Public Sphere in Eighteenth-Century America.* Cambridge, Mass: Harvard, 1990.

Wharam, Alan. *The Treason Trials, 1794.* Leicester: Leicester University Press, 1992.

Ziff, Larzer. "A Silent Revolution: Benjamin Franklin and Print Culture" *Publishing and Readership. In Revolutionary France and America.* Ed. Carol Armbruster. Westport, Conn.: Greenwood, 1993.

EXPELLING *HUCK FINN*

Nat Hentoff

1   The Pennsylvania State Conference of the NAACP has instructed its branches to file grievances with the state's human rights commission demanding that local school boards and district superintendents remove Mark Twain's *Adventures of Huckleberry Finn* from mandatory reading lists.

2   The charge, supported by the national NAACP, is that "tax dollars should not be used to perpetuate a stereotype that has psychologically damaging effects on the self-esteem of African American children."

3   Some years ago I was talking to African American eighth-graders in a Brooklyn public school who had been reading *Huckleberry Finn* in class—along with the history of racism in such towns as Hannibal, Mo., where Twain had grown up.

4   The students recently had been discussing the passage in which Huck, on the raft with Jim, was tormented by what he had been raised to believe—that he would go to hell if he did not report this runaway slave to the owner.

5   Huck wrote a note doing just that, but finally, destroying the note, he said to himself, "All right, then, I'll *go* to hell!"

6   "Do you think we're so dumb," one of the Brooklyn eighth-graders said to me, "that we don't know the difference between a racist book and an anti-racist book? Sure, the book is full of the word 'Nigger.' That's how those bigots talked back then."

7   As Twain said years later, Huck, after writing the note, was struggling between "a sound heart" and "a deformed conscience" that he had to make right.

8   "The people whom Huck and Jim encounter on the Mississippi"—Russell Baker wrote in the *New York Times* in 1982—"are drunkards, murderers, bullies, swindlers, lynchers, thieves, liars, frauds, child abusers, numskulls, hypocrites, windbags and

traders in human flesh. All are white. The one man of honor in this phantasmagoria is 'Nigger Jim,' as Twain called him to emphasize the irony of a society in which the only true gentleman was held beneath contempt."

Michael Meyers—assistant national director of the NAACP under Roy Wilkins from 1975 to 1984—wrote to Julian Bond, the present NAACP chairman, about the organization's desire to censor *Huck Finn.*

Calling the book "a great anti-slavery classic," Meyers—now the executive director of the New York Civil Rights Coalition— asked Bond whether there is an actual NAACP policy "that encourages NAACP branches to either support or seek book banning or censorship." Bond, as Meyers noted in his letter, is on the ACLU's national advisory council, as is the NAACP's president, Kweisi Mfume. If such a policy exists, Meyers wrote, "what are you doing—or what are you prepared to do—to change such a policy?"

Bond answered that "the NAACP does not have a policy for every occasion. Might I ask you for a policy we might adopt that could allow the NAACP to express outrage at racist expression while protecting free speech?"

Meyers was puzzled by the response because, he says, *Huckleberry Finn*—as the youngsters in Brooklyn emphatically understood—is *anti*-racist.

In 1998 Judge Stephen Reinhardt, writing for a unanimous three-judge panel of the 9th Circuit Court of Appeals, rejected a lawsuit by an African American parent, who is also a teacher, asking that *Huckleberry Finn* be removed from mandatory reading lists in the Phoenix, Ariz., schools.

"Words can hurt, particularly racist epithets," Reinhardt wrote, "but a necessary component of any education is learning to think critically about offensive ideas. Without that ability, one can do little to respond to them." Part of learning to think critically about offensive speech is to understand the context in which it is used.

Bond might consider sending Judge Reinhardt's decision (*Kathy Monteiro v. the Tempe Union High School District*) to the Pennsylvania State Conference of the NAACP. He might also inform it of "The Jim Dilemma: Reading Race in *Huckleberry Finn*" by Jocelyn Chadwick-Joshua, an African American who has been instructing black and white teachers about the book for years.

16   She writes: "Without the memory of what a word once meant and what it can continue to mean, we as a society are doomed to repeat earlier mistakes about ourselves, each other, and serious issues involving us all."

WHAT LIMITS SHOULD CAMPUS NETWORKS PLACE ON PORNOGRAPHY?

Robert O'Neil

1 What if you were about to present a PowerPoint lecture to a large undergraduate class, but found instead on your computer a series of sexually explicit ads and material from pornographic Web sites? That's essentially what happened recently to Mary Pedersen, a nutrition-science professor at California Polytechnic State University at San Luis Obispo. That incident and the increasing presence of such imagery at Cal Poly have led to a novel, although undoubtedly predictable, struggle over computer content—one that is quite likely to be replicated at countless campuses in the coming months.

2   A concerned faculty group at Cal Poly has announced its intention to bring before the Academic Senate, sometime this spring, a "Resolution to Enhance Civility and Promote a Diversity-Friendly Campus Climate." Specifically, the measure would prohibit using the university's computers or network to access or download digital material generally described as "pornography." The resolution would also forbid the "transmission" of hate literature and obscenity on the Cal Poly network.

3   The sponsoring faculty members have offered several reasons for proposing such drastic action. First and foremost, they contend that the ready availability of sexually explicit imagery can create occasional but deeply disturbing encounters like Pedersen's discovery of unwelcome and unexpected material on her classroom computer. The pervasive presence of such images, proponents of the resolution argue, is inherently demeaning to female faculty members, administrators, and students.

Indeed, they suggest that the university might even be legally 4 liable for creating and maintaining a "hostile workplace environment" if it fails to take steps to check the spread of such offensive material. That concern has been heightened by a putative link to a growing number of sexual assaults in the environs of the university.

Those who call for tighter regulation cite several others factors 5 to support anti-pornography measures. In their view, a college or university must maintain the highest of standards, not only in regard to the integrity of scholarship and relations between teachers and students, but also in the range of material to which it provides electronic access. The clear implication is that the ready availability of sexually explicit and deeply offensive imagery falls below "the ethical standards that the university claims to uphold."

Critics of easy access to such material also claim that it can 6 divert time, talent, and resources from the university's primary mission. Kimberly Daniels, a local lawyer who is advising the resolution's sponsors, told the student newspaper that "it is offensive that Cal Poly is taking the position that it is acceptable for professors to view pornography during work hours in their work office." That risk is not entirely conjectural. In fact, one professor left the institution last year after being convicted on misdemeanor charges for misusing a state-owned computer, specifically for the purpose of downloading in his office thousands of sexually explicit images. Local newspapers have also reported that the FBI is investigating another former Cal Poly professor who allegedly used a campus computer to view child pornography.

Finally, the concerned faculty group insists that the free flow of 7 pornographic materials may expose the Cal Poly computer network to a greater risk of virus infection. They cite a student's recent experience in opening a salacious virus-bearing attachment that the student mistakenly believed had been sent by one of his professors.

The proposed Academic Senate resolution has touched off an 8 intense debate. The university's existing computer-use policy presumes that access and choice of material are broadly protected, although it adds that "in exceptional cases, the university may decide that such material directed at individuals presents such a hostile environment under the law that certain restrictive actions are warranted." The new proposal would focus more sharply on sexually explicit imagery, and would require those who wish to view such material through the campus network to obtain the express permission of the university's president.

9   Defenders of the current approach, including the senior staff of the university's office of information technology, insist that a public university may not banish from its system material that is offensive, but legal, without violating First Amendment rights. Those familiar with the operations of such systems also cite practical difficulties in the enforcement of any such restrictions, given the immense volume of digital communications that circulate around the clock at such a complex institution.

10   The debate at Cal Poly echoes what occurred some six years ago in Virginia. The General Assembly enacted what remains as the nation's only ban on public employees' use of state-owned or state-leased computers to access sexually explicit material—at least without express permission of a "superior" for a "bona fide research purpose." Six state university professors immediately challenged the law on First Amendment grounds. A district judge struck down the statute, but the U.S. Court of Appeals for the Fourth Circuit reversed that ruling. The law had been modified before that judgment, and many Virginia professors have since received exemptions or dispensations, but the precedent created by the appeals-court decision remains troubling for advocates of free and open electronic communications.

11   The Virginia ruling complicates the Cal Poly situation. The First Amendment challenge of those who oppose the Academic Senate resolution is less clear than it might at first appear. Two premises underlying that resolution—the need to protect government-owned hardware and the imperative to combat sexual hostility in the public workplace—contributed both to the passage of the Virginia ban, and to its eventual success in the federal courts. What's more, the U.S. Equal Employment Opportunity Commission some months ago gave its blessing to a hostile-workplace complaint filed by Minneapolis Public Library staff members who were offended by persistent display of graphic sexual images on reading-room terminals.

12   Thus, there is more than a superficial basis for the claims of Cal Poly's pornbanishers that (in the words of one faculty member) "the First Amendment doesn't protect . . . subjecting others to inappropriate material in the workplace." Even the information-technology consultant who has championed the current computer-

use policy at the university has conceded that access to controversial material is fully protected only "as long as it isn't offending others."

Although the desire to reduce the potential for offense and 13 affront to other users of a campus computer network seems unobjectionable, its implications deserve careful scrutiny. In the analogous situation of public terminals in a library reading room, it is one thing to ask a patron who wishes to access and display sexually explicit material—or racially hateful material, for that matter—to use a terminal facing away from other users and staff members. It is quite another matter to deny access to such material altogether on the plausible premise that, if it can be obtained at all, there is a palpable risk that its visible display will offend others. To invoke an analogy that is now before the U.S. Supreme Court in a challenge to the Children's Internet Protection Act: It is one thing for a library to provide—even be compelled to provide—filtered access for parents who wish it for their children, but quite another to deny all adult patrons any unfiltered access.

What Cal Poly should seek to do, without impairing free expres- 14 sion, is to protect people from being gratuitously assaulted by digital material that may be deeply offensive, without unduly restricting access of those who, for whatever reason, may wish to access and view such material without bothering others. The proposal in the resolution that permission may be obtained from the university's president, for bona-fide research purposes, is far too narrow. Among other flaws, such a precondition might well deter sensitive or conscientious scholars, whether faculty members or students, who are understandably reluctant to reveal publicly their reasons for wishing to access sexually explicit images or hate literature.

A responsible university, seeking to balance contending inter- 15 ests of a high order, might first revisit and make more explicit its policies that govern acceptable computer use and access, by which all campus users are presumably bound. Such policies could condemn the flaunting of thoughtless dissemination of sexually explicit material and digital hate literature, expressing institutional abhorrence of such postings, without seeking to ban either type of material. The computer network might also establish a better warning system through which to alert sensitive users to the occasional and inevitable presence of material that may offend. Finally, a broader disclaimer might be in order, recognizing the limited practical capacity of a university server to control (or even enable users to avoid) troubling material.

16   What is needed is a reasonable balance that avoids, as Justice William O. Douglas warned a half-century ago, "burning down the house to roast the pig." That aphorism has special felicity here; in the offensive flaunting of sexually explicit imagery, there is a "pig" that doubtless deserves to be roasted. But there is also a house of intellect that must remain free and open, even to those with aberrant tastes and interests.

Censorship Wins Out

Andrew Stroehlein

1   A decade or so ago, it was all clear: the Internet was believed to be such a revolutionary new medium, so inherently empowering and democratizing, that old authoritarian regimes would crumble before it. What we've learned in the intervening years is that the Internet does not inevitably lead to democracy any more than it inevitably leads to great wealth.

2   The idea that the Internet itself is a threat to authoritarian regimes was a bit of delusional post–Cold War optimism. It is true that many activists and journalists have brought their struggle for democracy, the rule of law and freedom of expression to the new medium, but they have not been blessed by inevitable victory, and plenty of nasty regimes have learned how to co-exist with the Internet in one way or another. In country after country, the same old struggle goes on: hard-line regimes and their opponents remain locked in battle, and the Internet has become simply one more forum for their fight.

PARANOID REGIMES

3   Repressive regimes are paranoid by nature. Those in power see enemies everywhere and encourage mass paranoia, overemphasizing threats to national security in order to justify their draconian rule. When early Web-heads equated the Internet with inevitable

democracy, paranoia-prone regimes were natural suckers for the idea. "The Web really does scare these regimes," Veronica Forwood told me. Forwood is the UK Representative for Reporters without Borders, the publisher of the excellent "Enemies of the Internet" report, outlining the situation in many regimes around the world: "They want to control everything, and the Web seems so nebulous and unknowable to them, they are just frightened by it."

Indeed, many repressive states see the Internet as such a 4 threat that they simply ban it altogether. The former regime in Taliban-controlled Afghanistan and North Korea are two cases of a complete ban, though it is known that a few very high-ranking ministers in each regime have had access to e-mail at least.

Another particularly harsh example is Burma. A. Lin Neu- 5 mann, Asia Consultant for the Committee to Protect Journalists (CPJ) and author of an excellent recent report on press freedom in Burma, explained to me that the military junta in Rangoon effectively prevents public Internet access in the country. One needs a permit for a modem, and though a few people have them illegally, long-distance calls for foreign access are prohibitively expensive. The tiny number of government-approved e-mail accounts are all monitored by censors, and the high price of those accounts again keeps most ordinary citizens away in any case.

Relying on high access costs as a *de facto* censor is an easy 6 trick for regimes, as they generally lord over desperately poor countries. As we previously discussed here in the Online Journalism Review (OJR), Uzbekistan is a perfect example. In true Soviet style, the authorities in Tashkent have set up the technical infrastructure so that they have the capability to monitor e-mails and Web browsing, but it seems they don't actually interfere that much just yet, because they know the price of access means that only a tiny fraction of the population are online, an insignificant fraction apparently in the authorities' view.

But an all-out ban and relying on high access costs are hardly 7 the only methods of keeping control over online information. Despite the theory behind the Internet's built-in anti-censorship architecture, official control is actually very possible in practice, especially as the regimes run the telecommunications infrastructure when the country comes online.

8   In Iraq the regime is trying to use the Internet to its own advantage while cutting off access to the public. The Internet is accessible from some government ministries, but since, like Burma, one needs special permission to own a modem, home access is limited to the most trusted members of the ruling elite.

9   The situation in Cuba is little better. The government allows access at approved institutions, including trusted firms and universities. Private access at home is nearly non-existent, and the government is setting up a Cuba-only intranet for young people, to keep their activity corralled in an easily controlled space. The overall effect of these efforts, according to a detailed report by the Carnegie Endowment for International Peace, is that, "there is essentially no legal, commercially available public access to the Internet" in Cuba.

10   Some repressive regimes, however, realizing that the new technology can have some positive benefits for society at large, have developed a more sophisticated approach to the Internet, attempting to allow widespread access and yet maintain control over it. China has tens of millions of Internet users and has easily one of the fastest growing online populations in the world. Still, the authorities' control points are several. Chinese chatrooms, for example, are monitored and comments offensive to the regime are removed quickly by the moderators.

11   Much more importantly, though, is the Chinese government's ability to censor material coming in from outside China. All external information runs through government servers, so the authorities can and do block outside Web sites they deem potentially dangerous. A report by CPJ in January of 2001 notes that the main targets for blocking are Western news sites, Chinese dissident sites, Taiwanese media and sites of the banned religious group, Falun Gong. But the CPJ Report also observed how inconsistent the blocking can be, and this point is backed up by this writer's experience. On a recent trip to China, I did a little test of my own in an Internet cafe: US sites cnn.com and time.com were blocked, but UK sites for *The Guardian* and *The Independent* newspapers, both with plenty of articles critical of Beijing, were easily accessible.

12   It is, however, probably not as random as it appears, and the Chinese authorities have blocked a huge number of sites, most

likely paying more attention to those sites they feel are better known to Chinese users. Certainly, the authorities' overall control can be in no doubt, exemplified by the fact that their blocking can be turned on and off at will: during last October's APEC meeting in Shanghai, the Chinese authorities temporarily lifted their blocks of some American Web sites as a sop to foreign delegates.

As CPJ's A. Lin Neumann told me: "Chinese blocking is rea- 13 sonably effective on their part. It takes some determination to get around it, and I doubt that many people want to really play the game. Most of the students I talked with, quite frankly, were more interested in sex, computer games and English proficiency (in that order) than they were in politics on the Internet."

While it's true some editors try to stay one step ahead of the 14 blockers by constantly setting up new proxy sites, that kind of cat-and-mouse routine, forcing the reader to waste time keeping up with frequent address changes, only benefits the censors.

While access to the outside world is significantly limited in 15 China through extensive and complex blocking, the authorities have a much easier time controlling what is published within China. As in many heavy-handed regimes, self-censorship is the key factor in China: editors of Web sites inside China know well the limits of what is acceptable and what is not, and it only takes a few tough arrests and harsh crackdowns to send a clear signal to Web journalists and activists everywhere. The infamous perse-cution of online publisher Huang Qi is probably enough to keep most Chinese Web editors in line.

This "let that be a lesson to you all" tactic is as old as man, 16 but even with the newest technology it still works—and is a typ-ical ploy even in regimes that are generally considered less repres-sive than China. Umit Ozturk, vice-chair of Amnesty Interna-tional's Journalists' Network, explained to me how this works in Turkey. In Turkey, if a Web site publishes something the military-dominated state finds unacceptable, the ISPs will receive a quick visit or a phone call from someone "suggesting" the immediate removal of that site. Failure to do so would be very detrimental to one's health, so the ISPs naturally comply.

When the optimists spoke of inevitable freedom through the 17 Internet a few years back, they forgot about such crude and effec-tive methods of information control.

VIRTUALLY IN EXILE

18 With such personal threats at home, it's not difficult to see why some online journalists and activists chose to work in exile. There are problems with this approach, obviously—their online information might be blocked at home, many potential readers will not be able to afford access to their site and their critics will always accuse them of being stooges of foreign governments—but for some the benefit of being able to tell the truth outweighs these concerns.

19   The main problem of running a Web site in exile is maintaining local relevance and authenticity when writing from abroad; specifically, the site needs regular, up-to-date information from within the country. The only way to do this is to develop a network of reliable correspondents on the ground and to develop efficient channels for getting their information out of the country.

20   In the worst cases this means either heavily working the phones to your contacts on the ground, or, where phone-tapping is a concern, the smuggling of documentation out of the country. On the face of it, that would seem to be little advancement on the tedious and dangerous methods of the Communist-era dissidents. Still, when it works, it can bring the only non-regime-sponsored information to the outside world and offers a unique eye on closed societies. The work of the Revolutionary Association of the Women of Afghanistan in Taliban-controlled Afghanistan was certainly one of the best examples of such activity the Internet has ever seen.

21   In less restrictive situations, the Internet itself is the networking tool, and e-mail allows émigré publishing to be current from the ground in a way that Iron Curtain dissidents never could be. Even then, however, expanding a network of correspondents on the ground is not always straightforward, and the specifics of the local culture and local regime need to be considered.

22   My own Institute for War and Peace Reporting is familiar with this problem. The editors of our online publications covering post–Soviet Central Asia, Afghanistan and the Balkans are all émigré journalists in London who develop their networks on the ground according to the possibilities in individual countries. In Uzbekistan, for example, the situation is relaxed enough for us to

have a physical office in Tashkent and a rather normal network of correspondents radiating out from it. In Turkmenistan, however, the situation is significantly more complicated for us. Forget a physical office: all our reporters on the ground communicate directly via e-mail with our central office in London. Trying to build a normal network there would only attract informants who would turn in all our associates, so we keep our correspondents on the ground isolated from one another. They wouldn't recognize each other if they sat next to one another on a bus in downtown Ashghabat.

But even if you have a developed network of correspondents 23 on the ground, that doesn't mean that people will feel comfortable talking to them. When fear so thoroughly permeates society, mouths stay closed.

In some cases, however, the subject matter is so potentially 24 damaging to people's lives that they are able to overcome their fear of the authorities. The work of the Three Gorges Probe, a Web-site in Canada dedicated to discussing the controversial Three Gorges dam project in China, provides an interesting example of this. Publisher Patricia Adams was reluctant to discuss the details of her network on the ground, but she told me that ordinary people in the region are very eager to talk to TGP correspondents about the dam, as they genuinely hope their concerns will be addressed. Their willingness to talk is understandable; after all, many of them are the ones being resettled by the dam project.

The Three Gorges Probe Web site highlights another particular 25 problem of this genre: oftentimes, the line between journalism and activism becomes fuzzy—to the detriment of the reader seeking objective information. Adams insists Three Gorges Probe is pure journalism, but it is pretty clear that the site offers a mostly critical view of the project. While that may be a justifiable editorial policy intended to counter all the official information on the dam project, many émigré sites have very serious problems with balance.

Amnesty International's Umit Ozturk sees this as unfortunate 26 in the Turkish case but admits, "It couldn't be any other way." Most Turkish and Kurdish émigré sites are run by "activist reporters," people who care so passionately about their cause that objectivity takes a back seat in their online efforts.

27   Veronica Forwood of Reporters without Borders, however, says it depends on the background of the editors. Those who come from a strong journalism background usually try to maintain a sense of balance and concentrate on on-the-ground reporting rather than commentary.

28   Interestingly, there is now serious talk in U.K. NGO circles of creating a non-profit project specifically designed to help émigré journalists establish Web sites with local correspondent networks for the people in their repressive regimes back home. The idea is to provide start-up funds as well as the technical expertise and journalism training needed to run an émigré Web site with real impact on the ground.

REAL CHANGE IS NOT VIRTUAL

29 That impact is the heart of the problem for all Web sites working within and around repressive regimes. For all the excited talk about the Internet bringing freedom, actual examples of online publishing bringing about change in these countries are few.

30   In many ways, the Internet seems to fulfill the same role as *samizdat* did in Communist Czechoslovakia. Like that old dissident literature, the Internet in authoritarian regimes offers the only place for critical voices, but, sadly, it has little effect on the ground. Remember, despite the international fame of writers like Vaclav Havel, outside of a small circle of intellectuals in Prague, hardly anyone ever read *samizdat* within Communist Czechoslovakia. The Velvet Revolution emerged from direct action within a changed geo-political atmosphere; decades of dissident carping had nothing to do with real change when the regime finally fell.

31   As it was with *samizdat,* most people in authoritarian regimes never get a chance to see Internet publications, and the whole enterprise, both the publishing of banned information and official attempts to stop it, is more a game for elites: elite dissident intellectuals criticize elite rulers, and they argue back and forth in a virtual space. The opponents can score a few victories in that virtual space, but meanwhile, back in reality, little changes for the people on the ground.

Some may find such a conclusion a bit pessimistic, especially   32
coming from someone who works in the field of online journalism in these countries. But it is important to keep one's feet on
the ground and neither underestimate the scope of the problem
nor overestimate the ability of the medium.

And there is some reason for cautious optimism. CPJ's A. Lin   33
Neumann, for example, reminded me that, "elites, generally, tend
to lead the movement toward change so the fact that the Internet
is somewhat confined to elite communication in some places does
not disqualify it as a change agent." Neumann points to China,
saying that the Internet has had an effect on the ground there,
leading, for instance, to greater impact of stories on corruption.

Neumann also told me that the nature of the Internet means,   34
"It is simply harder, even for the Burmese bad guys, to keep
secrets from the world, because once information gets out it cir-
culates widely."

"Twenty years ago," he noted, "that information—such as a   35
secret arrest that is revealed through an underground contact—
would have to circulate by newsletters sent in the post; now it is
on the desks of journalists and others within minutes."

Ice-T: The Issue Is Creative Freedom

Barbara Ehrenreich

Ice-T's song "Cop Killer" is as bad as they come. This is black   1
anger—raw, rude, and cruel—and one reason the song's so shocking is that in postliberal America, black anger is virtually taboo.
You won't find it on TV, not on the *McLaughlin Group* or *Crossfire,*
and certainly not in the placid features of Arsenio Hall or Bernard
Shaw. It's been beaten back into the outlaw subcultures of rap and
rock, where, precisely because it is taboo, it sells. And the nastier
it is, the faster it moves off the shelves. As Ice-T asks in another
song on the same album, "Goddamn what a brotha gotta do / To
get a message through / To the red, white, and blue?"

But there's a gross overreaction going on, building to a veri-   2
table paroxysm of white denial. A national boycott has been

called, not just of the song or Ice-T, but of all Time Warner products. The president himself has denounced Time Warner as "wrong" and Ice-T as "sick." Ollie North's Freedom Alliance has started a petition drive aimed at bringing Time Warner executives to trial for "sedition and anarchy."

3   Much of this is posturing and requires no more courage than it takes to stand up in a VFW hall and condemn communism or crack. Yes, "Cop Killer" is irresponsible and vile. But Ice-T is as right about some things as he is righteous about the rest. And ultimately, he's not even dangerous—least of all to the white power structure his songs condemn.

4   The "danger" implicit in all the uproar is of empty-headed, suggestible black kids, crouching by their boom boxes, waiting for the word. But what Ice-T's fans know and his detractors obviously don't is that "Cop Killer" is just one more entry in pop music's long history of macho hyperbole and violent boast. Flip to the classic-rock station, and you might catch the Rolling Stones announcing "the time is right for violent revoloo-shun!" from their 1968 hit "Street Fighting Man." And where were the defenders of our law-enforcement officers when a white British group, the Clash, taunted its fans with the lyrics: "When they kick open your front door / How you gonna come / With your hands on your head / Or on the trigger of your gun?"

5   "Die, Die, Die Pig" is strong speech, but the Constitution protects strong speech, and it's doing so this year more aggressively than ever. The Supreme Court has just downgraded cross burnings to the level of bonfires and ruled that it's no crime to throw around verbal grenades like "nigger" and "kike." Where are the defenders of decorum and social stability when prime-time demagogues like Howard Stern deride African Americans as "spear chuckers"?

6   More to the point, young African Americans are not so naive and suggestible that they have to depend on a compact disc for their sociology lessons. To paraphrase another song from another era, you don't need a rap song to tell which way the wind is blowing. Black youths know that the police are likely to see them through a filter of stereotypes as miscreants and potential "cop killers." They are aware that a black youth is seven times as likely to be charged with a felony as a white youth who has committed the same offense, and is much more likely to be imprisoned.

They know, too, that in a shameful number of cases, it is the 7
police themselves who indulge in "anarchy" and violence. The
U.S. Justice Department has received 47,000 complaints of police
brutality in the past six years, and Amnesty International has just
issued a report on police brutality in Los Angeles, documenting
forty cases of "torture or cruel, inhuman, or degrading treatment."

Menacing as it sounds, the fantasy in "Cop Killer" is the 8
fantasy of the powerless and beaten down—the black man who's
been hassled once too often ("A pig stopped me for nothin'!"),
spread-eagled against a police car, pushed around. It's not a
"responsible" fantasy (fantasies seldom are). It's not even a very
creative one. In fact, the sad thing about "Cop Killer" is that it
falls for the cheapest, most conventional image of rebellion that
our culture offers: the lone gunman spraying fire from his AK-47.
This is not "sedition"; it's the familiar, all-American, Hollywood-
style pornography of violence.

Which is why Ice-T is right to say he's no more dangerous 9
than George Bush's pal Arnold Schwarzenegger, who wasted an
army of cops in *Terminator 2*. Images of extraordinary cruelty and
violence are marketed every day, many of far less artistic merit
than "Cop Killer." This is our free market of ideas and images,
and it shouldn't be any less free for a black man than for other
purveyors of "irresponsible" sentiments, from David Duke to
Andrew Dice Clay.

Just, please, don't dignify Ice-T's contribution with the word 10
sedition. The past masters of sedition—men like George Washington,
Toussaint L'Ouverture, Fidel Castro, or Mao Zedong, all of whom
led and won armed insurrections—would be unimpressed by
"Cop Killer" and probably saddened. They would shake their
heads and mutter words like "infantile" and "adventurism." They
might point out that the cops are hardly a noble target, being, for
the most part, honest working stiffs who've got stuck with the job
of patrolling ghettos ravaged by economic decline and official
neglect.

There is a difference, the true seditionist would argue, 11
between a revolution and a gesture of macho defiance. Gestures
are cheap. They feel good, they blow off some rage. But revolutions, violent or otherwise, are made by people who have learned
how to count very slowly to ten.

Ideological Videogames: Press Left Button to Dissent

Gonzalo Frasca

1   "Videogames do not necessarily need to be entertaining." Such a statement is still likely to trigger passionate debates (albeit less likely than a few years ago). Who would play a game that is not fun? The answer, of course, relies on how you define fun and entertainment.

2   The question is trivial in other media, such as books or films. Certainly, thousands of movies and novels are made every year with the sole goal of entertaining their audience, while a similar amount supposedly aim at more serious goals such as generating debate, making a point, explaining something or sharing knowledge. The latter are not fun under the broader definition of the term, even if they do provide certain pleasures.

3   The question should be trivial in games, too. Actually, videogames were born for non-entertaining uses, as military simulators designed for training. There is also an extensive history of educational videogames with an explicit pedagogical agenda. These examples, which exist since the very beginning of the genre, should suffice to make the point that videogames can certainly have non-entertaining purposes. However, in my experience, most players react negatively to the idea of games that do not just aspire at being fun.

4   If videogames are indeed persuasive tools, then they can be used for conveying passionate ideas. If you want to know if a medium is ready to deliver an ideological message, simply ask if somebody would be willing to endanger her life for it. There are multiple cases of this in literature (i.e. Salman Rushdie) and it certainly happens in films, even though on a minor degree (Martin Scorsese's *Last Temptation of Christ* was violently boycotted).

5   Would somebody be willing to die for a videogame? I guess the answer is still no. Currently, it is more likely that games can simply trigger passionate arguments and some foul language. As a matter of fact, the moment I knew that my game *September 12th* had succeeded at conveying its ideas was when the first piece of hate mail arrived to my inbox.

Ideological videogames are games that you can agree or dis- 6
agree with. Certainly, nobody disagrees with *Tetris*. However, as
games started dealing with more realistic simulations of human
life, the situation changed. A clear example is *The Sims*, which has
been criticized for its supposed consumerist ideology (and
defended by its author as anti-consumerist). Still, I think *The Sims*
was clearly designed primarily as entertainment. Of course, there
is nothing wrong with that, but personally I would also love to
see more games with a clear agenda.

Before professionally working as a game designer, I worked in 7
advertising and journalism. The connection between videogames
and ads was clear for me since I saw a Budweiser banner displayed
in *Tapper,* the classic bartender game. It was while working at CNN
that I started daydreaming about creating games that would complement news with editorial statements, like political cartoons do.
A few years later, I was finally able to launch Newsgaming.com
with the help of a group of collaborators.

Newsgames, or games based on news events, are certainly not 8
new. There are countless examples of games based on political
and social events, as well as many created after the events of 9-11.
It is on this tradition that I created *September 12th,* a game (even
if its instructions provocatively claim that it is not a game) that
tries to make a point about the war on terror.

Basically, the game models a Middle Eastern town showcas- 9
ing mostly civilians and some terrorists. The player controls a
crosshair with which it is possible to launch missiles. It is almost
impossible to kill the terrorists without generating "collateral
damage." Every time that a civilian dies, others will mourn him
or her and, suddenly, become terrorists. After a few minutes of
play, the number of terrorists is out of control.

September 12th was conceived with two goals in mind. One 10
was conveying a simple idea through a simple model: violence
will create more violence. It was my hope that this idea would
contribute to generate debate around the issue of the civilian casu-
alties of the war on terror. The other goal was exploring the problems of creating actual ideological videogames instead of just
writing about them from my nice and tall ivory tower.

The game certainly generated debate. A few weeks after its 11
launch, more than 100 thousand people from all over the world

have played *September 12th*. More importantly, half of the links pointing to it came from online forums and weblog comments, where both the game and its topic were discussed.

12   The game also generated criticism and was very often dismissed as too simplistic (which, of course, it obviously is). In part, this rejection may be due to what Sherry Turkle identifies in her book *Life on the Screen* as "simulation denial": some people believe that simulations cannot help us in understanding reality because they always offer a limited model of it. However, I think that a big part of this critique is due to the fact that political videogaming is not yet a well-established genre. Nobody would ever criticize a printed political cartoon on the basis of being too simplistic: caricatures are simplifications by definition. In spite of this, cartoons make a point and this is why they remain a useful journalistic tool.

13   We need more games that make statements. Surely, games and simulations will always be limited. Games will always be biased. Games will always be interpreted (and manipulated) in ways that its authors never foresaw. However, I agree with Sherry Turkle that games could also provide great insight:

> Understanding the assumptions that underlie simulation is a key element of political power. People who understand the distortions imposed by simulations are in a position to call for more direct economic and political feedback, new kinds of representation, more channels of information.

14   In order to accomplish this, we academics must join forces with developers and provide them with practical game theory or, even better, start making our own games. Personally, I see *September 12th* as a small experiment on game rhetoric. But the potential of videogames for critical thinking and debate is, I believe, much larger. It lies, I think, in providing players with tools to contest the game's ideological assumptions by designing their own games. Eventually, games will allow us to model our ideas and let others play with them and vice versa.

15   One of my most vivid childhood memories was witnessing my mother and aunt crying together as they burned most of their books in our backyard. This was during my home country's military dictatorship, when owning certain books was enough reason

for being imprisoned and/or tortured. I wonder if some day somebody would hold a match in front of a pile of videogames and seriously consider burning them down in order to maintain their freedom. If that ever happens, it would mean that our civilization would have been able to turn a supposedly trivial medium into something that really matters. Thanks to Ray Bradbury, we know that books flame at 451 degrees Fahrenheit. Who knows how much heat is needed to burn videogames?

Pop Culture and the Media: Do We Cover Events or Invent Them?

A Flood of Pseudo-Events

Daniel Boorstin

ADMIRING FRIEND: "My, that's a beautiful baby you have there"
MOTHER: "Oh, that's nothin—you should see his photograph!"

1 The simplest of our extravagant expectations concerns the amount of novelty in the world. There was a time when the reader of an unexciting newspaper would remark, "How dull is the world today!" Nowadays he says, "What a dull newspaper!" When the first American newspaper, Benjamin Harris' *Publick Occurrences Both Forreign and Domestick*, appeared in Boston on September 25, 1690, it promised to furnish news regularly once a month. But, the editor explained, it might appear oftener "if any Glut of Occurrences happen." The responsibility for making news was entirely God's—or the Devil's. The newsman's task was only to give "an Account of such considerable things as have arrived unto our Notice."

2 Although the theology behind this way of looking at events soon dissolved, this view of the news lasted longer. "The skilled and faithful journalist," James Parton observed in 1866, "recording with exactness and power the thing that has come to pass, is Providence addressing men." The story is told of a Southern Baptist clergyman before the Civil War who used to say, when a newspaper was brought in the room, "Be kind enough to let me have it a few minutes, till I see how the Supreme Being is governing

the world." Charles A. Dana, one of the great American editors of the nineteenth century, once defended his extensive reporting of crime in the New York *Sun* by saying, "I have always felt that whatever the Divine Providence permitted to occur I was not too proud to report."

Of course, this is now a very old-fashioned way of thinking. 3 Our current point of view is better expressed in the definition by Arthur MacEwen, whom William Randolph Hearst made his first editor of the San Francisco *Examiner:* "News is anything that makes a reader say, 'Gee whiz!'" Or, put more soberly, "News is whatever a good editor chooses to print."

We need not be theologians to see that we have shifted 4 responsibility for making the world interesting from God to the newspaperman. We used to believe there were only so many "events" in the world. If there were not many intriguing or startling occurrences, it was no fault of the reporter. He could not be expected to report what did not exist.

Within the last hundred years, however, and especially in the 5 twentieth century, all this has changed. We expect the papers to be full of news. If there is no news visible to the naked eye, or to the average citizen, we still expect it to be there for the enterprising newsman. The successful reporter is one who can find a story, even if there is no earthquake or assassination or civil war. If he cannot find a story, then he must make one—by the questions he asks of public figures, by the surprising human interest he unfolds from some commonplace event, or by "the news behind the news." If all this fails, then he must give us a "think piece"—an embroidering of well-known facts, or a speculation about startling things to come.

This change in our attitude toward "news" is not merely a basic 6 fact about the history of American newspapers. It is a symptom of a revolutionary change in our attitude toward what happens in the world, how much of it is new, and surprising, and important. Toward how life can be enlivened, toward our power and the power of those who inform and educate and guide us, to provide synthetic happenings to make up for the lack of spontaneous events. Demanding more than the world can give us, we require that something be fabricated to make up for the world's deficiency. This is only one example of our demand for illusions.

7   Many historical forces help explain how we have come to our present immoderate hopes. But there can be no doubt about what we now expect, nor that it is immoderate. Every American knows the anticipation with which he picks up his morning newspaper at breakfast or opens his evening paper before dinner, or listens to the newscasts every hour on the hour as he drives across country, or watches his favorite commentator on television interpret the events of the day. Many enterprising Americans are now at work to help us satisfy these expectations. Many might be put out of work if we should suddenly moderate our expectations. But it is we who keep them in business and demand that they fill our consciousness with novelties, that they play God for us.

8   The new kind of synthetic novelty which has flooded our experience I will call "pseudo-events." The common prefix "pseudo" comes from the Greek word meaning false, or intended to deceive. Before I recall the historical forces which have made these pseudo-events possible, have increased the supply of them and the demand for them, I will give a commonplace example.

9   The owners of a hotel, in an illustration offered by Edward L. Bernays in his pioneer *Crystallizing Public Opinion* (1923), consult a public relations counsel. They ask how to increase their hotel's prestige and so improve their business. In less sophisticated times, the answer might have been to hire a new chef, to improve the plumbing, to paint the rooms, or to install a crystal chandelier in the lobby. The public relations counsel's technique is more indirect. He proposes that the management stage a celebration of the hotel's thirtieth anniversary. A committee is formed, including a prominent banker, a leading society matron, a well-known lawyer, an influential preacher, and an "event" is planned (say a banquet) to call attention to the distinguished service the hotel has been rendering the community. The celebration is held, photographs are taken, the occasion is widely reported, and the object is accomplished. Now this occasion is a pseudo-event, and will illustrate all the essential features of pseudo-events.

10   This celebration, we can see at the outset, is somewhat—but not entirely—misleading. Presumably the public relations counsel would not have been able to form his committee of prominent citizens if the hotel had not actually been rendering service to the

community. On the other hand, if the hotel's services had been all that important, instigation by public relations counsel might not have been necessary. Once the celebration has been held, the celebration itself becomes evidence that the hotel really is a distinguished institution. The occasion actually gives the hotel the prestige to which it is pretending.

It is obvious, too, that the value of such a celebration to the 11 owners depends on its being photographed and reported in newspapers, magazines, newsreels, on radio, and over television. It is the report that gives the event its force in the minds of potential customers. The power to make a reportable event is thus the power to make experience. One is reminded of Napoleon's apocryphal reply to his general, who objected that circumstances were unfavorable to a proposed campaign: "Bah, I make circumstances!" The modern public relations counsel—and he is, of course, only one of many twentieth-century creators of pseudo-events—has come close to fulfilling Napoleon's idle boast. "The counsel of public relations," Mr. Bernays explains, "not only knows what news value is, but knowing it, he is in a position to *make news happen*. He is a creator of events."

The intriguing feature of the modern situation, however, 12 comes precisely from the fact that the modern news makers are not God. The news they make happen, the events they create, are somehow not quite real. There remains a tantalizing difference between man-made and God-made events.

A pseudo-event, then, is a happening that possesses the 13 following characteristics:

1. It is not spontaneous, but comes about because someone has 14 planned, planted, or incited it. Typically, it is not a train wreck or an earthquake, but an interview.
2. It is planted primarily (not always exclusively) for the immedi- 15 ate purpose of being reported or reproduced. Therefore, its occurrence is arranged for the convenience of the reporting or reproducing media. Its success is measured by how widely it is reported. Time relations in it are commonly fictitious or factitious; the announcement is given out in advance "for future release" and written as if the event had occurred in the past. The question, "Is it real?" is less important than, "Is it newsworthy?"

16   **3.** Its relation to the underlying reality of the situation is ambiguous. Its interest arises largely from this very ambiguity. Concerning a pseudo-event the question, "What does it mean?" has a new dimension. While the news interest in a train wreck is in *what* happened and in the real consequences, the interest in an interview is always, in a sense, in *whether* it really happened and in what might have been the motives. Did the statement really mean what it said? Without some of this ambiguity a pseudo-event cannot be very interesting.

17   **4.** Usually it is intended to be a self-fulfilling prophecy. The hotel's thirtieth-anniversary celebration, by saying that the hotel is a distinguished institution, actually makes it one.

18   In the last half century a larger and larger proportion of our experience, of what we read and see and hear, has come to consist of pseudo-events. We expect more of them and we are given more of them. They flood our consciousness. Their multiplication has gone on in the United States at a faster rate than elsewhere. Even the rate of increase is increasing every day. This is true of the world of education, of consumption, and of personal relations. It is especially true of the world of public affairs which I describe in this chapter.

19   A full explanation of the origin and rise of pseudo-events would be nothing less than a history of modern America. For our present purposes it is enough to recall a few of the more revolutionary recent developments.

20   The great modern increase in the supply and the demand for news began in the early nineteenth century. Until then newspapers tended to fill out their columns with lackadaisical secondhand accounts or stale reprints of items first published elsewhere at home and abroad. The laws of plagiarism and of copyright were undeveloped. Most newspapers were little more than excuses for espousing a political position, for listing the arrival and departure of ships, for familiar essays and useful advice, or for commercial or legal announcements.

21   Less than a century and a half ago did newspapers begin to disseminate up-to-date reports of matters of public interest written by eyewitnesses or professional reporters near the scene. The telegraph was perfected and applied to news reporting in the 1830's

and '40's. Two newspapermen, William M. Swain of the Philadelphia *Public Ledger* and Amos Kendall of Frankfort, Kentucky, were founders of the national telegraphic network. Polk's presidential message in 1846 was the first to be transmitted by wire. When the Associated Press was founded in 1848, news began to be a salable commodity. Then appeared the rotary press, which could print on a continuous sheet and on both sides of the paper at the same time. The New York *Tribune's* highspeed press, installed in the 1870's, could turn out 18,000 papers per hour. The Civil War, and later the Spanish-American War, offered raw materials and incentive for vivid up-to-the-minute, on-the-spot reporting. The competitive daring of giants like James Gordon Bennett, Joseph Pulitzer, and William Randolph Hearst intensified the race for news and widened newspaper circulation.

These events were part of a great, but little-noticed, revolution—   22 what I would call the Graphic Revolution. Man's ability to make, preserve, transmit, and disseminate precise images—images of print, of men and landscapes and events, of the voices of men and mobs—now grew at a fantastic pace. The increased speed of printing was itself revolutionary. Still more revolutionary were the new techniques for making direct images of nature. Photography was destined soon to give printed matter itself a secondary role. By a giant leap Americans crossed the gulf from the daguerreotype to color television in less than a century. Dry-plate photography came in 1873; Bell patented the telephone in 1876; the phonograph was invented in 1877; the roll film appeared in 1884; Eastman's Kodak No. 1 was produced in 1888; Edison's patent on the radio came in 1891; motion pictures came in and voice was first transmitted by radio around 1900; the first national political convention widely broadcast by radio was that of 1928; television became commercially important in 1941, and color television even more recently.

Verisimilitude took on a new meaning. Not only was it now   23 possible to give the actual voice and gestures of Franklin Delano Roosevelt unprecedented reality and intimacy for a whole nation, vivid image came to overshadow pale reality. Sound motion pictures in color led a whole generation of pioneering American movie-goers to think of Benjamin Disraeli as an earlier imitation of George Arliss, just as television has led a later generation of television watchers to see the Western cowboy as an inferior replica of John Wayne. The Grand Canyon itself became a disappointing reproduction of the Kodachrome original.

24   The new power to report and portray what had happened was a new temptation leading newsmen to make probable images or to prepare reports in advance of what was expected to happen. As so often, men came to mistake their power for their necessities. Readers and viewers would soon prefer the vividness of the account, the "candidness" of the photograph, to the spontaneity of what was recounted.

25   Then came round-the-clock media. The news gap soon became so narrow that in order to have additional "news" for each new edition or each new broadcast it was necessary to plan in advance the stages by which any available news would be unveiled. After the weekly and the daily came the "extras" and the numerous regular editions. The Philadelphia *Evening Bulletin* soon had seven editions a day. No rest for the newsman. With more space to fill, he had to fill it ever more quickly. In order to justify the numerous editions, it was increasingly necessary that the news constantly change or at least seem to change. With radio on the air continuously during waking hours, the reporters' problems became still more acute. News every hour on the hour, and sometimes on the half hour. Programs interrupted any time for special bulletins. How to avoid deadly repetition, the appearance that nothing was happening, that news gatherers were asleep, or that competitors were more alert? As the costs of printing and then of broadcasting increased, it became financially necessary to keep the presses always at work and the TV screen always busy. Pressures toward the making of pseudo-events became ever stronger. News gathering turned into news making.

26   The "interview" was a novel way of making news which had come in with the Graphic Revolution. Later it became elaborated into lengthy radio and television panels and quizzes of public figures, and the three-hour-long, rambling conversation programs. Although the interview technique might seem an obvious one—and in a primitive form was as old as Socrates—the use of the word in its modern journalistic sense is a relatively recent Americanism. The Boston *News-Letter's* account (March 2,

1719) of the death of Blackbeard the Pirate had apparently been based on a kind of interview with a ship captain. One of the earliest interviews of the modern type—some writers call it the first—was by James Gordon Bennett, the flamboyant editor of the New York *Herald* (April 16, 1836), in connection with the Robinson-Jewett murder case. Ellen Jewett, inmate of a house of prostitution, had been found murdered by an ax. Richard P. Robinson, a young man about town, was accused of the crime. Bennett seized the occasion to pyramid sensational stories and so to build circulation for his *Herald;* before long he was having difficulty turning out enough copies daily to satisfy the demand. He exploited the story in every possible way, one of which was to plan and report an actual interview with Rosina Townsend, the madam who kept the house and whom he visited on her own premises.

Historians of journalism date the first full-fledged modern 27 interview with a well-known public figure from July 13, 1859, when Horace Greeley interviewed Brigham Young in Salt Lake City, asking him questions on many matters of public interest, and then publishing the answers verbatim in his New York *Tribune* (August 20, 1859). The common use of the word "interview" in this modern American sense first came in about this time. Very early the institution acquired a reputation for being contrived. "The 'interview,'" *The Nation* complained (January 28, 1869), "as at present managed, is generally the joint product of some humbug of a hack politician and another humbug of a reporter." A few years later another magazine editor called the interview "the most perfect contrivance yet devised to make journalism an offence, a thing of ill savor in all decent nostrils." Many objected to the practice as an invasion of privacy. After the American example it was used in England and France, but in both those countries it made much slower headway.

Even before the invention of the interview, the news-making 28 profession in America had attained a new dignity as well as a menacing power. It was in 1828 that Macaulay called the gallery where reporters sat in Parliament a "fourth estate of the realm." But Macaulay could not have imagined the prestige of journalists in the twentieth-century United States. They have long since made themselves the tribunes of the people. Their supposed detachment and lack of partisanship, their closeness to the sources of information, their articulateness, and their constant and direct access to the whole citizenry have made them also the counselors of the people. Foreign observers are now astonished by the almost constitutional—perhaps we should say supra-constitutional— powers of our Washington press corps.

29   Since the rise of the modern Presidential press conference, about 1933, capital correspondents have had the power regularly to question the President face-to-face, to embarrass him, to needle him, to force him into positions or into public refusal to take a position. A President may find it inconvenient to meet a group of dissident Senators or Congressmen; he seldom dares refuse the press. That refusal itself becomes news. It is only very recently, and as a result of increasing pressures by newsmen, that the phrase "No comment" has become a way of saying something important. The reputation of newsmen—who now of course include those working for radio, TV, and magazines—depends on their ability to ask hard questions, to put politicians on the spot; their very livelihood depends on the willing collaboration of public figures. Even before 1950 Washington had about 1,500 correspondents and about 3,000 government information officials prepared to serve them.

30   Not only the regular formal press conferences, but a score of other national programs—such as *Meet the Press* and *Face the Nation*—show the power of newsmen. In 1960 David Susskind's late-night conversation show, *Open End,* commanded the presence of the Russian Premier for three hours. During the so-called "Great Debates" that year between the candidates in the Presidential campaign, it was newsmen who called the tune.

31   The live television broadcasting of the President's regular news conferences, which President Kennedy began in 1961, immediately after taking office, has somewhat changed their character. Newsmen are no longer so important as intermediaries who relay the President's statements. But the new occasion acquires a new interest as a dramatic performance. Citizens who from homes or offices have seen the President at his news conference are then even more interested to hear competing interpretations by skilled commentators. News commentators can add a new appeal as dramatic critics to their traditional role as interpreters of current

history. Even in the new format it is still the newsmen who put the questions. They are still tribunes of the people. . . .

In many subtle ways, the rise of pseudo-events has mixed up our 32 roles as actors and as audience—or, the philosophers would say, as "object" and as "subject." Now we can oscillate between the two roles. "The movies are the only business," Will Rogers once remarked, "where you can go out front and applaud yourself." Nowadays one need not be a professional actor to have this satisfaction. We can appear in the mob scene and then go home and see ourselves on the television screen. No wonder we become confused about what is spontaneous, about what is really going on out there!

New forms of pseudo-events, especially in the world of poli- 33 tics, thus offer a new kind of bewilderment to both politician and newsman. The politician (like F.D.R. in our example, or any holder of a press conference) himself in a sense composes the story; the journalist (like the wire service reporter we have quoted, or any newsman who incites an inflammatory statement) himself generates the event. The citizen can hardly be expected to assess the reality when the participants themselves are so often unsure who is doing the deed and who is making the report of it. Who is the history, and who is the historian?

An admirable example of this new intertwinement of subject 34 and object, of the history and the historian, of the actor and the reporter, is the so-called news "leak." By now the leak has become an important and well-established institution in American politics. It is, in fact, one of the main vehicles for communicating important information from officials to the public.

A clue to the new unreality of the citizen's world is the 35 perverse new meaning now given to the word "leak." To leak, according to the dictionary, is to "let a fluid substance out or in accidentally: as, the ship leaks." But nowadays a news leak is one of the most elaborately planned ways of emitting information. It is, of course, a way in which a government official, with some clearly defined purpose (a leak, even more than a direct announcement, is apt to have some definite devious purpose behind it) makes an announcement, asks a question, or puts a suggestion. It might more accurately be called a "sub rosa announcement," an "indirect statement," or "cloaked news."

36   The news leak is a pseudo-event par excellence. In its origin and growth, the leak illustrates another axiom of the world of pseudo-events: pseudo-events produce more pseudo-events. I will say more on this later.

37   With the elaboration of news-gathering facilities in Washington—of regular, planned press conferences, of prepared statements for future release, and of countless other practices—the news protocol has hardened. Both government officials and reporters have felt the need for more flexible and more ambiguous modes of communication between them. The Presidential press conference itself actually began as a kind of leak. President Theodore Roosevelt for some time allowed Lincoln Steffens to interview him as he was being shaved. Other Presidents gave favored correspondents an interview from time to time or dropped hints to friendly journalists. Similarly, the present institution of the news leak began in the irregular practice of a government official's helping a particular correspondent by confidentially giving him information not yet generally released. But today the leak is almost as well organized and as rigidly ruled by protocol as a formal press conference. Being fuller of ambiguity, with a welcome atmosphere of confidence and intrigue, it is more appealing to all concerned. The institutionalized leak puts a greater burden of contrivance and pretense on both government officials and reporters.

38   In Washington these days, and elsewhere on a smaller scale, the custom has grown up among important members of the government of arranging to dine with select representatives of the news corps. Such dinners are usually preceded by drinks, and beforehand there is a certain amount of restrained conviviality. Everyone knows the rules: the occasion is private, and any information given out afterwards must be communicated according to rule and in the technically proper vocabulary. After dinner the undersecretary, the general, or the admiral allows himself to be questioned. He may recount "facts" behind past news, state plans, or declare policy. The reporters have confidence, if not in the ingenuousness of the official, at least in their colleagues' respect of the protocol. Everybody understands the degree of attribution permissible for every statement made: what, if anything, can be directly quoted, what is

"background," what is "deep background," what must be ascribed to "a spokesman," to "an informed source," to speculation, to rumor, or to remote possibility.

Such occasions and the reports flowing from them are loaded 39 with ambiguity. The reporter himself often is not clear whether he is being told a simple fact, a newly settled policy, an administrative hope, or whether perhaps untruths are being deliberately diffused to allay public fears that the true facts are really true. The government official himself (who is sometimes no more than a spokesman) may not be clear. The reporter's task is to find a way of weaving tines, threads of unreality into a fabric that the reader will not recognize as entirely unreal. Some people have criticized the institutionalized leak as a form of domestic counter-intelligence inappropriate in a republic. It has become more and more important and is the source today of many of the most influential reports of current politics.

One example will be enough. On March 26, 1955, *The New* 40 *York Times* carried a three-column headline on the front page: "U.S. Expects Chinese Reds to Attack Isles in April; Weighs All-Out Defense." Three days later a contradictory headline in the same place read: "Eisenhower Sees No War Now Over Chinese Isles." Under each of these headlines appeared a lengthy story. Neither story named any person as a source of the ostensible facts. The then-undisclosed story (months later recorded by Douglass Cater) was this. In the first instance, Admiral Robert B. Carney, Chief of Naval Operations, had an off-the-record "background" dinner for a few reporters. There the Admiral gave reporters what they (and their readers) took to be facts. Since the story was "not for attribution," reporters were not free to mention some very relevant facts—such as that this was the opinion only of Admiral Carney, that this was the same Admiral Carney who had long been saying that war in Asia was inevitable, and that many in Washington (even in the Joint Chiefs of Staff) did not agree with him. Under the ground rules the first story could appear in the papers only by being given an impersonal authority, an atmosphere of official unanimity which it did not merit. The second, and contradictory, statement was in fact made not by the President himself, but by the President's press secretary, James Hagerty, who, having been alarmed by what he saw in the papers, quickly called a second "background" meeting to deny the stories that had sprouted from the first. What, if anything, did it all mean? Was there any real news here at all except that there was disagreement between Admiral Carney and James Hagerty? Yet this was the fact newsmen were not free to print.

41   Pseudo-events spawn other pseudo-events in geometric progression. This is partly because every kind of pseudo-event (being planned) tends to become ritualized, with a protocol and a rigidity all its own. As each type of pseudo-event acquires this rigidity, pressures arise to produce other, derivative, forms of pseudo-event which are more fluid, more tantalizing, and more interestingly ambiguous. Thus, as the press conference (itself a pseudo-event) became formalized, there grew up the institutionalized leak. As the leak becomes formalized still other devices will appear. Of course the shrewd politician or the enterprising newsman knows this and knows how to take advantage of it. Seldom for outright deception; more often simply to make more "news," to provide more "information," or to "improve communication."

42   For example, a background off-the-record press conference, if it is actually a mere trial balloon or a diplomatic device (as it sometimes was for Secretary of State John Foster Dulles), becomes the basis of official "denials" and "disavowals," of speculation and interpretation by columnists and commentators, and of special interviews on and off television with Senators, Representatives, and other public officials.

43   Any statement or non-statement by anyone in the public eye can become the basis of counter-statements or refusals to comment by others. All these compound the ambiguity of the occasion which first brought them into being.

44   Nowadays the test of a Washington reporter is seldom his skill at precise dramatic reporting, but more often his adeptness at dark intimation. If he wishes to keep his news channels open he must accumulate a vocabulary and develop a style to conceal his sources and obscure the relation of a supposed event or statement to the underlying facts of life, at the same time seeming to offer hard facts. Much of his stock in trade is his own and other people's speculation about the reality of what he reports. He lives in a penumbra between fact and fantasy. He helps create that very obscurity without which the supposed illumination of his reports would be unnecessary. A

deft administrator these days must have similar skills. He must master "the technique of denying the truth without actually lying."

These pseudo-events which flood our consciousness must be 45 distinguished from propaganda. The two do have some characteristics in common. But our peculiar problems come from the fact that pseudo-events are in some respects the opposite of the propaganda which rules totalitarian countries. Propaganda—as prescribed, say, by Hitler in *Mein Kampf*—is information intentionally biased. Its effect depends primarily on its emotional appeal. While a pseudo-event is an ambiguous truth, propaganda is an appealing falsehood. Pseudo-events thrive on our honest desire to be informed, to have "all the facts," and even to have more facts than there really are. But propaganda feeds on our willingness to be inflamed. Pseudo-events appeal to our duty to be educated, propaganda appeals to our desire to be aroused. While propaganda substitutes opinion for facts, pseudo-events are synthetic facts which move people indirectly, by providing the "factual" basis on which they are supposed to make up their minds. Propaganda moves them directly by explicitly making judgments for them.

In a totalitarian society, where people are flooded by pur- 46 poseful lies, the real facts are of course misrepresented, but the representation itself is not ambiguous. The propaganda is asserted as if it were true. Its object is to lead people to believe that the truth is simpler, more intelligible, than it really is. "Now the purpose of propaganda," Hitler explained "is not continually to produce interesting changes for a few blasé little masters, but to convince; that means to convince the masses. The masses, however, with their inertia, always need a certain time before they are ready even to notice a thing, and they will lend their memories only to the thousandfold repetition of the most simple ideas." But in our society, pseudo-events make simple facts seem more subtle, more ambiguous, and more speculative than they really are. Propaganda oversimplifies experience, pseudo-events overcomplicate it.

At first it may seem strange that the rise of pseudo-events has 47 coincided with the growth of the professional ethic which obliges newsmen to omit editorializing and personal judgments from their news accounts. But now it is in the making of pseudo-events that newsmen find ample scope for their individuality and creative imagination.

48   In a democratic society like ours—and more especially in a highly literate, wealthy, competitive, and technologically advanced society—the people can be flooded by pseudo-events. For us, freedom of speech and of the press and of broadcasting includes freedom to create pseudo-events. Competing politicians, competing newsmen, and competing news media contest in this creation. They vie with one another in offering attractive, "informative" accounts and images of the world. They are free to speculate on the facts, to bring new facts into being, to demand answers to their own contrived questions. Our "free marketplace of ideas" is a place where people are confronted by competing pseudo-events and are allowed to judge among them. When we speak of "informing" the people this is what we really mean.

Propaganda in a Democratic Society

Aldous Huxley

1   "The doctrines of Europe," Jefferson wrote, "were that men in numerous associations cannot be restrained within the limits of order and justice, except by forces physical and moral wielded over them by authorities independent of their will. . . . We (the founders of the new American democracy) believe that man was a rational animal, endowed by nature with rights, and with an innate sense of justice, and that he could be restrained from wrong, and protected in right, by moderate powers, confided to persons of his own choice and held to their duties by dependence on his own will." To post-Freudian ears, this kind of language seems touchingly quaint and ingenuous. Human beings are a good deal less rational and innately just than the optimists of the eighteenth century supposed. On the other hand they are neither so morally blind nor so hopelessly unreasonable as the pessimists of the twentieth would have us believe. In spite of the Id and the Unconscious, in spite of endemic neurosis and the prevalence of low IQ's, most men and women are probably decent enough and sensible enough to be trusted with the direction of their own destinies.

Democratic institutions are devices for reconciling social order 2 with individual freedom and initiative, and for making the immediate power of a country's rulers subject to the ultimate power of the ruled. The fact that, in Western Europe and America, these devices have worked, all things considered, not too badly is proof enough that the eighteenth century optimists were not entirely wrong. Given a fair chance, I repeat; for the fair chance is an indispensible prerequisite. No people that passes abruptly from a state of subservience under the rule of a despot to the completely unfamiliar state of political independence can be said to have a fair chance of being able to govern itself democratically. Liberalism flourishes in an atmosphere of prosperity and declines as declining prosperity makes it necessary for the government to intervene ever more frequently and drastically in the affairs of its subjects. Over-population and over-organization are two conditions which . . . deprive a society of a fair chance of making democratic institutions work effectively. We see, then, that there are certain historical, economic, demographic and technological conditions which make it very hard for Jefferson's rational animals, endowed by nature with inalienable rights and an innate sense of justice, to exercise their reason, claim their rights and act justly within a democratically organized society. We in the West have been supremely fortunate in having been given a fair chance of making the great experiment in self-government. Unfortunately, it now looks as though, owing to recent changes in our circumstances, this infinitely precious fair chance were being, little by little, taken away from us. And this, of course, is not the whole story. These blind impersonal forces are not the only enemies of individual liberty and democratic institutions. There are also forces of another, less abstract character, forces that can be deliberately used by power-seeking individuals whose aim is to establish partial or complete control over their fellows. Fifty years ago, when I was a boy, it seemed completely self-evident that the bad old days were over, that torture and massacre, slavery, and the persecution of heretics, were things of the past. Among people who wore top hats, traveled in trains, and took a bath every morning such horrors were simply out of the question. After all, we were living in the twentieth century. A few years later these people who took daily baths and went to church in top hats were committing atrocities on a scale undreamed of by the benighted Africans and Asiatics. In the light of recent history it would be foolish to suppose that this sort of thing cannot happen again. It can and, no doubt, it will. But in the immediate future there is some reason to believe that the punitive measures of *1984* will give place to the reinforcements and manipulations of *Brave New World*.

3   There are two kinds of propaganda—rational propaganda in favor of action that is consonant with the enlightened self-interest of those who make it and those to whom it is addressed, and non-rational propaganda that is not consonant with anybody's enlightened self-interest, but is dictated by, and appeals to, passion. Where the actions of individuals are concerned there are motives more exalted than enlightened self-interest, but where collective action has to be taken in the fields of politics and economics, enlightened self-interest is probably the highest of effective motives. If politicians and their constituents always acted to promote their own or their country's long-range self-interest, this world would be an earthly paradise. As it is, they often act against their own interests, merely to gratify their least credible passions; the world, in consequence, is a place of misery. Propaganda in favor of action that is consonant with enlightened self-interest appeals to reason by means of logical arguments based upon the best available evidence fully and honestly set forth. Propaganda in favor of action dictated by the impulses that are below self-interest offers false, garbled or incomplete evidence, avoids logical argument and seeks to influence its victims by the mere repetition of catchwords, by the furious denunciation of foreign or domestic scapegoats, and by cunningly associating the lowest passions with the highest ideals, so that atrocities come to be perpetrated in the name of God and the most cynical kind of *Realpolitik* is treated as a matter of religious principle and patriotic duty.

4   In John Dewey's words, "a renewal of faith in common human nature, in its potentialities in general, and in its power in particular to respond to reason and truth, is a surer bulwark against totalitarianism than a demonstration of material success or a devout worship of special legal and political forms." The power to respond to reason and truth exists in all of us. But so, unfortunately, does the tendency to respond to unreason and

falsehood—particularly in those cases where falsehood evokes some enjoyable emotion, or where the appeal to unreason strikes some answering chord in the primitive, subhuman depths of our being. In certain fields of activity men have learned to respond to reason and truth pretty consistently. The authors of learned articles do not appeal to the passions of their fellow scientists and technologists. They set forth what, to the best of their knowledge, is the truth about some particular aspect of reality, they use reason to explain the facts they have observed and they support their point of view with arguments that appeal to reason in other people. All this is fairly easy in the fields of physical science and technology. It is much more difficult in the fields of politics and religion and ethics. Here the relevant facts often elude us. As for the meaning of the facts, that of course depends upon the particular system of ideas, in terms of which you choose to interpret them. And these are not the only difficulties that confront the rational truth-seeker. In public and in private life, it often happens that there is simply no time to collect the relevant facts or to weigh their significance. We are forced to act on insufficient evidence and by a light considerably less steady than that of logic. With the best will in the world, we cannot always be completely truthful or consistently rational. All that is in our power is to be as truthful and rational as circumstances permit us to be, and to respond as well as we can to the limited truth and imperfect reasoning offered for our consideration by others.

"If a nation expects to be ignorant and free," said Jefferson, 5 "it expects what never was and never will be. . . . The people cannot be safe without information. Where the press is free, and every man able to read, all is safe." Across the Atlantic another passionate believer in reason was thinking about the same time, in almost precisely similar terms. Here is what John Stuart Mill wrote of his father, the utilitarian philosopher, James Mill: "So complete was his reliance upon the influence of reason over the minds of mankind, whenever it is allowed to reach them, that he felt as if all would be gained, if the whole population were able to read, and if all sorts of opinions were allowed to be addressed to them by word or in writing, and if by the suffrage they could nominate a legislature to give effect to the opinions they had adopted." *All is safe, all would be gained!* Once more we hear the note of eighteenth-century optimism. Jefferson, it is true, was a realist as well as an optimist. He knew by bitter experience that the freedom of the press can be shamefully abused. "Nothing," he declared, "can now be believed which is seen in a newspaper." And yet, he insisted (and we can only agree with him), "within the pale of truth, the press is a noble institution, equally the friend of science and civil liberty." Mass communication, in a word, is neither good nor bad; it is simply a force and, like any other force, it can be used either well or ill. Used in one way, the press, the radio and the cinema are indispensable to the survival of democracy. Used in another way, they are among the most powerful weapons in the dictator's armory. In the field of mass communications as in almost every other field of enterprise, technological progress has hurt the Little Man and helped the Big Man. As lately as fifty years ago, every democratic country could boast a great number of small journals and local newspapers. Thousands of country editors expressed thousands of independent opinions. Somewhere or other almost anybody could get almost anything printed. Today the press is still legally free, but most of the little papers have disappeared. The cost of wood pulp, of modern printing machinery and of syndicated news is too high for the Little Man. In the totalitarian East there is political censorship, and the media of mass communication are controlled by the State. In the democratic West there is economic censorship and the media of mass communication are controlled by members of the Power Elite. Censorship by rising costs and the concentration of communication power in the hands of a few big concerns is less objectionable than State ownership and government propaganda; but certainly it is not something of which a Jeffersonian democrat could possibly approve.

6   In regard to propaganda the early advocates of universal literacy and a free press envisaged only two possibilities: the propaganda might be true, or it might be false. They did not forsee what in fact has happened, above all in our Western capitalist democracies—the development of a vast mass communications industry, concerned in the main neither with the true nor the false, but with the unreal, the more or less totally irrelevant. In a word, they failed to take into account man's almost infinite appetite for distractions.

In the past most people never got a chance of fully satisfying 7 this appetite. They might long for distractions, but the distractions were not provided. Christmas came but once a year, feasts were "solemn and rare," there were few readers and very little to read, and the nearest approach to a neighborhood movie theater was the parish church, where the performances, though infrequent, were somewhat monotonous. For conditions even remotely comparable to those now prevailing we must return to imperial Rome, where the populace was kept in good humor by frequent, gratuitous doses of many kinds of entertainment—from poetical dramas to gladitorial fights, from recitations of Virgil to all-out boxing, from concerts to military reviews and public executions. But even in Rome there was nothing like the non-stop distraction now provided by newspapers and magazines, by radio, television and the cinema. In *Brave New World* non-stop distractions of the most fascinating nature (the feelies, orgy-porgy, centrifugal bumblepuppy) are deliberately used as instruments of policy, for the purpose of preventing people from paying too much attention to the realities of the social and political situation. The other world of religion is different from the other world of entertainment; but they resemble one another in being most decidedly "not of this world." Both are distractions and, if lived in too continuously, both can become, in Marx's phrase, "the opium of the people" and so a threat to freedom. Only the vigilant can maintain their liberties, and only those who are constantly and intelligently on the spot can hope to govern themselves effectively by democratic procedures. A society, most of whose members spend a great part of their time, not on the spot, not here and now and in the calculable future, but somewhere else, in the irrelevant other worlds of sport and soap opera, of mythology and metaphysical fantasy, will find it hard to resist the encroachments of those who would manipulate and control it.

In their propaganda today's dictators rely for the most part 8 on repetition, supression and rationalization—the repetition of catchwords which they wish to be accepted as true, the suppression of facts which they wish to be ignored, the arousal and rationalization of passions which may be used in the interests of the Party or the State. As the art and science of manipulation come to be better understood, the dictators of the future will doubtless learn to combine these techniques with the non-stop distractions which, in the West, are now threatening to drown in a sea of irrelevance the rational propaganda essential to the maintenance of individual liberty and the survival of democratic institutions.

TV Isn't Violent Enough

Mike Oppenheim

1   Caught in an ambush, there's no way our hero (Matt Dillon, Eliot Ness, Kojak, Hoss Cartwright . . .) can survive. Yet, visibly weakening, he blazes away, and we suspect he'll pull through. Sure enough, he's around for the final clinch wearing the traditional badge of the honorable but harmless wound: a sling.

2   As a teenager with a budding interest in medicine, I knew this was nonsense and loved to annoy my friends with the facts.

3   "Aw, the poor guy! He's crippled for life!"

4   "What do you mean? He's just shot in the shoulder."

5   "That's the worst place! Vital structures everywhere. There's the blood supply for the arm: axillary artery and vein. One nick and you can bleed to death on the spot."

6   "So he was lucky."

7   "OK. If it missed the vessels it hit the brachial plexus: the nerve supply. Paralyzes his arm for life. He's gotta turn in his badge and apply for disability."

8   "So he's *really* lucky."

9   "OK. Missed the artery. Missed the vein. Missed the nerves. Just went through the shoulder joint. But joint cartilage doesn't heal so well. A little crease in the bone leaves him with traumatic arthritis. He's in pain the rest of his life—stuffing himself with codeine, spending his money on acupuncture and chiropractors, losing all his friends because he complains all the time. . . . Don't ever get shot in the shoulder. It's the end. . . ."

10 Today, as a physician, I still sneer at TV violence, though not because of any moral objection. I enjoy a well-done scene of gore and slaughter as well as the next viewer, but "well-done" is something I rarely see on a typical evening in spite of the plethora of shootings, stabbings, muggings, and brawls. Who can believe the

stuff they show? Anyone who remembers high-school biology knows the human body can't possibly respond to violent trauma as it's usually portrayed.

On a recent episode, Matt Houston is at a fancy resort, on the trail of a vicious killer who specializes in knifing beautiful women in their hotel rooms in broad daylight. The only actual murder sequence was in the best of taste: all the action off screen, the flash of a knife, moans on the sound track.   11

In two scenes, Matt arrives only minutes too late. The hotel is alerted, but the killer's identity remains a mystery. Absurd! It's impossible to kill someone instantly with a knife thrust—or even render him unconscious. Several minutes of strenuous work are required to cut enough blood vessels so the victim bleeds to death. Tony Perkins in *Psycho* gave an accurate, though abbreviated, demonstration. Furthermore, anyone who has watched an inexperienced farmhand slaughter a pig knows that the resulting mess must be seen to be believed.   12

If consulted by Matt Houston, I'd have suggested a clue: "Keep your eyes peeled for someone panting with exhaustion and covered with blood. That might be your man."   13

Many Americans were puzzled at the films of the assassination attempt on President Reagan. Shot in the chest, he did not behave as TV had taught us to expect ("clutch chest, stagger backward, collapse"). Only after he complained of a vague chest pain and was taken to the hospital did he discover his wound. Many viewers assumed Mr. Reagan is some sort of superman. In fact, there was nothing extraordinary about his behavior. A pistol is certainly a deadly weapon, but not predictably so. Unlike a knife wound, one bullet can kill instantly—provided it strikes a small area at the base of the brain. Otherwise, it's no different: a matter of ripping and tearing enough tissue to cause death by bleeding. Professional gangland killers understand the problem. They prefer a shotgun at close range.   14

The trail of quiet corpses left by TV's good guys, bad guys, and assorted ill-tempered gun owners is ridiculously unreal. Firearms reliably produce pain, bleeding, and permanent, crippling injury (witness Mr. Reagan's press secretary, James Brady: shot directly in the brain but very much alive). For a quick, clean death, they are no match for Luke Skywalker's light saber.   15

16   No less unreal is what happens when T. J. Hooker, Magnum, or a Simon brother meets a bad guy in manly combat. Pow! Our hero's fist crashes into the villain's head. Villain reels backward, tipping over chairs and lamps, finally falling to the floor, unconscious. Handshakes all around. . . . Sheer fantasy! After hitting the villain, our hero would shake no one's hand. He'd be too busy waving his own about wildly, screaming with the pain of a shattered fifth metacarpal (the bone behind the fifth knuckle), an injury so predictable it's called the "boxer's fracture." The human fist is far more delicate than the human skull. In any contest between the two, the fist will lose.

17   The human skull is tougher than TV writers give it credit. Clunked with a blunt object, such as the traditional pistol butt, most victims would not fall conveniently unconscious for a few minutes. More likely, they'd suffer a nasty scalp laceration, be stunned for a second or two, then be extremely upset. I've sewn up many. A real-life, no-nonsense criminal with a blackjack (a piece of iron weighing several pounds) has a much better success rate. The result is a large number of deaths and permanent damage from brain hemorrhage.

18   Critics of TV violence claim it teaches children sadism and cruelty. I honestly don't know whether or not TV violence is harmful, but if so the critics have it backward. Children can't learn to enjoy cruelty from the neat, sanitized mayhem on the average series. There isn't any! What they learn is far more malignant: that guns or fists are clean, efficient, exciting ways to deal with a difficult situation. Bang!—you're dead! Bop!—you're unconscious (temporarily)!

19   "Truth-in-advertising" laws eliminated many absurd commercial claims. I often daydream about what would happen if we had "truth in violence"—if every show had to pass scrutiny by a board of doctors who had no power to censor but could insist that any action scene have at least a vague resemblance to medical reality ("Stop the projector! . . . You have your hero waylaid by three Mafia thugs who beat him brutally before he struggles free. The next day he shows up with this cute little Band-aid over his eyebrow. We can't pass that. You'll have to add one eye swollen shut, three missing front teeth, at least twenty stitches over the lips and eyes, and a wired jaw. Got that? Roll 'em . . . ").

Seriously, real-life violence is dirty, painful, bloody, disgusting. 20
It causes mutilation and misery, and it doesn't solve problems. It
makes them worse. If we're genuinely interested in protecting our
children, we should stop campaigning to "clean up" TV violence.
It's already too antiseptic. Ironically, the problem with TV violence
is: It's not violent enough.

"But First, a Word from Our Sponsor"

James B. Twitchell

Whenever a member of my paunchy fifty-something set pulls me 1
aside and complains of the dumbing down of American culture,
I tell him that if he doesn't like it, he should quit moaning and
go buy a lot of Fast-Moving Consumer Goods. And every time he
buys soap, toothpaste, beer, gasoline, bread, aspirin, and the like,
he should make it a point to buy a different brand. He should
implore his friends to do likewise. At the same time, he should
quit giving so much money to his kids. That, I'm sorry to say, is
his only hope.

Here's why. The culture we live in is carried on the back of 2
advertising. Now I mean that literally. If you cannot find commercial support for what you have to say, it will not be transported. Much of what we share, and what we know, and even
what we treasure, is carried to us each second in a plasma of elec-
trons, pixels, and ink, underwritten by multinational advertising
agencies dedicated to attracting our attention for entirely nonal-
truistic reasons. These agencies, gathered up inside worldwide
conglomerates with weird, sci-fi.names like WPP, Omnicom,
Saatchi & Saatchi, Dentsu, and Euro RSCG, are usually collections
of established shops linked together to provide "full service" to
their global clients. Their service is not moving information or creating entertainment, but buying space and inserting advertising.
They essentially rent our concentration to other companies—
sponsors—for the dubious purpose of informing us of something

that we've longed for all our lives even though we've never heard of it before. Modern selling is not about trading information, as it was in the 19th century, as much as about creating an infotainment culture with sufficient allure to enable other messages—commercials—to get through. In the spirit of the enterprise, I call this new culture Adcult.

3   Adcult is there when we blink, it's there when we listen, it's there when we touch, it's even there to be smelled in scent strips when we open a magazine. There is barely a space in our culture not already carrying commercial messages. Look anywhere: in schools there is Channel One; in movies there is product placement; ads are in urinals, played on telephone hold, in alphanumeric displays in taxis, sent unannounced to fax machines, inside catalogs, on the video in front of the Stairmaster at the gym, on T-shirts, at the doctor's office, on grocery carts, on parking meters, on tees at golf holes, on inner-city basketball backboards, piped in along with Muzak . . . ad nauseam (and yes, even on airline vomit bags). We have to shake magazines like rag dolls to free up their pages from the "blow-in" inserts and then wrestle out the stapled- or glued-in ones before reading can begin. We now have to fast-forward through some five minutes of advertising that opens rental videotapes. President Bill Clinton's inaugural parade featured a Budweiser float. At the Smithsonian, the Orkin Pest Control Company sponsored an exhibit on exactly what it advertises it kills: insects. No venue is safe. Is there a blockbuster museum show not decorated with corporate logos? The Public Broadcasting Service is littered with "underwriting announcements" that look and sound almost exactly like what PBS claims they are not: commercials.

4   Okay, you get the point. Commercial speech is so powerful that it drowns out all other sounds. But sounds are always conveyed in a medium. The media of modern culture are these: print, sound, pictures, or some combination of each. Invariably, conversations about dumbing down focus on the supposed corruption of these media, as demonstrated by the sophomoric quality of most movies, the fall from the golden age of television, the mindlessness of most best-sellers, and the tarting-up of the news, be it in or on *USA Today, Time,* ABC, or *Inside Edition.* The media make especially convenient whipping boys because they are now all

conglomerated into huge worldwide organizations such as Time Warner, General Electric, Viacom, Bertelsmann, and Sony. But, alas, as much fun as it is to blame the media, they have very little to do with the explanation for whatever dumbing down has occurred.

The explanation is, I think, more fundamental, more economic 5 in nature. These media are delivered for a price. We have to pay for them, either by spending money or by spending time. Given a choice, we prefer to spend time. We spend our time paying attention to ads, and in exchange we are given infotainment. This trade is central to Adcult. Economists call this "cost externalization." If you want to see it at work, go to McDonald's. You order. You carry your food to the table. You clean up. You pay less. Want to see it elsewhere? Buy gas. Just as the "work" you do at the self-service gas station lowers the price of gas, so consuming ads is the "work" you do that lowers the price of delivering the infotainment. In Adcult, the trade is more complex. True, you are entertained at lower cost, but you are also encultured in the process.

So far, so good. The quid pro quo of modern infotainment cul- 6 ture is that if you want it, you'll get it—no matter what it is—as long as there are enough of you who (1) are willing to spend some energy along the way hearing "a word from our sponsor" and (2) have sufficient disposable income possibly to buy some of the advertised goods. In Adcult you pay twice: once with the ad and once with the product. So let's look back a step to examine these products because—strange as it may seem—they are at the center of the dumbing down of American culture.

Before all else, we must realize that modern advertising is tied 7 primarily to things, and only secondarily to services. Manufacturing both things *and* their meanings is what American culture is all about. If Greece gave the world philosophy, Britain drama, Austria music, Germany politics, and Italy art, then America gave mass-produced objects. "We bring good things to life" is no offhand claim. Most of these "good things" are machine made and hence interchangeable. Such objects, called parity items, constitute most of the stuff that surrounds us, from bottled water to toothpaste to beer to cars. There is really no great difference between Evian and Mountain Spring, Colgate and Crest, Miller and

Budweiser, Ford and Chevrolet. Often, the only difference is in the advertising. Advertising is how we talk about these fungible things, how we know their supposed differences, how we recognize them. We don't consume the products as much as we consume the advertising.

8   For some reason, we like it this way. Logically, we should all read *Consumer Reports* and then all buy the most sensible product. But we don't. So why do we waste our energy (and billions of dollars) entertaining fraudulent choice? I don't know. Perhaps just as we drink the advertising, not the beer, we prefer the illusion of choice to the reality of decision. How else to explain the appearance of so much superfluous choice? A decade ago, grocery stores carried about 9,000 items; they now stock about 24,000. Revlon makes 158 shades of lipstick. Crest toothpaste comes in 36 sizes and shapes and flavors. We are even eager to be offered choice where there is none to speak of. AT&T offers "the right choice"; Wendy's asserts that "there is no better choice"; Pepsi is "the choice of a new generation"; Taster's Choice is "the choice for taste." Even advertisers don't understand the phenomenon. Is there a relationship between the number of soft drinks and television channels—about 27? What's going to happen when the information pipe carries 500?

9   I have no idea. But I do know this: human beings like things. We buy things. We like to exchange things. We steal things. We donate things. We live through things. We call these things "goods," as in "goods and services." We do not call them "bads." This sounds simplistic, but it is crucial to understanding the power of Adcult. The still-going-strong Industrial Revolution produces more and more things, not because production is what machines do and not because nasty capitalists twist their handlebar mustaches and mutter, "More slop for the pigs," but because we are powerfully attracted to the world of things. Advertising, when it's lucky, supercharges some of this attraction.

10   This attraction to the inanimate happens all over the world. Berlin Walls fall because people want things, and they want the culture created by things. China opens its doors not so much because it wants to get out, but because it wants to get things in. We were not suddenly transformed from customers to consumers by wily manufacturers eager to unload a surplus of products. We have created a surfeit of things because we enjoy the process of "getting and

spending." The consumption ethic may have started in the early 1900s, but the desire is ancient. Kings and princes once thought they could solve problems by amassing things. We now join them.

The Marxist balderdash of cloistered academics aside, human   11 beings did not suddenly become materialistic. We have always been desirous of things. We have just not had many of them until quite recently, and, in a few generations, we may return to having fewer and fewer. Still, while they last, we enjoy shopping for things and see both the humor and the truth reflected in the aphoristic "born to shop," "shop 'til you drop," and "when the going gets tough, the tough go shopping." Department store windows, whether on the city street or inside a mall, did not appear by magic. We enjoy looking through them to another world. It is voyeurism for capitalists. Our love of things is the *cause* of the Industrial Revolution, not the consequence. We are not only *homo sapiens,* or *homo ludens,* or *homo faber,* but also *homo emptor.*

Mid-20th-century American culture is often criticized for being   12 too materialistic. Ironically, we are not too materialistic. We are not materialistic enough. If we craved objects *and* knew what they meant, there would be no need to add meaning through advertising. We would gather, use, toss out, or hoard based on some *inner* sense of value. But we don't. We don't know what to gather, we like to trade what we have gathered, and we need to know how to evaluate objects of little practical use. What is clear is that most things in and of themselves simply do not mean enough. In fact, what we crave may not be objects at all but their meaning. For whatever else advertising "does," one thing is certain: by adding value to material, by adding meaning to objects, by branding things, advertising performs a role historically associated with religion. The Great Chain of Being, which for centuries located value above the horizon in the world Beyond, has been reforged to settle value into the objects of the Here and Now . . .

We are now closing in on why the dumbing down of American   13 culture has occurred with such startling suddenness in the last 30 years. We are also closing in on why the big complainers about dumbing down are me and my paunchy pals. The people who want things the most and have the best chance to acquire them are the young. They are also the ones who have not yet decided which brands of objects they wish to consume. In addition, they have a surplus of two commodities: time and money, especially the former. If you can make a sale to these twentysome-things, if you can "brand" them with your product, you may have them for life. But to do this you have to be able to speak to them, and to do that you have to go to where you will be heard.

14   The history of mass media can be summarized in a few words: if it can't carry advertising, it won't survive . . .

15   We need not be reminded of what is currently happening to television to realize the direction of the future. MTV, the infomercial, and the home-shopping channels are not flukes but the predictable continuation of this medium. Thanks to the remote-control wand and the coaxial (soon to be fiber-optic) cable, commercials will disappear. They will become the programming. Remember, the first rule of Adcult is this: given the choice between paying money or paying attention, we prefer to pay attention.

16   What all this means is that if you think things are bad now, just wait. There are few gatekeepers left. Most of them reside on Madison Avenue. Just as the carnival barker doesn't care what is behind the tent flap, only how long the line is in front, the poobahs of Adcult care only about who's looking, not what they are looking at. The best-seller lists, the box office, the Nielsens, the various circulation figures for newspapers and magazines, are the meters. They decide what gets through. Little wonder that so much of our popular culture is derivative of itself, that prequels and sequels and spin-offs are the order of the day, that celebrity is central, and that innovation is the cross to the vampire. Adcult is recombinant culture. This is how it has to be if advertisers are to be able to direct their spiels at the appropriate audiences for their products. It's simply too expensive to be any other way.

17   Will Adcult continue? Will there be some new culture to "afflict the comfortable and comfort the afflicted"? Will advertising, on its own terms, lose *it*? Who knows? Certainly, signs of stress are showing. Here are a few: (1) The kids are passing through "prime-branding time" like a rabbit in the python, and as they get older things may settle down. The supposedly ad-proof Generation X may be impossible to reach and advertisers will turn

to older audiences by default. (2) The media are so clogged and cluttered that companies may move to other promotional highways, such as direct mail, point-of-purchase displays, and couponing, leaving the traditional avenues targeted at us older folks. (3) Branding, the heart of advertising, may become problematic if generics or store brands become as popular in this country as they have in Europe. After all, the much-vaunted brand extension whereby Coke becomes Diet Coke which becomes Diet Cherry Coke does not always work, as Kodak Floppy Disks, Milky Way Ice Cream, Arm & Hammer antiperspirant, Life Saver Gum, and even EuroDisney have all shown. And (4)—the unthinkable—mass consumption may become too expensive. Advertising can flourish only in times of surplus, and no one can guarantee that our society will always have more than it needs.

But by no means am I predicting Adcult's imminent demise. As 18 long as goods are interchangeable and in surplus quantities, as long as producers are willing to pay for short-term advantages (especially for new products), and as long as consumers have plenty of disposable time and money so that they can consume both the ad and the product, Adcult will remain the dominant meaning-making system of modern life. I don't think you can roll this tape backwards. Adcult is the application of capitalism to culture: dollars voting. And so I say to my melancholy friends who bemoan the passing of a culture once concerned with the arts and the humanities that the only way they can change this situation is if they buy more Fast-Moving Consumer Goods, change brands capriciously, and cut the kids' allowances. Good luck.

Money, Power, Elect: Where's the Hip-Hop Agenda?

Raquel Cepeda

Hip-hop culture has given my generation its tag line, if not its very 1 identity: For more than 20 years, rap—hip-hop's sometimes furious, sometimes laid-back, rhythmic spoken-word expression—has provided a mesmerizing sound track for the lives of many young African-American and Latino people. Spawned from humble beginnings in New York City's South Bronx, hip-hop style spread like wildfire, while rap rocked our neighborhood block parties, turntables and boom boxes, and then White suburban headphones all over the country. Eventually rap would generate a $1.3 billion industry in the United States, exclusive of its still-growing global influences.

2   But consider how rap music, back at the end of the catastrophic Reagan administration, was also identified as *the* platform to educate *and* entertain the nation on the realties of what was going on socially and politically in Black and Latino America. Only a decade ago, rapper KRS-One and his crew BDP (Boogie Down Productions) proclaimed in the title track to their 1990 album *Edutainment:* "Every time a Black man speaks up, KA-POW!/ See people concentrate on the leader. . . ." Other groups such as Public Enemy, Brand Nubian, Poor Righteous Teachers and even such West Coast pioneers as Compton, California's gangsta-rappers N.W.A (Niggas With Attitude) penned tracks that depicted and responded to the political agendas brewing in their communities—namely, racial profiling, police brutality, the state of public education and the prison system, Black-on-Black crime and predatory drug peddling and abuse.

3   Compare that to the music that dominates the top of the charts today: Rap is now a sample-heavy, benjamin-raking, crudely individualistic pop-culture phenomenon that is very far from its earlier countercultural and activist impulses. "There's no spiritual content to the majority of records being made today," says cultural critic Nelson George, 42, author of *Hip-Hop America.* Icons like Jay-Z, Puffy and Lil' Kim now compare themselves to high-profile White celebrity entrepreneurs like Donald Trump, Donatella Versace and Martha Stewart. Ironically, traditional Black community leaders like the Reverend Jesse L. Jackson, Sr., NAACP president and CEO Kweisi Mfume, and even the Reverend Al Sharpton have been far less successful at appealing politically to these hip-hop megastars and the young people who follow them than folks like Trump and *Playboy* monarch Hugh Hefner have been in *partying* with them.

4   Meanwhile, today's post–civil-rights hip-hop civilian masses seem politically inert. Just as the rise of gangsta rap overwhelmed

message rap, hip-hop's social energies have also been redirected by commercial success and corporate marketing. The popular mind, seduced by the ethic of getting paid, became preoccupied with rap's shiny, platinum-dipped dreams. Mogul Sean "Puffy" Combs almost single-handedly steered the sound of rap music into mainstream pop. Predictably, other popular hip-hop artists have followed suit.

Foxy Brown and Lil' Kim, in particular, enjoy new status as glam celebrity spokespeople-for-hire, successfully marketing luxury goods. But the media power this trend represents is rarely put to use for the benefit of our communities. "The so-called Black celebrities are created by companies to be advertisements for what companies promote." observes Public Enemy's Chuck D. "These celebrities lose focus and think it's all about them; that's individual instead of collective thought."

But now, as we face the first national election season of the new century, will the hip-hop generation *stay* obsessed with living the ghetto-fabulons life? Will we remain unorganized and politically unresponsive to racism and police brutality, bad schools, economic gaps and other persistent problems in our communities? After all, this generation, however flaccid its political muscle may seem to be is heir to the Black Power era. We have witnessed two Republican administrations, the 1992 Los Angeles riots, the 1999 murder of our immigrant brother Amadou Diallo and most recently, California's passing of Proposition 21, which disproportionately criminalizes urban youth. So why haven't we been galvanized into an articulate and activist political movement by such events? Could the star power in merchandising and marketing, for example, ever be used successfully as a coalescing political force to get out our vote?

In fact, with the possible exceptions of Lauryn Hill and Queen Latifah, few platinum-level artists have ever considered moving beyond conscious rhetoric and rhyme to organize our people. Many ask, why even expect a celebrity to take a particular political stand? The answer is simple: There's a long-standing tradition in our communities that unites the arts and activism (Paul Robeson is a historic example, as are Ossie Davis, Ruby Dee and Harry Belafonte). But cultural commentators agree that while our rap celebrities have an enormous influence on urban-youth culture, there's little interest in transferring it to politics. "What hip-hop has done is taken the strategies of grass-roots organizing and used it to sell records and images," explains Nelson George. "The same kind of kids who used to canvass a neighborhood door-to-door to get people registered to vote now give parties."

8   A similar observation comes from another older "hip-hop head." Bill Stephney, 38, president of StepSun Music, board member of the National Urban League and founder of New York City's Families Organized for Liberty and Action (FOLA): "As Vernon Reid [musician and Black Rock Coalition founder] once said, the nineties were just the sixties turned upside down," recalls Stephney. "During the sixties, you had a generation of Black folks who were socially active and politically conscious. We wanted to change the world, but we really didn't have an idea, beyond the romance of revolution, how we were going to finance or set up any economic systems for Black and Latino people to survive. By the nineties, you have the kids of the sixties generation, who know how to make money, but who don't have the sociopolitical orientation their predecessors had. Imagine, if you will, having the social and political heart of Fannie Lou Hamer, Rosa Parks, Medgar Evers and Dr. King combined with the financial brains of Puffy."

9   Still, there *are* activist forces stirring within the twenty-first–century hip-hop community. I'm not talking about well-publicized, star-sponsored operations like Puffy's Daddy's House (which finances camps and other activities for inner-city youth) and Lauryn Hill's Refugee Project (which also works with at-risk urban youth); even these operations have been criticized—perhaps unjustly—for being vanity charity activities, not really informed by an overall social or political strategy. No, I'm talking about a largely unnoticed grass-roots hip-hop movement that is persistently making its way through urban neighborhoods all over the country. Most of this so-called hip-hop activism began in New York, just as rap did, but it has also cropped up among youths in Los Angeles, San Francisco, Washington, D.C., Atlanta and cyberspace, according to Angela Ards, a senior associate editor at *Ms.* magazine. Ards investigated hip-hop activism last year as a fellow at the Nation Institute (the independent nonprofit organization dedicated to protecting First Amendment freedoms and affiliated with *The Nation* magazine).

These local groups identify with hip-hop expression but tap 10 into the energies of performers who are less well known than our stars. One example: Last year Mos Def and Talib Kweli—Brooklyn-based rappers–entrepreneurs who record individually and together as the duo Black Star—rescued a local landmark Black bookstore from going out of business by buying it. Black Star is also known for spearheading anti–police brutality campaigns in the hip-hop industry, and other conscious artists like Common, OutKast and dead prez have joined them in representing and working with the urban neighborhoods they came from.

Such activity certainly deserves more recognition and support 11 from the hip-hop nation's everyday citizens. Although many of our young adults seem to have little interest, or aspiration to participate, in politics or activism, a strident few, whom you will meet below, show that the hip-hop generation has untapped potential to become a serious political force. The question is, how do we pump up the volume?

VOTER REGISTRATION AND PARTICIPATION

In this election year, young Black people are at best skeptical about 12 the political mainstream, and a few hardworking Black political organizers are trying to change that. Donna Frisby-Greenwood, former executive director of Rock the Vote (a nonpartisan, non-profit organization dedicated to motivating young people to participate in the political process) and a political organizer who has worked with urban youth for more than a decade, points out that in the last Presidential election only about half the 8,928,000 eligible Black voters 18–34 registered to vote, and only 3.5 million of them—or about 72 percent—voted. (By comparison, about 68 percent of the 10,932,000 eligible Black voters 34–65 registered, and nearly 84 percent of them voted.) At Rock the Vote, Frisby-Greenwood organized the Hip-Hop Coalition for Political Power to reach out to the young Black voter. Artists like Public Enemy's Chuck D, Queen Latifah, LL Cool J and The Roots took an active role in the effort. Of the more than 500,000 voters Rock the Vote registered in 1996, at least 150,000 were registered through the efforts of the now-defunct Coalition.

13   Today, Frisby-Greenwood, 35, lives and works in Philadelphia and cochairs the Black Youth Vote (BYV) Coalition—part of the National Coalition on Black Civic Participation, Inc., in Washington, D.C.—with BET talk-show host Tavis Smiley, 34, and Chuck D, 39. "We are now registering voters on-line, in the streets and on college campuses," says Frisby-Greenwood. "We've planned summer workshops to train young people to organize, educate and register voters in Pennsylvania, North Carolina, Alabama, Florida, D.C., Los Angeles, Ohio, Georgia, Texas and California."

14   The BYV works with an advisory committee of 21–to–40-year-old leaders, including author and syndicated columnist Farai Chideya, 31; activists Conrad Muhammad, 35, and Ras Baraka, 31; and journalists Angela Ards, 31, and Kevin Powell, 34. "One of the things we emphasize in the BYV manifesto is awakening the sleeping giant of the hip-hop generation," says Chideya. "Black youths are such a force—I mean, we run American pop culture." Hoping to motivate at least 10 percent of young Black people between 18 and 29 to participate in the 2000 political process, BYV has been training local coordinators around the country. (For further information, see www.bigvote.com.)

15   These education and registration efforts are certainly needed, according to my sample of attitudes. "*Politics* is a dangerous word," says Black Star's Kweli, 24, "because what it means to me is just a bunch of lies and rhetoric, not anything concrete." Still, Kweli, like many of his contemporaries, is motivated to do *something* about the issues that Black youths encounter every day in their own lives: police brutality and racial profiling, gun control, education and welfare reform, Black-on-Black crime and the racially slanted prison system, to name a few. But he feels neither elected politicians nor candidates speak to these issues directly in a language that makes sense to hip-hop youths. In fact, Black youths simply don't respond to politicians, including Black ones who, for the most part, have also made only token attempts to reach out to them.

16   One Black leader who insists that responsible Blacks in positions of authority can't give up on politically apathetic young people is Congresswoman Maxine Waters (D–CA). "I've tried to make the connection between rappers, young people and the Congressional Black Caucus," says Waters. "My main agenda is to

connect to the hip-hop generation—more than to actual rappers—and close the communication gap between them and older adults." Freedom of speech and censorship issues have split the generations in Black communities. Some White politicians gleefully supported longtime Black political activist C. Delores Tucker in her 1996 campaign against gangsta rap, says Waters, "because they didn't like rap *or* young Black people." She also recalls the highly publicized congressional hearings, headed by then-Senator Carol Moseley Braun (D–IL): "I had to literally read lyrics from Snoop Dogg's records to show that all the words were not simply vulgar curse words. They were oftentimes deeply meaningful in describing young people's experiences, and they connected to many others who felt left outside of the system."

For the past few years at the annual Congressional Black Caucus Week in Washington, D.C., Waters has sponsored and moderated a workshop called Young, Gifted and Black, in which young people and rappers are given a platform before lawmakers to define themselves and their issues. But a surprising number of Black politicians have essentially thrown up their hands. Congressman Jesse L. Jackson, Jr. (D–IL), himself a member of the hip-hop generation at age 35, points out that he didn't see any rappers in Decatur, Illinois, "when my father was fighting to get six young African-Americans back in school." (The young Black men, who got into a fistfight at a local high-school football game in September 1999, were expelled because of the school district's zero-tolerance policy on school violence, which the young men argue has been disproportionately applied to Decatur's Black students.) When Congressman Jackson was pressed to detail the extent of Rev. Jackson's previous outreach efforts to the hip-hop community, he replied, "They probably wouldn't have shown up. I ain't blaming them. I'm just simply saying people are busy."

True. "Most rappers who say they're spokesmen for the generation generally are spokesmen only as it relates to social and cultural trends," says Conrad Muhammad, former minister of the Nation of Islam's Mosque No. 7 in Harlem and founder of A Movement for CHHANGE (Conscious Hip-Hop Activism Necessary for Global Empowerment), a national organization aimed at educating urban youth about the political process and registering young people to vote. CHHANGE aims to put 1 million Black young people on the rolls this November and Muhammad has also targeted several popular rappers to groom as candidates for local political office. Although he reports "opening the minds" of rappers like Fat Joe, DJ Kool Here and Vinnie and Treach of Naughty by Nature, no actual campaigns have moved beyond the talking stage.

19   Similarly, in a 1998 *Essence* cover story, Sean "Puffy" Combs himself expressed interest in political activism and maybe even running for office. So far he has committed, along with LL Cool J, Mary J. Blige and Rosie Perez, to appear in public-service announcements for Rap the Vote 2000. A joint project of rap mogul Russell Simmons's new Web site, 360HipHop.com, and Rock the Vote, Rap the Vote 2000 aims to get 850,000 new young voters to the polls this year under the slogan "Register. Vote. Represent."

POLICE BRUTALITY AND RACIAL PROFILING

20 The death of the 22-year-old West African immigrant Amadou Diallo—an unarmed man shot 41 times by four New York Police Department officers who were later acquitted of all charges—forced the ever-present issue of police brutality and racial profiling to the top of urban America's political agenda. The Hip-Hop for Respect Foundation (HHFRF) project was one activist response from the community of hip-hop artists. "Most of the people that got killed by police this year and in the past have probably been some of your fans" wrote rapper Mos Def, 26, in an open letter to the rap-music industry. "We are the senators and the congressmen of our communities. We come from communities that don't have anybody to speak for them and that's why they love us." As fund-raisers for the foundation, which supports activist groups that effectively deal with police brutality issues, Mos Def and Talib Kweli went on to organize the recording session for the maxisingle "One for Love, Pt. 1," which also features Common, Rah Digga, Pharoahe Monch, Pos (from De La Soul) and others.

21   But the acquittal of the four officers charged with the Diallo shooting elicited strong statements from the hip-hop elite, like Russell Simmons (largely covered in the Black press and rap-music magazines), and, more important, thrust thousands of

young protesters from a mix of races into the streets of Manhattan and the Bronx neighborhood where the killing took place. Some marchers replaced the slogans of yesteryear with a popular chorus from a Nas track: "I wanna talk to the mayor, to the governor and the muthaf—king President/I wanna talk to the FBI and the CIA and the muthaf—king congressmen." Here hip-hoppers took their music back to the streets to make a pointed political statement.

JUVENILE JUSTICE AND PROPOSITION 21

Another grassroots organization spawned by the hip-hop gener-   22
ation is San Francisco's Third Eye Movement. This collective of 40 members became a major force in making the antigang–crime-prevention initiative Proposition 21 a centerpiece debate in California's elections last spring. A campaign spearheaded by former Republican governor Pete Wilson put Prop 21 on the ballot. The measure gives police the right to make arrests under a number of questionable charges that disproportionately target young people of color. It's possible for a young woman and two of her friends, dressed similarly, to be classified as a gang and therefore arrested. "If I happen to be on the basketball court playing ball with somebody, and that person leaves and commits a crime, the doors are open for me to be put in jail under conspiracy charges because of my association," says Davey D. 35, a community-affairs director and on-air radio personality at 106 KMEL in Oakland. Prop 21 also allows courts to try juveniles as adults for felonies, as well as permit police surveillance and phone taps without a court order.

Jasmin de la Rosa, 24, coordinator and founder of Third Eye,   23
organized school walkouts, free concerts, rallies and sit-ins to protest the initiative. But Prop 21 was ultimately passed last March in the statewide count, although it was defeated in several districts, including San Francisco and Oakland, where young protesters were active. More than 170 hip-hop heads were arrested after more than 500 people staged a sit-in at the San Francisco Hilton because they believed a Hilton family member pumped money into the "Yes on Prop 21" campaign. Here hip-hop aficionados customized

a chant from an old-school rap song: "Hotel, motel and the Hilton, say what/If you fund the war on youth, you ain't gonna win." Bay Area rappers, including Digital Underground, Boots, Money B. and Sugar T., joined the anti–Prop 21 rallies. But the biggest impact was at the grass-roots level, according to De la Rosa. "The cultural events and hip-hop parties—getting young people to organize those events was very effective in calling them to action," she says. "The people who organize the shows get skills in political organizing."

24   Davey D, who is also the Web master for the popular Internet site Davey D's Hip-Hop Corner (www.daveyd.com), concludes: "The best way to bring people under one umbrella is for them to engage in politics on a local level first."

SCHOOLS, NOT JAILS

25 How can we cultivate strong leadership when the prison-industrial complex has an obscene percentage of our generation on lockdown? If you are imprisoned for a felony, depending on the state, your voting rights may be revoked for life. Marc Maurer, expert analyst and author of *Race to Incarcerate* (New Press), points out that three out of every ten Black males and one in six Latinos born today can expect to do time in prison if current trends continue. African-Americans make up half the prison population, with an increasing number of drug arrests made among nonviolent offenders. Maurer also argues that the $40-billion prison-industrial complex has encroached on funds for higher education.

26   There is also the concern that the educational system teaches young people a racially slanted, warped history of themselves and their place in society. "Next on Third Eye's agenda." says De la Rosa, "is exploring educational reform and reinforcing the allies we've made with teachers, principals and prison activists. We're studying how to frame these issues to have the most statewide appeal." (See its Web site, www.thirdeyemovement.org.)

27   Is the hip-hop generation going to do something effective to coalesce around these issues? The outlook is still uncertain. "Artists, whether we accept it or not, are more representative of

their labels than they are of a community," says Angela Ards. But she adds, "The sixties generation saw power as a political thing, and our generation has come to understand that power is also economic. Mainstream artists could be using their capital to finance grass-roots movements."

But Bill Stephney puts it another way: "To think that the 28 NAACP, the Urban League and other civil-rights organizations emerged in environments that, particularly for Black people, had nowhere near the level of capital finance and marketing the hip-hop generation has." In the final analysis, Stephney says, "It's never from the top down, anyway. It's always from the bottom up. That's the great thing about 'street' and 'neighborhood Black culture'—it grows like a beautiful flower, from the ground up." So it must be with the hip-hop agenda.

The Media and Its Representation of Islam and Muslim Women

Sairra Patel

In June of 1995 an event seen as an international tragedy took 1 place in that an American government building in Oklahoma City was bombed. This atrocious act of terrorism killed many innocent people, including children. The following day a British newspaper, *Today*, carried the headline "In the name of Islam", accompanied by a picture of a fireman carrying the charred remains of a dead baby. It was then very quickly established that the bombing had, in fact, been carried out by Christian militants. This incident illustrates a trend which has emerged in the media—the demonisation of Islam and Muslims. The word "Islam" means "Peace," and also "Submission to the will of God." The Islamic religion and way of life is essentially one which provides total harmony and fulfilment to its followers, yet the media does not portray this image. In television, films, books, newspapers and magazines Islam is presented as being a backward and barbaric religion. It is seen as oppressive and unjust; and more then this it is seen as being most oppressive to women. These various forms of media misrepresent Islam in different ways, but overall achieve the same negative result—the creation of "otherness," and from this a growing barrier of misunderstanding and hostility between Islam and its followers, and the West.

2   The form of media which reaches most people in Britain on a daily basis is television. It therefore has the power to communicate with and influence people at all levels of society. Television offers a source of information which viewers often accept as being factual, and thus use as a basis to form their own ideas. Therefore it should provide an accurate picture of what it seeks to portray. With regards to Islam this is rarely the case, instead only two stereotypical images of Muslims are offered. On the one hand we have characters from films and dramas, such as BBC 1s *Eastenders* and BBC 2s *This Life,* who are Muslim, though only by name. These characters are Western conformists, totally adopting Western values and culture. There remains no sign of their religious or ethnic identity, and should the issue of their cultural background be mentioned it is treated as a cause for embarrassment. The other, and more common stereotype is that of the violent religious fanatic. In current affairs programmes we are constantly offered the image of Muslims as savage terrorists, killing innocent people with no remorse. No insight is given as to why some Muslim organisations carry out acts of violence. What results from this is that the common people, the viewers of these programmes, recognise and accept only the labels—and therefore with "Islam" they immediately associate negative images. As can be seen, two extremes emerge, and with this the question arises of whether these are the only types of Muslims that are acceptable to the Western media. One upholds the status quo while the other provides sensationalism, neither being a true reflection of the majority of Muslims. Myself as an example, I am a practising Muslim women with all my values stemming from Islam, yet I also adopt some Western ideas and institutions, having been born and brought up in the West. I therefore represent many Muslims who are rarely depicted in the media; proud of my Islamic identity though aware of my position in the West. Directly related to this, an issue which is close to my heart, is how the media depicts Muslim women.

Rana Kabbani, in the introduction to *Imperial Fictions: Europe's* 3
Myths of the Orient, discusses how a journalist from the magazine
Vanity Fair came to her for material on an article about Islam.
When this article was published Kabbani was disappointed to say
the least:

> It was one more unrelieved catalogue of horrors about Islam . . .
> it ignored any of the important debates within Islam about the
> rights of women. It distorted every sentence I had uttered . . .

She concludes that the article was "intellectually dishonest", 4
but that "the whole Western debate about Muslim women is a
dishonest one". Being a Muslim woman, I am hurt most by this
misrepresentation. With no insight into Islam, journalists and
writers condemn the religion's attitude to women. Only recently,
in July of this year, an article in the newspaper *The Telegraph*
claimed that an Islamic school of great influence in Deoband,
India, believed and taught that women are the source of evil. I am
acquainted with the ideas of this school, and know that it does
not make such a claim—to the contrary it teaches men to respect
women, and to know their rights. In newspaper and magazine
articles and on television in general, we are portrayed as being
weak and submissive to a religion which seeks to oppress and
dominate. Muslim women who choose to cover themselves are
pitied, and are thought the victims of a patriarchal and misogynistic religion. However, for a large proportion of women this
simply is not the case. In Islam we have a place of respect and
equality. Despite the beliefs advocated by the Media, our religion
does not offer us a lower status than men, as the *Noble Qur'an*
clearly illustrates:

> And for women are rights over men/similar to those of men
> over women. (2:226)

And as the Prophet Mohammed (peace be upon him) stated, 5
"Women are the twin halves of men." Over fourteen hundred
years ago Islam gave women rights which women in the West
have only been given during this century, such as the right to own
property, the right to inherit and the right to make a contract in
one's own name. Annie Besant, who was writing in the 1930's,
observed that, "It is only in the last twenty years that Christian

England has recognised the right of woman to property, while Islam has allowed this right from all times. It is a slander to say that Islam preaches that women have no souls." Women are seen as the spiritual and intellectual equals of men, though again this is not the image presented. The *hijab* (the garment worn by Muslim women to cover the hair), is another issue of contention. The media presents it as being an enforced condition, though for most Muslim women it is a voluntary act which signifies their allegiance to Islam, acting as well as a symbol of their faith. The negative images built up around the Muslim way of life has influenced the ideas of many of my non-Muslim colleagues at University who have implied in conversation that I wear the *hijab* because I am forced to by my community. Many have been surprised and enlightened when I have spoken about my true reasons, and furthermore that I chose to convert to Islam from another faith. Where the public believes that they are being presented with educational material about Islam from a reputable and reliable source, all that they are being provided with are the confused opinions of individual producers and journalists—many of whom begin their research with preconceived ideas and aims.

6   Islam is the fastest growing religion in the World. To this fact the media has again managed to attach a negative stigma. It claims that this spread has taken place in the Third World, and in deprived communities in the West, such as the black people in the inner-city areas of Britain and the USA (documentaries have been made in Brixton and the Bronx following this theme). It is therefore, according to them, an isolated phenomenon amongst people of lower standing in the larger community, which does not affect the majority of those in the West. Such a presentation is again untrue. Although it does appeal to the sections of the community mentioned above (who are just as important as any other section), Islam appeals to many different people from many different walks of life. Islam is able to provide satisfactory answers to every question posed by the individual, and thus provides them with total peace of mind; something which many Muslims would argue no other religion can provide. Islam's appeal is universal, illustrated by the book *Islam—Our Choice*, in which testaments are given by people of many different professions (Lords and Barons, statesmen, diplomats, scientists, doctors, scholars, writers, social workers,

preachers) from all over the World (England, the USA, Austria, Germany, Hungary, Holland, Australia, Japan, Poland, Canada, Ireland, Sweden) as to why they chose to convert to Islam. Importantly, within these people are also women. If Islam is the misogynistic religion which the media claims it is, then this conversion to Islam by women brought up in the West would not make any sense. This supports my claim that the debate within the media regarding Muslim women is indeed an unfair one.

In the past some influential figures of the West have attempted 7 to provide an account of Islam without prejudice. In his writings in the 1770s the great German writer and philosopher Goethe concluded that "If this be Islam, do we not all live in Islam?" Another authority in the literary field, Thomas Carlyle, gave a lecture in 1840 to the "intellectual elite" of London entitled "The Hero as Prophet. Mohomet: Islam." This also did a lot to dispel myths associated with Islam in an age where the religion was thought of as savage and barbaric. Countless other less influential figures within the West have also documented fair and unbiased presentations of Islam, yet in the current climate such open minded investigation seemingly no longer exists. Many young British Muslims are coming to the conclusion that Western discourse, of which they believe the media to be a large player, is set against them, only satisfied when documenting them in a distorted light. The term "Islamophobia" has emerged within these circles, and can be used to summarise the collective feeling of rejection and alienation that is being experienced by Muslims within Britain. At the hands of the Western media British Muslims face marginalisation, having their beliefs and practices ridiculed and degraded on a regular basis.

Salman Rushdie's novel, *The Satanic Verses*, and the Rushdie 8 Affair that followed its publication demonstrates this marginalisation. Rushdie's novel makes a crude play with the sacred beliefs of Muslims; in effect he laughs at what he considers an irrational and ignorant people. Muslims world-wide were unsurprisingly deeply shocked, insulted and angered by the novel. In London a peaceful march in protest took place, in which many of my close friends participated—however, a small handful of youths became unruly, resulting in clashes with the police. Again the media chose to give the event a negative image, with news programmes giving coverage only to the small minority who became violent. The focus also turned to Ayatollah Komeini's *fatwa* (simply translated as "ruling," and not as the "death sentence" as the media has claimed) for Rushdie to be executed. The idea of Muslims as an irrationally violent people was again put across by the media, yet no mention was made of the fact that Khomeini's *fatwa* only applied to Shi'ite Muslims, who make up less then twenty percent of the Muslim population in the World. Throughout the Rushdie affair the media came down heavily against Muslims; journalists and writers spoke out in support of Rushdie, and his right to freedom of expression. No voices lent support to the hurt suffered by the Muslims—to my memory only one writer, Roald Dahl, spoke out against Rushdie and his insensitivity in insulting the beliefs of Muslims. Another sharp lesson was also learnt by Muslims within Britain due to the affair: the limitations of the law in providing them with protection, and therefore the limitations of equality for all in Britain. When Abdul Husain Choudary attempted to bring summonses against Rushdie and his publishers, the Chief Metropolitan Magistrate in London ruled that the law of blasphemy in England and Wales protected only the Christian religion.

9   Why does the media choose to misrepresent Islam and Muslims in such a manner? The question is one with no defined answer. Many, myself included, may first consider that ignorance is at its roots—that those in control of the media simply are not well informed on Islam, and that this comes through in the articles and programmes they produce. However, on further reflection this argument can easily be dismissed. There are too many good sources from which the true Islam can be researched, and found. There are books written within the West by Muslims, by converts to Islam, even some by non-Muslims that reflect fairly on the religion. There are monthly magazines published by Muslim organisations in Britain, and now there are even web-sites and CD-ROMs available with Islamic themes, and these show what Islam really is. With all this information it would be impossible to simply believe that the researchers are ignorant with regards to Islam. Many Muslims now have an alternative and more sceptical answer, that the media purposely misrepresents Islam as it challenges the order of the West. It commands an allegiance which

goes beyond boundaries of wealth, nationality, sex, race or culture. It is a threat, and as such, it is treated as the enemy. Many have associated the rise of anti–Islamic sentiments in the media to the end of the Cold War—Muslims will now argue that with the fall of the USSR, Islam is the new common enemy of the West. Such ideas reflect the extent of the damage done to the Muslim community. The media has a great power, and how it chooses to exercise this power directly affects people. It is a propaganda machine of the highest order. The way in which this powerful organisation has mistreated and misrepresented Islam and Muslims is unjust, but furthermore dangerous. This subject warrants and desperately deserves further debate and investigation, which I sincerely hope it will receive in the near future.

Globalization and Culture: Should Slow Invasions Be Stopped?

A Discourse on the Love of Our Country

Richard Price

1 The love of our country has in all times been a subject of warm commendations; and it is certainly a noble passion; but, like all other passions, it requires regulation and direction. There are mistakes and prejudices by which, in this instance, we are in particular danger of being misled. I will briefly mention some of these to you, and observe,

2   First, that by our country is meant, in this case, not the soil or the spot of earth on which we happen to have been born; not the forests and fields, but that community of which we are members; or that body of companions and friends and kindred who are associated with us under the same constitution of government, protected by the same laws, and bound together by the same civil polity.

3   Secondly, it is proper to observe, that even in this sense of our country, that love of it which is our duty, does not imply any conviction of the superior value of it to other countries, or any particular preference of its laws and constitution of government. Were this implied, the love of their country would be the duty of only a very small part of mankind; for there are few countries that

164

enjoy the advantage of laws and governments which deserve to be preferred. To found, therefore, this duty on such a preference, would be to found it on error and delusion. It is, however, a common delusion. There is the same partiality in countries to themselves, that there is in individuals. All our attachments should be accompanied, as far as possible, with right opinions. We are too apt to confine wisdom and virtue within the circle of our own acquaintance and party. Our friends, our country, and in short everything related to us, we are disposed to overvalue. A wise man will guard himself against this delusion. He will study to think of all things as they are, and not suffer any partial affections to blind his understanding. In other families there may be as much worth as in our own. In other circles of friends there may be as much wisdom; and in other countries as much of all that deserves esteem; but, notwithstanding this, our obligation to love our own families, friends, and country, and to seek, in the first place, their good, will remain the same.

Thirdly, it is proper I should desire you particularly to distinguish between love of our country and that spirit of rivalship and ambition which has been common among nations. What has the love of their country hitherto been among mankind? What has it been but a love of domination; a desire of conquest, and a thirst for grandeur and glory, by extending territory, and enslaving surrounding countries? What has it been but a blind and narrow principle, producing in every country a contempt of other countries, and forming men into combinations and factions against their common rights and liberties? This is the principle that has been too often cried up as a virtue of the first rank: a principle of the same kind with that which governs clans of Indians or tribes of Arabs, and leads them out to plunder and massacre. As most of the evils which have taken place in private life, and among individuals, have been occasioned by the desire of private interest overcoming the public affections; so most of the evils which have taken place among bodies of men have been occasioned by the desire of their own interest overcoming the principle of universal benevolence: and leading them to attack one another's territories, to encroach on one another's rights, and to endeavor to build their own advancement on the degradation of all within the reach of their power. What was the love of their country among the Jews, but a wretched partiality to themselves, and a proud contempt of all other nations? What was the love of their country among the old Romans? We have heard much of it; but I cannot hesitate in saying that, however great it appeared in some of its exertions, it was in general no better than a principle holding together a band of robbers in their attempts to crush all liberty but their own. What is now the love of his country in a Spaniard, a Turk, or a Russian? Can it be considered as anything better than a passion for slavery, or a blind attachment to a spot where he enjoys no rights, and is disposed of as if he were a beast?

5   Let us learn by such reflections to correct and purify this passion, and to make it a just and rational principle of action.

6   It is very remarkable that the founder of our religion has not once mentioned this duty, or given us any recommendation of it; and this has, by unbelievers, been made an objection to Christianity. What I have said will entirely remove this objection. Certain it is, that, by inculcating on men an attachment to their country, Christianity would, at the time it was propagated, have done unspeakably more harm than good. Among the Jews, it would have been an excitement to war and insurrections; for they were then in eager expectation of becoming soon (as the favorite people of Heaven) the lords and conquerors of the earth, under the triumphant reign of the Messiah. Among the Romans, likewise, this principle had, as I have just observed, exceeded its just bounds, and rendered them enemies to the peace and happiness of mankind. By inculcating it, therefore, Christianity would have confirmed both Jews and Gentiles in one of the most pernicious faults. Our Lord and his Apostles have done better. They have recommended that UNIVERSAL BENEVOLENCE which is an unspeakably nobler principle than any partial affections. They have laid such stress on loving all men, even our enemies, and made an ardent and extensive charity so essential a part of virtue, that the religion they have preached may, by way of distinction from all other religions, be called the Religion of Benevolence. Nothing can be more friendly to the general rights of mankind; and were it duly regarded and practiced every man would consider every other man as his brother, and all the animosity that now takes place among contending nations would be abolished. . . .

But I am digressing from what I had chiefly in view, which 7
was, after noticing that love of our country which is false and spu-
rious, to explain the nature and effects of that which is just and
reasonable. With this view I must desire you to recollect that we
are so constituted that our affections are more drawn to some
among mankind than to others, in proportion to their degrees of
nearness to us, and our power of being useful to them. It is obvious that this is a circumstance in the constitution of our natures
which proves the wisdom and goodness of our Maker; for had
our affections been determined alike to all our fellow-creatures,
human life would have been a scene of embarrassment and distraction. Our regards, according to the order of nature, begin with
ourselves; and every man is charged primarily with the care of
himself. Next come our families, and benefactors, and friends; and
after them our country. We can do little for the interest of mankind
at large. To this interest, however, all other interests are subordinate. The noblest principle in our nature is the regard to general
justice, and that good will which embraces all the world. I have
already observed this; but it cannot be too often repeated. Though
our immediate attention must be employed in promoting our own
interest and that of our nearest connections: yet we must remember, that a narrower interest ought always to give way to a more
extensive interest. In pursuing particularly the interest of our
country, we ought to carry our views beyond it. We should love
it ardently, but not exclusively. We ought to seek its good, by all
the means that our different circumstances and abilities will allow;
but at the same time we ought to consider ourselves as citizens
of the world, and take care to maintain a just regard to the rights
of other countries. . . .

Our first concern, as lovers of our country, must be to 8
enlighten it. Why are the nations of the world so patient under
despotism? Why do they crouch to tyrants, and submit to be
treated as if they were a herd of cattle? Is it not because they
are kept in darkness, and want knowledge? Enlighten them and
you will elevate them. Show them they are men, and they will
act like men. Give them just ideas of civil government, and let
them know that it is an expedient for gaining protection against
injury and defending their rights, and it will be impossible for
them to submit to governments which, like most of those now

in the world, are usurpations on the rights of men, and little better than contrivances for enabling the few to oppress the many. Convince them that the Deity is a righteous and benevolent as well as omnipotent being, who regards with equal eye all his creatures, and connects his favor with nothing but an honest desire to know and do his will; and that zeal for mystical doctrines which has led men to hate and harass one another will be exterminated. Set religion before them as a rational service, consisting not in rites and ceremonies, but in worshipping God with a pure heart and practicing righteousness from the fear of his displeasure and the apprehension of a future righteous judgment, and that gloomy and cruel superstition will be abolished which has hitherto gone under the name of religion, and to the support of which civil government has been perverted. Ignorance is the parent of bigotry, intolerance, persecution, and slavery. Inform and instruct mankind; and these evils will be excluded. Happy is the person who, himself raised above vulgar errors, is conscious of having aimed at giving mankind this instruction. Happy is the scholar or philosopher who at the close of life can reflect that he has made this use of his learning and abilities: but happier far must he be, if at the same time he has reason to believe he has been successful, and actually contributed, by his instructions, to disseminate among his fellow-creatures just notions of themselves, of their rights, of religion, and the nature and end of civil government. Such were Milton, Locke, Sidney, Hoadley, etc. in this country; such were Montesquieu, Fenelon, Turgot, etc. in France. They sowed a seed which has since taken root, and is now growing up to a glorious harvest. To the information they conveyed by their writings we owe those revolutions in which every friend of mankind is now exulting. What an encouragement is this to us all in our endeavors to enlighten the world? Every degree of illumination which we can communicate must do the greatest good. It helps to prepare the minds of men for the recovery of their rights, and hastens the overthrow of priestcraft and tyranny. In short, we may, in this instance, learn our duty from the conduct of the oppressors of the world. They know that light is hostile to them, and therefore they labor to keep men in the dark. With this intention they have appointed licensers of the press; and, in

Popish countries, prohibited the reading of the Bible. Remove the darkness in which they envelope the world, and their usurpations will be exposed, their power will be subverted, and the world emancipated.

The next great blessing of human nature which I have men- 9 tioned is VIRTUE. This ought to follow knowledge, and to be directed by it. Virtue without knowledge makes enthusiasts: and knowledge without virtue makes devils; but both united elevates to the top of human dignity and perfection. We must, therefore, if we would serve our country, make both these the objects of our zeal. We must discourage vice in all its forms; and our endeavors to enlighten must have ultimately in view a reformation of manners and virtuous practice. . . .

LIBERTY is the next great blessing, which I have mentioned 10 as the object of patriotic zeal. It is inseparable lrom knowledge and virtue, and together completes the glory of a community. An enlightened and virtuous country must be a free country. It cannot suffer invasions of its rights, or bend to tyrants. . . .

The observations I have made include our whole duty to our 11 country; for by endeavoring to liberalize and enlighten it, to discourage vice and to promote virtue in it, and to assert and support its liberties, we shall endeavor to do all that is necessary to make it great and happy. . . .

The Culture Blockade

James Ledbetter

The Bush Administration seems to be gunning to make history as 1 the first great unilateralist government of the twenty-first century. But if the notion of going it alone appeals to the American public, it's partly because America routinely practices a less-noticed *cultural* unilateralism: If a work of art wasn't made in America, chances are Americans will never know about it.

Consider: 2

§ Approximately 92 percent of the US music market in the 3 year 2000 consisted of music from domestic acts. That makes

America the most insular music market in the world except for Pakistan. The inward listening trend survives even though most of the big labels—Sony, Universal and BMG—are now controlled by non-US companies.

4   § This summer the bestseller lists in both France and Argentina included novels from the American author Paul Auster. (The top spot on France's list, however, was captured by our own Mary Higgins Clark.) Jonathan Franzen's *The Corrections* made the bestseller lists in Italy and Germany. English-language authors J.K. Rowling, Jean Auel, Stephen King and John Grisham were all represented on Germany's, Italy's and Spain's bestseller lists. And in Poland, the late suspense writer Robert Ludlum hit No. 1.

5   Yet try finding a book on the *New York Times* bestseller list that wasn't originally written in English. OK, a few times a year one crops up, usually at the lower end of the nonfiction list. But the point holds: The rest of the world reads what Americans write, but rarely vice versa. If you don't believe this, ask yourself: How many top-selling, living French, Russian or Japanese novelists can you name?

6   § Theoretically, cable television represents one of the most diverse forms of American communication. But during one of the most news-heavy periods of recent memory, has a single American cable operator decided to run the Qatar-based Al Jazeera, even for a few hours a day? Why aren't the cable news channels following the lead of satellite-channel WorldLink TV, which provides a daily digest of what is broadcast on Arab networks? That's a decision made for reasons that have nothing to do with popularity; it's hard to imagine that a condensed Al Jazeera would get lower ratings than the Golf Channel.

7   Of course, cultural taste is cyclical. There's been, for example, a complete absence of British acts on the US music charts this year (for the first time in forty years). That vacuum derives partly from the current British vogue of prepackaged groups who manufacture an audience by appearing on *Pop Idol* or other television programs little seen outside Britain.

8   Still, the overall trend is clear. The strongest recent performance from non-US cultural works has been in cinema: 2002 has been a promising year for non-American filmmakers. Yet it's indisputable that foreign cinema occupies a smaller portion of

American intellectual life today than it did in the 1960s and '70s. Despite a recent renaissance in European cinema (especially in France), fewer than 15 percent of the films made in France and Italy make it to US screens. As filmmaker David Lynch said during this year's Cannes festival: "If Fellini made $8\frac{1}{2}$ today, I'm not sure that it would be distributed in America."

Even one year's relatively successful hits from overseas, like 9 *Amélie, Monsoon Wedding* and *Y Tu Mamá También* don't begin to compare to the supremacy of *Star Wars* or *Spiderman* abroad.

Americans tend to rationalize such discrepancies by saying: 10 "Well, consumers have a choice; if they want to buy these books, etc., they can find them." But that's a naïve view: Marketing plays an essential role in determining hits versus also-rans. For example, record labels pay at least $200,000 per song to get music on the playlists of the major radio chains (and sometimes up to $1 million per song). It is self-evident that smaller, non-US labels lack the resources to compete on that level. Similarly, even if a small, nonconglomerate American publisher is willing to go to the expense of translating a work by a non-American writer, promotion dollars are scarce, review space at a premium and, without a guarantee of profitability, book orders are difficult to secure. This is what André Schiffrin and others have referred to as "market censorship."

Moreover, the US market remains just as structurally protec- 11 tionist as many of those it criticizes. The United States may preach the virtues of a free information market, but it rarely practices it. It's still illegal, for example, for a non-US citizen to own a US radio or TV license. Foreign film producers face massive distribution hurdles to get their products on American screens or television. CDs imported from Europe are still subject to a 1.8 percent tariff, and from certain other nations one as high as 30 percent.

And as with any trade war, protectionism on one side breeds 12 retaliation on the other. The steady encroachment of US culture into European markets makes the French, for example, push all the harder to maintain their government film subsidies.

All of which makes recent debate about piracy and 13 unwarranted digital distribution seem beside the point. Movie and record executives can drone on incessantly about the billions they lose to unauthorized copies. But those words ring hollow in countries that have little hope of exporting culture to the world's largest media market. It's far from clear that the American culture industry wants to compete on a level playing field—any more than the steel industry does. Closing off borders to terrorists is one thing; closing off borders to the world's culture is quite another.

As American As . . .

David Van Biema with reporting by Nadia Mustafa, Mitch Frank, David E. Thigpen, Cathy Booth Thomas, and David Schwartz

1   He wanted a congenial space where people might gather, which is why Balbir Singh Sodhi was outside his Chevron station in Mesa, Ariz., two Saturdays ago, surveying the vinca and sage he had just planted. Says Guru Roop Kaur Khalsa, one of Sodhi's ministers: "Even though it was just a gas station, he saw it as a center of the community. He looked for innocence and sweetness and tried to capture it." Then, police allege, a man named Frank Silva Roque drove by in a black Chevy pickup and pumped three bullets into Sodhi, killing him almost instantly, mocking innocence and sweetness. Sodhi appears to have died because he looked Muslim. He was not. He was a Sikh, and his religion was born as a reform of Hinduism. But to some, the turban and beard that most Sikhs wear look like Osama bin Laden's. When the police caught Roque, they claim he explained his actions by saying, "I'm an American."

2   Imagine this: you wake up every morning nervous, stalked by faceless enemies. It is nothing personal; they just hate what they think you represent. The attack could come at any time, and there is virtually no defense. If that seems to describe all America at the moment, there is one group for whom the unbearable tension since the World Trade Center attack is doubled. If you are a Muslim or an Arab, or look like one to someone focused primarily on his own rage, you must fear not only bin Laden-style terrorism but also the insults, blows and bullets of your countrymen.

3   Last Thursday someone threw stone after stone through the windshields of cabs in Manhattan's Central Park, apparently

targeting dark-skinned drivers. "A lot of cabdrivers are not driving," says Ali Agha Abba, a Pakistani-American taxi driver in New York City. "I can't afford to not work. So I have to take a chance." Last Monday a man drove a Mustang through the front entrance of the Grand Mosque in Parma, Ohio, the largest in the state. The Sunday before, a Muslim woman in Memphis was beaten on her way to worship. The day before that, a Pakistani Muslim store owner was shot and killed. The FBI called it a hate crime.

True, George Bush spoke out for Muslims at a mosque and 4 before Congress last week, telling them, "We respect your faith. Its teachings are good and peaceful." Last Tuesday FBI agents began a round of bureau meetings with local Muslim and Arab leaders in various states, asking for their help with investigations and assuring their protection. Said a relieved participant: "We know we have the FBI behind us."

And yet . . . on Monday Louisiana Congressman John Cooksey 5 told a radio show, "If I see someone come in that's got a diaper on his head, that guy needs to be pulled over." (He later apologized.) On that same day, the pilot of a Delta flight in Texas had a Pakistani American removed before takeoff because he said his crew did not feel comfortable with the man aboard. Delta offered him a new ticket—on another carrier. (It later apologized.) In Lincoln, R.I., someone hit a pregnant woman wearing a hijab (head scarf) with a stone. She has been calling midwives to avoid giving birth in the hospital because "I don't want to go to any public place." A CNN/*USA Today*/Gallup poll of 1,032 adults indicated that 49% thought all Arabs—American citizens included— should have to carry special ID cards.

All told, the Council on American-Islamic Relations counts 6 more than 600 "incidents" since Sept. 11 victimizing people thought to be Arab or Muslim, including four murders, 45 people assaulted and 60 mosques attacked. Thousands were intimidated into not going to work, their mosques, their schools. Some 200 Muslims are estimated to have died in the Twin Towers. Yet, says C.A.I.R.'s Nihad Awad, "Muslims are being accused of something that the community has not done, and it's really an awkward and unfair position to be in." Thousands of answering machines—and actual people—fielded calls like the one that came into the offices of a Muslim organization in Santa Clara, Calif.: "We should bomb your ass and blow you back home." The caller was apparently unaware that "home" is here.

7   There is no God but Allah, and Muhammad is his prophet. Pray five times a day. Give alms. Fast during the month of Ramadan. If you are capable, make a pilgrimage to Mecca. If these "five pillars" seem foreign to you, you may not be talking with your neighbors. Islam is an American religion. There are some 7 million Muslims in the U.S. That's more than the number of Jews and more than twice the number of Episcopalians. Thirty years ago, the Islamic count was a mere 500,000. The number of mosques rose from 598 in 1986 to 1,372 this year. The number of American-born Muslims now far exceeds the count of immigrants.

8   Islam, the youngest of the major faiths, was influenced by Judaism and Christianity. Muslims are "people of the book," accepting the Jewish Bible and the New Testament as Holy Scripture while maintaining that the Koran's famously elegant and expressive Arabic is God's final and inerrant word. Similarly, followers of Islam believe Moses, John the Baptist and Jesus were prophets but the final messenger was Muhammad, to whom, they say, the angel Gabriel dictated the Koran. Like Christians and Jews, says Jamal Badawi, a religion professor at Saint Mary's University in Halifax, N.S., their core concerns are "moral behavior, love of neighbor, justice and compassion. We believe that we are created for a purpose, and we are going to be held responsible for our life on earth on the day of judgment." Muslims do not worship Muhammad (who, unlike Moses or Jesus, was a lavishly documented historical figure, dying in A.D. 632) but regard him as exemplary. It is upon the Koran and collections of his sayings (Hadiths) that Islamic law, or Sharia, is based.

9   Most Muslims resemble Protestants in that no priest mediates between the believer and God (although the 10% Shi'ite minority is more enamored of its imams). Like Christians, Muslims evangelize and look forward to the eventual conversion of the human race. The faith's directness, bright-line moral stances and the absence of hierarchy have proved attractive to converts in the U.S., while its role for women, who make up only 15% of average Friday mosque attendance, repels some seekers.

10   It is a point of Islamic pride that a Muslim can walk into any mosque anywhere in the world and participate in the service. That

said, the Islamic population in the U.S. is almost as varied as
Mecca's. The first Muslims here were African slaves, who were
forcibly Christianized, although some Muslim descendants still
live on the Georgia coast. Syrians and Lebanese began arriving in
the late 1800s. But the three largest groups in America are made
up of more recent additions.

The largest is African American, a group of almost 2 million   11
whose story is unknown to most of their countrymen. In the
1930s, Wallace D. Fard and his acolyte Elijah Muhammad founded
a group called the Nation of Islam. The Nation was misnamed: its
racialist views and unique theology cause most Muslims to see it
as non-Islamic. Elijah's son Wallace, however, was trained in classical Arabic and, following in the footsteps of his friend Malcolm X,
made a Meccan pilgrimage. After Malcolm's murder and Elijah
Muhammad's death, Wallace changed his name to Warith Deen
Muhammad and gradually led his flock to mainstream Sunni
Muslim observance. Although Louis Farrakhan eventually reacti-
vated the Nation name and attracted some 25,000 adherents, W.D.
Muhammad is the effective leader of 1.6 million believers. He is
regarded by many as a mujaddid, a once-in-a-century "renewer
of the faith."

African Americans are among America's most observant Mus-   12
lims. While Yvonne Haddad of Georgetown University's Center for
Muslim-Christian Understanding estimates the fraction of immigrants who attend mosque at a mere 10%, many American blacks,
with converts' zeal, memorize verse after verse of the Koran and
are extremely serious about Islamic injunctions against premarital
sex, abortion and alcohol. Most also shun MTV, Hollywood films,
hip-hop and dancing. Such social conservatism also translates
politically: the tally of Bush votes among African-American Muslims was 25% higher than in black America as a whole. The community is thoroughly patriotic: W.D. Muhammad sometimes leads
his flock in the Pledge of Allegiance before worship. And although
it has traditionally drawn from the poor and working classes (it
is immensely successful in prisons), the black middle class is
increasingly intrigued.

The remaining two large American Islamic blocs have roughly   13
parallel histories. The majority of Arab and South Asian (Indian
subcontinental) believers began arriving here in the late 1960s in

response to changes in immigration law and home-country programs that subsidized study here. The students became professionals and put down roots. They were joined by relatives and by refugees from various international upheavals. Most, while thrilled at America's free speech and its economic prospects, were shocked by the materialism, secularism and free morality that they encountered. Settling into lives as doctors, engineers or grocery-store owners, they contended with malls, disco and recurrent spasms of anti-Arab and -Muslim sentiment fueled by events such as the Arab oil boycott and the first World Trade Center bombing. Many also had vivid memories of American involvement in their home nations. A sizable faction was attracted to the Islamist movement, which argued for isolation from the American social and political system in favor of an eventual Muslim triumph. "The process of Americanization," wrote Georgetown's Haddad in 1987, "is impeded."

14   But 14 years later, Haddad reports, Islamist sympathy is below 10%. What happened? The new immigrants became more comfortable with the language and the culture around them. They realized that unlike many of their homelands, one could express political or cultural opposition here and still be regarded as a good American. And finally, they gave birth to a generation, now in its 20s and 30s, whose primary identification is American, albeit with a "Muslim" prefix. "The feeling is," paraphrases Haddad (who is not Muslim), "'We are American. We participate in this America. We cannot live off America and not be part of it, and we have something to contribute.'"

15   The burning issues in the average Muslim-American household are far less likely to be political than fairly standard sitcom fodder. A child refuses to wear a hijab. A mother suddenly realizes that despite the prohibition on premarital dating in most Muslim households, her daughter's "good friend" is really a boyfriend. A married couple notes bemusedly that while they attend mosque only once a month, or possibly twice a year, their college-age son, like many of his peers, seems to be returning to religious observance. Meanwhile, in his dorm room, that son is plying the Web in service of a human-rights organization, protesting American policies regarding Kashmir or Palestine or even Kabul—from within the American system.

That is not to say there may not be a tiny minority of mosques   16
in America whose congregants tilt toward the Taliban or even bin
Laden. At the Hazrat-I-Abubakr Sadiq mosque in Queens, after
the imam decried the World Trade attack to his 1,000-person
congregation, members of the Taliban's Pashtun clan moved to the
basement in apparent protest.

Omar Abdel Rahman, the jailed ringleader of the 1993 World   17
Trade Center bombing, used to preach at the Masjid al-Salaam
mosque in Jersey City, N.J. The day after the recent terror, two
men arrested on a train in Dallas with box cutters, hair dye and
more than $5,000 in cash are reported to have worshiped there
recently. Two cops now stand at the mosque door.

Two days before the attack, Moataz al-Hallak, the former   18
imam at the Center Street mosque in Arlington, Texas, returned
there to pray. It turns out that al-Hallak was close to Wadih
el-Hage, bin Laden's secretary who was recently found guilty
in the U.S. embassy bombings in East Africa. Al-Hallak's
name also reportedly showed up on a list at a Brooklyn refugee
center headed by several men convicted in the 1993 Trade
Center bombing. Al-Hallak, who has not been charged in either
World Trade plot, has denied connection to bin Laden and
claims to have counseled el-Hage only on religious matters.
Najam Khan, president of the group that runs the Arlington
mosque, says it fired al-Hallak last year for neglecting his
flock—before the bin Laden connections were known. "I don't
think he was preaching violence per se," Khan says, looking
mournful. "We feel this mosque is being targeted because of
individuals who may have had shady business somewhere,
but that has nothing to do with the mosque and the rest of the
community." He says the imam never talked politics from the
pulpit: "It doesn't make sense. No mosque wants that. It divides
people."

When Muslim immigrant groups first started arriving in the   19
'60s, says Professor Haddad, "they looked at each other and said,
'I have nothing to do with you.'" Today all that has changed.
C.A.I.R.'s Mosque in America project reports that only 7% of the
12,000 mosques surveyed serve a single ethnic group. Almost 90%
play host to a mix of African Americans, South Asian Americans
and Arab Americans.

20   Think about that: the Arabic word for all those who affirm Islam is ummah. It implies a sense of oneness and community. Around the world and over the centuries, as Islamic empires have collided, it has often been difficult to discern. But here in America, the country where Sunday is the most segregated day of the week, it flourishes. Balbir Singh Sodhi's killer would probably not have appreciated that. But Sodhi would have, despite not being a Muslim. And maybe there is something here for all Americans to learn, if we can only catch our breath.

The Ever-Expanding, Profit-Maximizing, Cultural-Imperialist, Wonderful World of Disney

Jonathan Weber

1   It's a sunny afternoon at the Window on the World theme park in the southern Chinese city of Shenzhen, and Chen Ping and Wei Qing Hua are strolling the grounds. A cheerful young couple from China's Hubei province, Chen and Wei migrated to this city, a remarkable symbol of the new capitalist China, to make money— he's a taxi driver and she works in a factory. They've come to the park this Tuesday to, well, see the sights.

2   "It's nothing special," concludes Chen as he surveys cheesy small-scale replicas of the Roman Colosseum and the Arc de Triomphe that anchor the "Europe" section of the park. The sprawling grounds feature dioramas of tourist attractions from five continents—including the Sphinx, Mount Rushmore, and a life-size African village—but there aren't many people around. Bored vendors hawk cheap trinkets, without much success.

3   Just a half hour train ride away, a rather more ambitious theme park is under construction. Slated to open in 2005, Hong Kong Disneyland will offer the sizzle, polish, and attention to

detail that's woefully lacking in Shenzhen. Chen and Wei, already well acquainted with Mickey and Donald, say they'll certainly visit, visas permitting. "It would be very brilliant," says Chen. "If it comes from outside China, it's going to be better than what comes from inside. You just know it."

There could hardly be a better summation of the opportunity 4 that American pop culture companies like Disney are enjoying overseas. With the end of the Cold War, the opening of China, and the worldwide triumph of American-style capitalism, the brand-name purveyors of American food, fashion, and entertainment have never had it so good. Hardly a city on the planet is without McDonald's and CNN and Levi's and MTV. American films are omnipresent and in some markets dominant, accounting for nearly three-quarters of movie admissions in Western Europe. *Who Wants to Be a Millionaire* is a hit in several Asian countries.

For many countries, especially in the developing world, the 5 ever-growing presence of the US culture industry is a mixed blessing. On the one hand, the pervasiveness of Americana can be seen as a sign of progress. US brands are symbols of wealth and modernity and freedom. Drinking coffee at Starbucks or taking the family to Disneyland signals the rise of a worldly middle class. On a more concrete level, Western companies often bring a measure of quality and service that are both a boon for local consumers and a prod for domestic firms to raise their standards.

At the same time, the enormous popularity of US brands over- 6 seas can pose a threat not only to a nation's domestic industries but to its cultural traditions and sense of identity. For decades now, intellectuals in Europe have lamented the Americanization of their societies. Euro Disney, now known as Disneyland Paris, was once famously denounced by the French theater director Ariane Mnouchkine as a "cultural Chernobyl." In the developing world, cultural imperialism has long been seen as the handmaiden of political domination, another way for strong countries to take advantage of the weak.

Even champions of globalization increasingly fret that 7 it may damage or destroy the diversity that makes the human race so fascinating, leaving nothing but homogenized, least-common-denominator forms of creativity. In the wake of

September 11, there is a new urgency to these concerns. The fury of the terrorists—and of the alarming number of people around the world who viewed the attacks as a deserved comeuppance for an arrogant, out-of-control superpower—is sparked in part by a sense that America is imposing its lifestyle on countries that don't want it. And one needn't condone mass murder to believe that a new world order that leaves every place on the globe looking like a California strip mall will make us all poorer.

8   No company conveys more powerfully the image of a conquering cultural army than Walt Disney. Its founder was a true-blue patriot who saw himself as a proselytizer for the values of the American heartland. The company's products and services—unlike, say, fast-food hamburgers or sugary soft drinks—are not merely symbolic of the American way of life, but contain as part of their essence a set of beliefs about good and evil and human aspiration. Disney, moreover, has throughout its history been extremely shrewd about building mutually reinforcing products across many different kinds of media, with theme parks and TV shows, movies and merchandise, all working together in service of the Disney way.

9   The company's drive for the China market shows how this machine can work overseas. Seen from the outside, the strategy seems quite savvy. It began with elemental Disney—its cartoons—which first aired on Chinese television in the mid–1980s, just as the country was opening up. Chinese entrepreneurs kicked in a flood of pirated videos and counterfeit merchandise, which did nothing for Disney's bottom line but had the effect of spreading its characters at viral speed.

10   In 1997, Disney's Miramax label released *Kundun,* a Martin Scorsese film about Tibet that angered the Chinese leadership. But behind the scenes the company was also working on *Mulan,* an animated blockbuster that brought a traditional Chinese fable to a global audience with classic Disney production values. In the wake of *Mulan*'s warm reception, Disney cut a deal with Hong Kong to build a theme park, and attendance there will no doubt get a boost from a major new television agreement, announced in December, under which Mickey Mouse cartoons will appear daily, in kids' prime time, on China's biggest television channel.

11   Disney executives, including CEO Michael Eisner and COO Bob Iger, make regular trips to China, meeting with top leadership

to pave the way for more deals. One possibility: a theme park in Shanghai. Meanwhile, China has become the world's largest producer of licensed Disney merchandise, which helps company executives when they push the government to crack down on the unlicensed variety.

Despite all this, the image of Disney—and of America in general—as an unstoppable cultural juggernaut is misleading. The truth is that selling American culture overseas is a tricky business. Disney and other big global brands are driven not by grand plans to promote American values, but rather by incremental, pragmatic, financially oriented, market research—based business decisions—and even then, the companies struggle mightily to make their initiatives work. Success depends on some rather mundane factors: Have you selected good local partners? Do your executives understand local traditions and speak the language? Have you developed an organization that allows for strategic coordination across far-flung locations? Have you earned the goodwill of citizens groups and government officials?

In most countries, media-related industries in particular are still dominated by domestic firms, and there is little reason to think that will change in the near future. Disney gets less than 20 percent of its revenue from overseas, a share that's been stagnant even though management has long cited the international market as a major growth area. The company's experience abroad suggests that even in this age of interconnection, where the combination of technology and American hegemony makes a shallow global monoculture a possibility, that dull new world won't be arriving anytime soon.

The Burbank, California, headquarters of the Walt Disney Company sits on the impeccably manicured Disney Studios lot, surrounded by paths with names like Mickey Avenue and Dopey Drive and featuring a roof held aloft by 19-foot-high statues of the Seven Dwarfs. In the sprawling executive suites, the ambience is high corporate rather than California casual, reflecting the relentlessly competitive, hierarchical style of the CEO Eisner.

It is Eisner who can claim credit for transforming Disney from a drifting, dated icon of American middle-class entertainment into a global media superpower, one that trails only AOL Time Warner in scope and scale. The ghost of Walt, the creative genius who invented most of the famous characters as well as the concept of Disneyland, still inhabits many corners of the company. But as befits a huge, publicly traded corporation, the true guiding spirit today is the bottom line. When Eisner took over in 1984, Disney had $1.7 billion in revenue, hardly any profits, and a miserable reputation both in Hollywood and on Wall Street. Today, thanks to aggressive exploitation of the signature characters, continued success in developing new animated hits, the revival of the movie studio, and the 1996 acquisition of Capital Cities/ABC Inc., Disney boasts revenue of more than $25 billion and employs 120,000 people worldwide. With its global outlook and willingness to experiment in multiple media, Disney is a member of the *Wired* Index, the 40 businesses charting the future of the economy.

16   Disney, in fact, can be a remarkable machine, and over the last decade it has been one of the few businesses of any kind that gives real meaning to the term *synergy*. Take a hit animated film like *The Lion King*. Released in 1994, it has grossed more than $765 million at the box office worldwide—and that's only the beginning. There was a best-selling record album, live stage shows, cartoons on the Disney Channel, a Toontown attraction at Disneyland, a vast array of merchandise, and extraordinarily lucrative home video and DVD sales.

17   What's more, much of the Disney empire is easy to export. The characters have long been popular overseas; Mickey Mouse is among the most recognized icons in the world. The animated feature films travel particularly well, since they can be seamlessly translated into other languages, and they are often big hits abroad. Disneyland Tokyo, opened in 1982, has been an unalloyed success, and the new Tokyo Disney Seas park, which debuted in September, appears poised to repeat that performance. Disneyland Paris had a terrible couple of years after opening in 1992, but it's now doing well enough that a Disney Studios park is about to move in next door. More than half of the sales of Disney merchandise come from outside the US. And because Disney stands for family entertainment and steers clear of political issues, it's even been mostly immune to a rising anti-American corporate backlash.

18   Yet with all of that, until a couple of years ago, the company had no real international strategy. "We had a couple hundred legal

entities overseas that needed to be consolidated—we were not world class in that," says Michael Johnson, a cheery veteran of the home entertainment division who now heads up the entity called Walt Disney International. "We were spending a huge amount of money. We didn't have a grip on some of our characters and how they were performing. It was a legacy of these huge silos."

The silos Johnson is referring to are Disney's five lines of busi- 19 ness: Media Networks, Parks and Resorts, Consumer Products, Studio Entertainment, and Internet. In principle, each business unit should constantly reinforce one another. In practice, each often goes its own way—especially overseas. To fix this problem, the company in 1999 created a system of country managers explicitly charged with coordinating brand strategy.

With its massive population and emerging economies, Asia is 20 the promised land for American culture merchants. And Japan, by far the richest country in Asia, is the logical first stop. Disneyland Tokyo has helped the company's animated movies and toys become staples for Japanese children. The new Disney Seas is one of the company's most innovative projects; aimed at adults as much as kids, it features beautifully crafted, self-contained environments such as the American Waterfront and the Mediterranean Harbor. A visit in November found both Tokyo parks mobbed, not just with families but with teens on dates, middle-aged couples, and even the occasional group of retirees. "We grew up with the Disney characters, so we feel comfortable with them," said repeat visitor Hideko Seki, a 36-year-old magazine designer from Kawasaki, Japan. The two Tokyo parks expect to draw some 25 million visitors in the first full year of Disney Seas operations.

Japan is famous for its willingness to adopt Western culture 21 even as it remains highly insular. One of Disney Internet's rare successes has been in the Japanese wireless market, where for reasons few understand, people are willing to pay to download cartoon characters onto their cell phones. But even here, Disney faces challenges. For one thing, Japan has its own strong tradition of animation. (Disney has even licensed the works of one top Japanese animator, *Princess Mononoke* creator Hayao Miyazaki, for international distribution.) It is also adept at creating its own pop culture characters: Think Pokémon and Power Rangers and Hello Kitty. Finally, there's the slumping Japanese economy. So while

Japan remains Disney's biggest market outside the US, it's still a niche player with limited growth prospects beyond the new theme park.

22   Which explains why Disney's been looking farther west, to China. There could hardly be a more enticing market: a billion people, rapidly getting richer, who turn to foreign brands both for symbolic value and superior quality, and who are devoted to their families. Disney products, moreover, are seen by the Chinese authorities as politically innocuous—unlike, say, how they view AOL Time Warner's CNN. Chairman Mao once referred to Western movies and art as "sugarcoated bullets" and sought to eradicate them during the Cultural Revolution. But the pragmatists who run the Chinese Communist Party today have no such qualms about Disney. "We're a family entertainment company, and that is pretty well understood by the government officials," says Jun Tang, Disney's vice president for China affairs. The characters, especially Mickey and Donald, are part of the fabric of Chinese culture. A hip teen wandering the Window on the World park in Shenzhen says Disney is no longer cool—and yet there's a battered Mickey Mouse doll hanging from her backpack.

23   For Disney, as for most Western companies, the China strategy begins in Hong Kong. In this citadel of commerce, the countless shopping malls could be straight out of an American suburb, and people snap up Western goods without a second thought. Tai-Lok Lui, a professor of sociology at the Chinese University of Hong Kong, attributes this to the fact that Hong Kong is a society of migrants who chose to leave their culture behind in order to pursue a new beginning. America, he says, has always represented "high tech, consumption, a comfortable way of life." Whether it was the moon landing or *Star Trek* or US soldiers coming ashore on leave, the image of America is of a distant but powerful and glamorous place. "We would watch *Bewitched*, and we'd be bewitched by the modern American kitchen," says Lui.

24   Disney began eyeing Hong Kong as a possible theme park location in the mid-'90s, just after it opened the Paris park. Asia was the obvious next market, and Hong Kong had the right mix of high per-capita income, solid infrastructure, and knowledge of the tourism business. And it had the hunger. The Hong Kong economy fell into the doldrums following the departure of the

British in 1997 and the Asian financial crisis in 1998; local leaders were terrified that it would be overwhelmed by a resurgent mainland China. Unemployment was rising, and tourism was hurting. Disney looked like a good fix for both of those things.

Just as it did in France, Disney squeezed a sweet deal out of the government—in part by threatening to build the park in Shanghai. Mike Rowse, the Hong Kong government's lead negotiator on the deal, quips: "They had the S-word and we had the U-word," referring to Disney's theme park rival Universal. It's not clear whether Shanghai was a real option; Steve Tight, a senior vice president in the Parks and Resorts group who leads Disney's Hong Kong project, says there still aren't enough people in China who can afford Disneyland. But sources say the deal almost collapsed when Disney insisted that Hong Kong promise it exclusivity—meaning no other foreign theme parks—but was unwilling to reciprocate with a promise not to build on the mainland. In the end, there is no exclusivity, and there may yet be a park in Shanghai someday.

The park is a key Disney wedge into the region—even though it's just part of a larger Asian strategy. At Disney's Asia Pacific headquarters off Hong Kong's Times Square, more than 20 different Disney entities are trying to build the brand. Jon Niermann, an ebullient young marketing maven, is charged with "bringing everyone together at one Disney table," as he puts it, persuading, say, Buena Vista Entertainment Asia Pacific to work with Consumer Products. There's a weekly meeting with all the regional line-of-business managers. There's a weekly conference call with all the country managers. There's a "synergy calendar" on Niermann's wall, charting the major film and video releases and the marketing programs that will go along with them. On this day, Niermann is excited about an initiative to roll out a new line of merchandise based on Marie, a cat, in local Disney stores. "Asians love cats," says Niermann. "Music came to the table, and we pulled in a local canto-pop duo" to help launch the promotion. "TV got behind it by giving local TV exposures. The people who worked on this all wore two hats."

Niermann has high hopes for Disney's new China Central Television deal, under which 142 episodes of Mickey Mouse cartoons will be featured on the leading children's TV program on a major Chinese station. The arrangement is something of a coup because the channel reaches 75 percent of all Chinese TV sets—a cool 225 million households—while most foreign programming is still relegated to satellite channels with far less reach. Disney's Jun Tang says it's just one in a range of brand-building initiatives, from book publishing to animated films to shows like *Disney on Ice* and the Broadway version of *Beauty and the Beast*, both of which recently played in China.

28   But all the synergy Disney can muster in China doesn't guarantee success. Plenty of Western companies have discovered this promising market to be a mirage. For Disney, the theme park is close to a can't-miss proposition; it needs to draw only 5.5 million people a year—just one-third of what the Tokyo park gets—to meet company projections. The market research shows that locals want the original Disneyland, not Sino-Disney, so there won't be a lot of execution risk on the creative side. Some wonder whether the impatient Chinese will put up with the lines, but if Americans are willing to wait two hours for a five-minute ride, the Chinese probably will be, too.

29   On other fronts, though, it's still an uphill battle. China Central Television has been making deals with most of the big Western broadcasters; Disney won't disclose the terms of its new arrangement, and it's not at all clear that it will be a significant moneymaker. In the merchandising business, China has been home to so many counterfeit Disney goods for so long that it may be tough for the real thing—at Disney-style prices—to make inroads. And with movies, China retains strict caps on the number of Western films it will allow to be screened. Disney has enjoyed more than its share, but China is still a rounding error in overall box office statistics.

30   China's love–hate relationship with the West dates to the arrival of European colonialists in the 19th century. Even today, the increasingly pro–Western sentiment can quickly melt away. When NATO bombs accidentally hit the Chinese embassy in Belgrade during the Kosovo war, furious anti–American protests erupted throughout China. KFC franchises were stoned, and MTV was yanked off the air. "China is enthralled by America, and repelled by it, and at the same time overwhelmed by it," says Orville Schell, a China scholar who is now dean of the Graduate School of Journalism at Berkeley. "It's an absolute contradiction."

Schell says the government tries from time to time to "curry popularity by surfing on anti–Western sentiment," but it's also eager to get the help of Western companies in building a more modern and prosperous country.

These contradictions exist in many countries; Islamic funda- 31 mentalists may denounce the Great Satan, but that doesn't stop them from drinking a Coke. In most industries, though, ambivalence about America doesn't much matter, because the products are basically value-neutral. A computer is a computer no matter who the manufacturer is, and while one might dislike modern multinationals, or believe that American computer imports are hurting local makers, IBM as a brand doesn't really represent anything other than good technology. Its machines don't speak any language other than binary.

But the culture industry is different. Disney and other media 32 brands are fraught with emotional and psychological undercurrents. Disney represents certain ideas: fun, family, personal freedom, optimism about life and about the future, confidence that good will triumph over evil. These are in many respects universal Western Enlightenment values, rather than specifically American ones, and company executives say their market research shows that people are not drawn to Disney because of its connection to the United States. Yet analysts of global branding—as well as every Disney customer interviewed for this story—affirm that those who buy Disney products overseas are keenly aware that the items are foreign. Indeed that is part of the appeal.

"American brands are about anything being possible—the 33 core value of all of them is optimism," says Martyn Straw, president of the consultancy Interbrand. "America is not a country, it's an idea; there is a distinction between America as a geopolitical entity and America as a concept, a place where you can be what you want to be. These themes play around the world, and the Disney brand is almost exclusively dependent on that."

The paradox, though, is that even as people are drawn to 34 American brands as symbols, when it comes to actual cultural content, they are looking for something more. They want the production values they associate with modernity and technology, whether it takes the form of a state-of-the-art theme park or a fast-food restaurant that is clean, air-conditioned, and offers good service. At the same time, they want things tailored to their tastes. Disneyland Hong Kong, for all its loyalty to the original, will feature a broad selection of Asian food as well as shows and special events that are built around local holidays. Even McDonald's, a symbol of monoculture if ever there was one, insists that its success overseas is due to the creativity and innovation of its local franchisees, who can modify menus to suit local tastes.

35   In the TV business, the need to localize is especially evident. For one thing, most people want to watch television in their own language, even if they speak English, and dubbing imported programs goes only so far. "If you want to create things, they have to be of that culture," says James Murdoch, son of the Aussie magnate and head of the Asian satellite broadcaster Star Television. He cites the development of more local programming as the key factor in improving the performance of Star, whose original model was based on Pan-Asian English-language programming. In China and India, Star's Mandarin and Hindi channels outdraw its English ones by huge margins. Almost by definition, television programming in Mandarin or Hindi is going to be a local product, even if it carries the patina of an international brand.

36   The same is true over at MTV, another successful purveyor of American culture. "Our product changes dramatically from region to region," says Bill Roedy, head of MTV Networks International. "We're all about different languages, different VJs, different themes. We are the antithesis of homogeneity." He says MTV's 33 channels around the world tend to have 50 to 80 percent local content. Harry Hui—until recently head of MTV Asia and soon to move to Universal Music—says the glamour of MTV is what brings people in, but the quality of the programming is what keeps them.

37   Even in the Internet business, which ought to be intrinsically the most global, the trend is toward localization. In China, Disney handed over management of its Mandarin site to a local company, Sea Rainbow. AOL, which has a presence in 17 countries, doesn't use the America Online branding anywhere except in the US and Latin America, and while the overseas operations piggyback on the mothership's technology, they are otherwise locally run, mostly with partners who own a substantial equity stake.

Iconic brands have enormous power, but they also impose 38 constraints. Disney is so closely identified with family entertainment that it can be difficult for the company to get outside that box. To grab its share of the teen and adult movie markets, for example, Disney produces films under the Touchstone, Hollywood Pictures, and Miramax labels. Likewise, Disney's biggest new international opportunity does not carry the Disney brand. Seeking to shore up its position in the fierce competition with the Cartoon Network and Nickelodeon, Disney recently spent $5.2 billion to buy the Fox Family Network from Rupert Murdoch. With 35 million viewers in Europe and Latin America, Fox Family has much greater penetration overseas than the Disney Channel. Its programming—edgier than Disney's, and thus in many ways more appealing to today's all-too-sophisticated kids—will be branded ABC Family, not Disney.

Even more critical to Disney's success abroad is its perfor- 39 mance in the US. After all, international customers are not going to be enamored of an American brand that's in decline at home. And Disney has had a tough few years. Network television is an increasingly difficult business as TV choices proliferate. The merchandising unit appears to be suffering from market saturation, and the company is closing about 100 of its roughly 750 Disney stores. Competitors are more powerful than ever, be they DreamWorks in animation or MGM/Universal in theme parks. The Internet business has been a fiasco—not only for Disney, to be sure, but it's been costly nonetheless. The current downturn in advertising and tourism will reverse itself eventually, but not before it takes a big bite out of profits. Eisner says the brand has never been stronger. But some analysts suggest that "age compression"—essentially kids growing up faster—poses a long-term threat.

Disney's challenges both at home and abroad illustrate just 40 how hard it is for even the biggest of American brands to keep growing—and give lie to many of the fears people have about cultural imperialism. Unlike other industries—oil, say, or agriculture, or even technology—culture businesses depend on giving people what they want, as opposed to what they need. It is true that the giant media conglomerates can sometimes suffocate competition and choice. But in television and theme parks in most of the world, there has never been much competition anyway, and in the sale of plush toys it is hardly an issue. For the most part, people will decide what elements of American culture they want. The Disneys of the world are slaves to the tastes of Chen Ping and Wei Qing Hua, not the other way around.

Globalization: The Super-Story

Thomas L. Friedman

1   I am a big believer in the idea of the super-story, the notion that we all carry around with us a big lens, a big framework, through which we look at the world, order events, and decide what is important and what is not. The events of 9/11 did not happen in a vacuum. They happened in the context of a new international system—a system that cannot explain everything but *can* explain and connect more things in more places on more days than anything else. That new international system is called globalization. It came together in the late 1980s and replaced the previous international system, the cold war system, which had reigned since the end of World War II. This new system is the lens, the super-story, through which I viewed the events of 9/11.

2   I define globalization as the inexorable integration of markets, transportation systems, and communication systems to a degree never witnessed before—in a way that is enabling corporations, countries, and individuals to reach around the world farther, faster, deeper, and cheaper than ever before, and in a way that is enabling the world to reach into corporations, countries, and individuals farther, faster, deeper, and cheaper than ever before.

3   Several important features of this globalization system differ from those of the cold war system in ways that are quite relevant for understanding the events of 9/11. I examined them in detail in my previous book, *The Lexus and the Olive Tree,* and want to simply highlight them here.

The cold war system was characterized by one overarching 4
feature—and that was *division*. That world was a divided-up,
chopped-up place, and whether you were a country or a company,
your threats and opportunities in the cold war system tended
to grow out of who you were divided from. Appropriately, this
cold war system was symbolized by a single word—*wall*, the
Berlin Wall.

The globalization system is different. It also has one overarch- 5
ing feature—and that is *integration*. The world has become an
increasingly interwoven place, and today, whether you are a company or a country, your threats and opportunities increasingly
derive from who you are connected to. This globalization system
is also characterized by a single word—*web*, the World Wide Web.
So in the broadest sense we have gone from an international system built around division and walls to a system increasingly built
around integration and webs. In the cold war we reached for the
hotline, which was a symbol that we were divided but at least
two people were in charge—the leaders of the United States and
the Soviet Union. In the globalization system we reach for the
Internet, which is a symbol that we are all connected and nobody
is quite in charge.

Everyone in the world is directly or indirectly affected by this 6
new system, but not everyone benefits from it, not by a long shot,
which is why the more it becomes diffused, the more it also produces a backlash by people who feel overwhelmed by it, homogenized by it, or unable to keep pace with its demands.

The other key difference between the cold war system and the 7
globalization system is how power is structured within them. The
cold war system was built primarily around nation-states. You
acted on the world in that system through your state. The cold
war was a drama of states confronting states, balancing states, and
aligning with states. And, as a system, the cold war was balanced
at the center by two superstates, two superpowers: The United
States and the Soviet Union.

The globalization system, by contrast, is built around three 8
balances, which overlap and affect one another. The first is the traditional balance of power between nation-states. In the globalization system, the United States is now the sole and dominant

superpower and all other nations are subordinate to it to one degree or another. The shifting balance of power between the United States and other states, or simply between other states, still very much matters for the stability of this system. And it can still explain a lot of the news you read on the front page of the paper, whether it is the news of China balancing Russia, Iran balancing Iraq, or India confronting Pakistan.

9   The second important power balance in the globalization system is between nation-states and global markets. These global markets are made up of millions of investors moving money around the world with the click of a mouse. I call them the Electronic Herd, and this herd gathers in key global financial centers—such as Wall Street, Hong Kong, London, and Frankfurt—which I call the Supermarkets. The attitudes and actions of the Electronic Herd and the Supermarkets can have a huge impact on nation-states today, even to the point of triggering the downfall of governments. Who ousted Suharto in Indonesia in 1998? It wasn't another state, it was the Supermarkets, by withdrawing their support for, and confidence in, the Indonesian economy. You also will not understand the front page of the newspaper today unless you bring the Supermarkets into your analysis. Because the United States can destroy you by dropping bombs, but the Supermarkets can destroy you by downgrading your bonds. In other words, the United States is the dominant player in maintaining the globalization game board, but it is hardly alone in influencing the moves on that game board.

10   The third balance that you have to pay attention to—the one that is really the newest of all and the most relevant to the events of 9/11—is the balance between individuals and nation-states. Because globalization has brought down many of the walls that limited the movement and reach of people, and because it has simultaneously wired the world into networks, it gives more power to *individuals* to influence both markets and nation-states than at any other time in history. Whether by enabling people to use the Internet to communicate instantly at almost no cost over vast distances, or by enabling them to use the Web to transfer money or obtain weapons designs that normally would have been controlled by states, or by enabling them to go into a hardware store now and buy a five-hundred-dollar global positioning device,

connected to a satellite, that can direct a hijacked airplane—globalization can be an incredible force-multiplier for individuals. Individuals can increasingly act on the world stage directly, unmediated by a state.

So you have today not only a superpower, not only Super- 11
markets, but also what I call "super-empowered individuals." Some of these super-empowered individuals are quite angry, some of them quite wonderful—but all of them are now able to act much more directly and much more powerfully on the world stage.

Osama bin Laden declared war on the United States in the 12
late 1990s. After he organized the bombing of two American embassies in Africa, the U.S. Air Force retaliated with a cruise missile attack on his bases in Afghanistan as though he were another nation-state. Think about that: on one day in 1998, the United States fired 75 cruise missiles at bin Laden. The United States fired 75 cruise missiles, at $1 million apiece, at a person! That was the first battle in history between a superpower and a super-empowered angry man. September 11 was just the second such battle.

Jody Williams won the Nobel Peace Prize in 1997 for help- 13
ing to build an international coalition to bring about a treaty outlawing land mines. Although nearly 120 governments endorsed the treaty, it was opposed by Russia, China, and the United States. When Jody Williams was asked, "How did you do that? How did you organize one thousand different citizens' groups and nongovernmental organizations on five continents to forge a treaty that was opposed by the major powers?" she had a very brief answer: "E-mail." Jody Williams used e-mail and the networked world to super-empower herself.

Nation-states, and the American superpower in particular, are 14
still hugely important today, but so too now are Supermarkets and super-empowered individuals. You will never understand the globalization system, or the front page of the morning paper—or 9/11—unless you see each as a complex interaction between all three of these actors: states bumping up against states, states bumping up against Supermarkets, and Supermarkets and states bumping up against super-empowered individuals—many of whom, unfortunately, are super-empowered angry men.

The Burka and the Bikini

Joan Jacobs Brumberg and Jacquelyn Jackson

1   The Female Body—covered in a burka or uncovered in a bikini—is a subtle subtext in the war against terrorism. The United States did not engage in this war to avenge women's rights in Afghanistan. However, our war against the Taliban, a regime that does not allow a woman to go to school, walk alone on a city street, or show her face in public, highlights the need to more fully understand the ways in which our own cultural "uncovering" of the female body impacts the lives of girls and women everywhere.

2   Taliban rule has dictated that women be fully covered when-ever they enter the public realm, while a recent U.S. television commercial for *Temptation Island 2* features near naked women. Although we seem to be winning the war against the Taliban, it is important to gain a better understanding of the Taliban's hatred of American culture and how women's behavior in our society is a particular locus of this hatred. The irony is that the images of sleek, bare women in our popular media that offend the Taliban also represent a major offensive against the health of American women and girls.

3   During the twentieth century, American culture has dictated a nearly complete uncovering of the female form. In Victorian America, good works were a measure of female character, while today good looks reign supreme. From the hair removal products that hit the marketplace in the 1920s to today's diet control mea-sures that seek to eliminate even healthy fat from the female form, American girls and women have been stripped bare by a sexually expressive culture whose beauty dictates have exerted a major toll on their physical and emotional health.

4   The unrealistic body images that we see and admire every day in the media are literally eating away at the female back-bone of our nation. A cursory look at women's magazines, pop-ular movies and television programs reveal a wide range of images modeling behaviors that directly assault the human skeleton. The ultra-thin woman pictured in a magazine sipping a martini or smoking a cigarette is a prime candidate for osteo-porosis later in life.

In fact, many behaviors made attractive by the popular media, 5
including eating disorders, teen smoking, drinking, and the
depression and anxiety disorders that can occur when one does
not measure up are taking a major toll on female health and well-
being. The American Medical Association last year acknowledged
a link between violent images on the screen and violent behavior
among children. In a world where eight-year-olds are on diets,
adult women spend $300 million a year to slice and laser their
bodies and legal pornography is a $56 billion industry, it is time
to note the dangers of unhealthy body images for girls and
women.

Now that the Taliban's horrific treatment of women is com- 6
mon knowledge, dieting and working out to wear a string bikini
might seem to be a patriotic act. The war on terrorism has certainly raised our awareness of the ways in which women's bodies are controlled by a repressive regime in a far away land, but
what about the constraints on women's bodies here at home, right
here in America?

In the name of good looks (and also corporate profits—the 7
Westernized image of the perfect body is one of our most successful exports) contemporary American women continue to engage in
behaviors that have created major public health concerns.

Although these problems may seem small in the face of the 8
threat of anthrax and other forms of bioterrorism, there is still a
need to better understand how American culture developed to the
point that it now threatens the health of its bikini-clad daughters
and their mothers.

Covered or uncovered, the homefront choice is not about moral- 9
ity but the physical and emotional health of future generations.

Whether it's the dark, sad eyes of a woman in purdah or the 10
anxious darkly circled eyes of a girl with anorexia nervosa, the
woman trapped inside needs to be liberated from cultural confines
in whatever form they take. The burka and the bikini represent
opposite ends of the political spectrum but each can exert a noose-
like grip on the psyche and physical health of girls and women.

Chapter

Security and Liberty: Are They Necessarily Opposed?

On Liberty

John Stuart Mill

1 The subject of this Essay is not the so-called Liberty of the Will, so unfortunately opposed to the misnamed doctrine of Philosophical Necessity; but Civil, or Social Liberty: the nature and limits of the power which can be legitimately exercised by society over the individual. A question seldom stated, and hardly ever discussed, in general terms, but which profoundly influences the practical controversies of the age by its latent presence, and is likely soon to make itself recognized as the vital question of the future. It is so far from being new, that, in a certain sense, it has divided mankind, almost from the remotest ages, but in the stage of progress into which the more civilized portions of the species have now entered, it presents itself under new conditions, and requires a different and more fundamental treatment.

2 The struggle between Liberty and Authority is the most conspicuous feature in the portions of history with which we are earliest familiar, particularly in that of Greece, Rome, and England. But in old times this contest was between subjects, or some classes of subjects, and the government. By liberty, was meant protection against the tyranny of the political rulers. The rulers were conceived (except in some of the popular governments of Greece) as

in a necessarily antagonistic position to the people whom they ruled. They consisted of a governing One, or a governing tribe or caste, who derived their authority from inheritance or conquest; who, at all events, did not hold it at the pleasure of the governed, and whose supremacy men did not venture, perhaps did not desire, to contest, whatever precautions might be taken against its oppressive exercise. Their power was regarded as necessary, but also as highly dangerous; as a weapon which they would attempt to use against their subjects, no less than against external enemies. To prevent the weaker members of the community from being preyed upon by innumerable vultures, it was needful that there should be an animal of prey stronger than the rest, commissioned to keep them down. But as the king of the vultures would be no less bent upon preying upon the flock than any of the minor harpies, it was indispensable to be in a perpetual attitude of defence against his beak and claws. The aim, therefore, of patriots, was to set limits to the power which the ruler should be suffered to exercise over the community; and this limitation was what they meant by liberty. It was attempted in two ways. First, by obtaining a recognition of certain immunities, called political liberties or rights, which it was to be regarded as a breach of duty in the ruler to infringe, and which, if he did infringe, specific resistance, or general rebellion, was held to be justifiable. A second, and generally a later expedient, was the establishment of constitutional checks; by which the consent of the community, or of a body of some sort supposed to represent its interests, was made a necessary condition to some of the more important acts of the governing power. To the first of these modes of limitation, the ruling power, in most European countries, was compelled, more or less, to submit. It was not so with the second; and to attain this, or when already in some degree possessed, to attain it more completely, became everywhere the principal object of the lovers of liberty. And so long as mankind were content to combat one enemy by another, and to be ruled by a master, on condition of being guaranteed more or less efficaciously against his tyranny, they did not carry their aspirations beyond this point.

A time, however, came in the progress of human affairs, when [3] men ceased to think it a necessity of nature that their governors should be an independent power, opposed in interest to themselves.

It appeared to them much better that the various magistrates of the State should be their tenants or delegates, revocable at their pleasure. In that way alone, it seemed, could they have complete security that the powers of government would never be abused to their disadvantage. By degrees, this new demand for elective and temporary rulers became the prominent object of the exertions of the popular party, wherever any such party existed; and superseded, to a considerable extent, the previous efforts to limit the power of rulers. As the struggle proceeded for making the ruling power emanate from the periodical choice of the ruled, some persons began to think that too much importance had been attached to the limitation of the power itself. That (it might seem) was a resource against rulers whose interests were habitually opposed to those of the people. What was now wanted was, that the rulers should be identified with the people; that their interest and will should be the interest and will of the nation. The nation did not need to be protected against its own will. There was no fear of its tyrannizing over itself. Let the rulers be effectually responsible to it, promptly removable by it, and it could afford to trust them with power of which it could itself dictate the use to be made. Their power was but the nation's own power, concentrated, and in a form convenient for exercise. This mode of thought, or rather perhaps of feeling, was common among the last generation of European liberalism, in the Continental section of which, it still apparently predominates. Those who admit any limit to what a government may do, except in the case of such governments as they think ought not to exist, stand out as brilliant exceptions among the political thinkers of the Continent. A similar tone of sentiment might by this time have been prevalent in our own country, if the circumstances which for a time encouraged it had continued unaltered.

4   But, in political and philosophical theories, as well as in persons, success discloses faults and infirmities which failure might have concealed from observation. The notion, that the people have no need to limit their power over themselves, might seem axiomatic, when popular government was a thing only dreamed about, or read of as having existed at some distant period of the past. Neither was that notion necessarily disturbed by such temporary aberrations as those of the French Revolution, the worst of

which were the work of an usurping few, and which, in any case, belonged, not to the permanent working of popular institutions, but to a sudden and convulsive outbreak against monarchical and aristocratic despotism. In time, however, a democratic republic came to occupy a large portion of the earth's surface, and made itself felt as one of the most powerful members of the community of nations; and elective and responsible government became subject to the observations and criticisms which wait upon a great existing fact. It was now perceived that such phrases as "self-government," and "the power of the people over themselves," do not express the true state of the case. The "people" who exercise the power, are not always the same people with those over whom it is exercised, and the "self-government" spoken of, is not the government of each by himself, but of each by all the rest. The will of the people, moreover, practically means, the will of the most numerous or the most active part of the people; the majority, or those who succeed in making themselves accepted as the majority; the people, consequently, may desire to oppress a part of their number; and precautions are as much needed against this, as against any other abuse of power. The limitation, therefore, of the power of government over individuals, loses none of its importance when the holders of power are regularly accountable to the community, that is, to the strongest party therein. This view of things, recommending itself equally to the intelligence of thinkers and to the inclination of those important classes in European society to whose real or supposed interests democracy is adverse, has had no difficulty in establishing itself; and in political speculations "the tyranny of the majority" is now generally included among the evils against which society requires to be on its guard.

Like other tyrannies, the tyranny of the majority was at first, 5 and is still vulgarly, held in dread, chiefly as operating through the acts of the public authorities. But reflecting persons perceived that when society is itself the tyrant—society collectively, over the separate individuals who compose it—its means of tyrannizing are not restricted to the acts which it may do by the hands of its political functionaries. Society can and does execute its own mandates: and if it issues wrong mandates instead of right, or any mandates at all in things with which it ought not to meddle, it practises a social tyranny more formidable than many kinds of political oppression, since, though not usually upheld by such extreme penalties, it leaves fewer means of escape, penetrating much more deeply into the details of life, and enslaving the soul itself. Protection, therefore, against the tyranny of the magistrate is not enough; there needs protection also against the tyranny of the prevailing opinion and feeling; against the tendency of society to impose, by other means than civil penalties, its own ideas and practices as rules of conduct on those who dissent from them; to fetter the development, and, if possible, prevent the formation, of any individuality not in harmony with its ways, and compel all characters to fashion themselves upon the model of its own. There is a limit to the legitimate interference of collective opinion with individual independence; and to find that limit, and maintain it against encroachment, is as indispensable to a good condition of human affairs, as protection against political despotism.

6   But though this proposition is not likely to be contested in general terms, the practical question, where to place the limit—how to make the fitting adjustment between individual independence and social control—is a subject on which nearly everything remains to be done. All that makes existence valuable to any one, depends on the enforcement of restraints upon the actions of other people. Some rules of conduct, therefore, must be imposed, by law in the first place, and by opinion on many things which are not fit subjects for the operation of law. What these rules should be, is the principal question in human affairs; but if we except a few of the most obvious cases, it is one of those which least progress has been made in resolving. No two ages, and scarcely any two countries, have decided it alike; and the decision of one age or country is a wonder to another. Yet the people of any given age and country no more suspect any difficulty in it, than if it were a subject on which mankind had always been agreed. The rules which obtain among themselves appear to them self-evident and self-justifying. This all but universal illusion is one of the examples of the magical influence of custom, which is not only, as the proverb says, a second nature, but is continually mistaken for the first. The effect of custom, in preventing any misgiving respecting the rules of conduct which mankind impose on one another, is all the more complete because the subject is one on which it is not

generally considered necessary that reasons should be given, either by one person to others, or by each to himself. People are accustomed to believe and have been encouraged in the belief by some who aspire to the character of philosophers, that their feelings, on subjects of this nature, are better than reasons, and render reasons unnecessary. The practical principle which guides them to their opinions on the regulation of human conduct, is the feeling in each person's mind that everybody should be required to act as he, and those with whom he sympathizes, would like them to act. No one, indeed, acknowledges to himself that his standard of judgment is his own liking; but an opinion on a point of conduct, not supported by reasons, can only count as one person's preference; and if the reasons, when given, are a mere appeal to a similar preference felt by other people, it is still only many people's liking instead of one. To an ordinary man, however, his own preference, thus supported, is not only a perfectly satisfactory reason, but the only one he generally has for any of his notions of morality, taste, or propriety, which are not expressly written in his religious creed; and his chief guide in the interpretation even of that. Men's opinions, accordingly, on what is laudable or blamable, are affected by all the multifarious causes which influence their wishes in regard to the conduct of others, and which are as numerous as those which determine their wishes on any other subject. Sometimes their reason—at other times their prejudices or superstitions: often their social affections, not seldom their anti-social ones, their envy or jealousy, their arrogance or contemptuousness: but most commonly, their desires or fears for themselves—their legitimate or illegitimate self-interest. Wherever there is an ascendant class, a large portion of the morality of the country emanates from its class interests, and its feelings of class superiority. The morality between Spartans and Helots, between planters and negroes, between princes and subjects, between nobles and roturiers, between men and women, has been for the most part the creation of these class interests and feelings: and the sentiments thus generated, react in turn upon the moral feelings of the members of the ascendant class, in their relations among themselves. Where, on the other hand, a class, formerly ascendant, has lost its ascendency, or where its ascendency is unpopular, the prevailing moral sentiments frequently bear the impress of an impatient dislike of superiority. Another grand determining principle of the rules of conduct, both in act and forbearance which have been enforced by law or opinion, has been the servility of mankind towards the supposed preferences or aversions of their temporal masters, or of their gods. This servility though essentially selfish, is not hypocrisy; it gives rise to perfectly genuine sentiments of abhorrence; it made men burn magicians and heretics. Among so many baser influences, the general and obvious interests of society have of course had a share, and a large one, in the direction of the moral sentiments: less, however, as a matter of reason, and on their own account, than as a consequence of the sympathies and antipathies which grew out of them: and sympathies and antipathies which had little or nothing to do with the interests of society, have made themselves felt in the establishment of moralities with quite as great force.

7   The likings and dislikings of society, or of some powerful portion of it, are thus the main thing which has practically determined the rules laid down for general observance, under the penalties of law or opinion. And in general, those who have been in advance of society in thought and feeling, have left this condition of things unassailed in principle, however they may have come into conflict with it in some of its details. They have occupied themselves rather in inquiring what things society ought to like or dislike, than in questioning whether its likings or dislikings should be a law to individuals. They preferred endeavouring to alter the feelings of mankind on the particular points on which they were themselves heretical, rather than make common cause in defence of freedom, with heretics generally. The only case in which the higher ground has been taken on principle and maintained with consistency, by any but an individual here and there, is that of religious belief: a case instructive in many ways, and not least so as forming a most striking instance of the fallibility of what is called the moral sense: for the odium theologicum, in a sincere bigot, is one of the most unequivocal cases of moral feeling. Those who first broke the yoke of what called itself the Universal Church, were in general as little willing to permit difference of religious opinion as that church itself. But when the heat of the conflict was over, without giving a complete victory to any party, and each church or sect was reduced to limit its hopes to retaining

possession of the ground it already occupied; minorities, seeing that they had no chance of becoming majorities, were under the necessity of pleading to those whom they could not convert, for permission to differ. It is accordingly on this battle-field, almost solely, that the rights of the individual against society have been asserted on broad grounds of principle, and the claim of society to exercise authority over dissentients openly controverted. The great writers to whom the world owes what religious liberty it possesses, have mostly asserted freedom of conscience as an indefeasible right, and denied absolutely that a human being is accountable to others for his religious belief. Yet so natural to mankind is intolerance in whatever they really care about, that religious freedom has hardly anywhere been practically realized, except where religious indifference, which dislikes to have its peace disturbed by theological quarrels, has added its weight to the scale. In the minds of almost all religious persons, even in the most tolerant countries, the duty of toleration is admitted with tacit reserves. One person will bear with dissent in matters of church government, but not of dogma; another can tolerate everybody, short of a Papist or an Unitarian; another, every one who believes in revealed religion; a few extend their charity a little further, but stop at the belief in a God and in a future state. Wherever the sentiment of the majority is still genuine and intense, it is found to have abated little of its claim to be obeyed.

In England, from the peculiar circumstances of our political 8 history, though the yoke of opinion is perhaps heavier, that of law is lighter, than in most other countries of Europe; and there is considerable jealousy of direct interference, by the legislative or the executive power with private conduct; not so much from any just regard for the independence of the individual, as from the still subsisting habit of looking on the government as representing an opposite interest to the public. The majority have not yet learnt to feel the power of the government their power, or its opinions their opinions. When they do so, individual liberty will probably be as much exposed to invasion from the government, as it already is from public opinion. But, as yet, there is a considerable amount of feeling ready to be called forth against any attempt of the law to control individuals in things in which they have not hitherto been accustomed to be controlled by it; and this with very little discrimination as to whether the matter is, or is not, within the legitimate sphere of legal control; insomuch that the feeling, highly salutary on the whole, is perhaps quite as often misplaced as well grounded in the particular instances of its application.

9   There is, in fact, no recognized principle by which the propriety or impropriety of government interference is customarily tested. People decide according to their personal preferences. Some, whenever they see any good to be done, or evil to be remedied, would willingly instigate the government to undertake the business; while others prefer to bear almost any amount of social evil, rather than add one to the departments of human interests amenable to governmental control. And men range themselves on one or the other side in any particular case, according to this general direction of their sentiments; or according to the degree of interest which they feel in the particular thing which it is proposed that the government should do; or according to the belief they entertain that the government would, or would not, do it in the manner they prefer; but very rarely on account of any opinion to which they consistently adhere, as to what things are fit to be done by a government. And it seems to me that, in consequence of this absence of rule or principle, one side is at present as often wrong as the other; the interference of government is, with about equal frequency, improperly invoked and improperly condemned.

10   The object of this Essay is to assert one very simple principle, as entitled to govern absolutely the dealings of society with the individual in the way of compulsion and control, whether the means used be physical force in the form of legal penalties, or the moral coercion of public opinion. That principle is, that the sole end for which mankind are warranted, individually or collectively in interfering with the liberty of action of any of their number, is self-protection. That the only purpose for which power can be rightfully exercised over any member of a civilized community, against his will, is to prevent harm to others. His own good, either physical or moral, is not a sufficient warrant. He cannot rightfully be compelled to do or forbear because it will be better for him to do so, because it will make him happier, because, in the opinions of others, to do so would be wise,

or even right. These are good reasons for remonstrating with him, or reasoning with him, or persuading him, or entreating him, but not for compelling him, or visiting him with any evil, in case he do otherwise. To justify that, the conduct from which it is desired to deter him must be calculated to produce evil to some one else. The only part of the conduct of any one, for which he is amenable to society, is that which concerns others. In the part which merely concerns himself, his independence is, of right, absolute. Over himself, over his own body and mind, the individual is sovereign.

It is, perhaps, hardly necessary to say that this doctrine is 11 meant to apply only to human beings in the maturity of their faculties. We are not speaking of children, or of young persons below the age which the law may fix as that of manhood or womanhood. Those who are still in a state to require being taken care of by others, must be protected against their own actions as well as against external injury. For the same reason, we may leave out of consideration those backward states of society in which the race itself may be considered as in its nonage. The early difficulties in the way of spontaneous progress are so great, that there is seldom any choice of means for overcoming them; and a ruler full of the spirit of improvement is warranted in the use of any expedients that will attain an end, perhaps otherwise unattainable. Despotism is a legitimate mode of government in dealing with barbarians, provided the end be their improvement, and the means justified by actually effecting that end. Liberty, as a principle, has no application to any state of things anterior to the time when mankind have become capable of being improved by free and equal discussion. Until then, there is nothing for them but implicit obedience to an Akbar or a Charlemagne, if they are so fortunate as to find one. But as soon as mankind have attained the capacity of being guided to their own improvement by conviction or persuasion (a period long since reached in all nations with whom we need here concern ourselves), compulsion, either in the direct form or in that of pains and penalties for non-compliance, is no longer admissible as a means to their own good, and justifiable only for the security of others.

It is proper to state that I forego any advantage which could 12 be derived to my argument from the idea of abstract right as a thing independent of utility. I regard utility as the ultimate appeal on all ethical questions; but it must be utility in the largest sense, grounded on the permanent interests of man as a progressive being. Those interests, I contend, authorize the subjection of individual spontaneity to external control, only in respect to those actions of each, which concern the interest of other people. If any one does an act hurtful to others, there is a prima facie case for punishing him, by law, or, where legal penalties are not safely applicable, by general disapprobation. There are also many positive acts for the benefit of others, which he may rightfully be compelled to perform; such as, to give evidence in a court of justice; to bear his fair share in the common defence, or in any other joint work necessary to the interest of the society of which he enjoys the protection; and to perform certain acts of individual beneficence, such as saving a fellow-creature's life, or interposing to protect the defenceless against ill-usage, things which whenever it is obviously a man's duty to do, he may rightfully be made responsible to society for not doing. A person may cause evil to others not only by his actions but by his inaction, and in neither case he is justly accountable to them for the injury. The latter case, it is true, requires a much more cautious exercise of compulsion than the former. To make any one answerable for doing evil to others, is the rule; to make him answerable for not preventing evil, is, comparatively speaking, the exception. Yet there are many cases clear enough and grave enough to justify that exception. In all things which regard the external relations of the individual, he is *de jure* amenable to those whose interests are concerned, and if need be, to society as their protector. There are often good reasons for not holding him to the responsibility; but these reasons must arise from the special expediencies of the case: either because it is a kind of case in which he is on the whole likely to act better, when left to his own discretion, than when controlled in any way in which society have it in their power to control him; or because the attempt to exercise control would produce other evils, greater than those which it would prevent. When such reasons as these preclude the enforcement of responsibility, the conscience of the agent himself should step into the vacant judgment-seat, and protect those interests of others which have no external protection; judging himself all the more rigidly, because the case does not admit of his being made accountable to the judgment of his fellow-creatures.

But there is a sphere of action in which society, as distin- 13
guished from the individual, has, if any, only an indirect interest; comprehending all that portion of a person's life and
conduct which affects only himself, or, if it also affects others,
only with their free, voluntary, and undeceived consent and participation. When I say only himself, I mean directly, and in the
first instance: for whatever affects himself, may affect others
through himself; and the objection which may be grounded on
this contingency, will receive consideration in the sequel. This,
then, is the appropriate region of human liberty. It comprises,
first, the inward domain of consciousness; demanding liberty of
conscience, in the most comprehensive sense; liberty of thought
and feeling; absolute freedom of opinion and sentiment on all
subjects, practical or speculative, scientific, moral, or theological.
The liberty of expressing and publishing opinions may seem to
fall under a different principle, since it belongs to that part of
the conduct of an individual which concerns other people; but,
being almost of as much importance as the liberty of thought
itself, and resting in great part on the same reasons, is practically inseparable from it. Secondly, the principle requires liberty
of tastes and pursuits; of framing the plan of our life to suit our
own character; of doing as we like, subject to such consequences
as may follow; without impediment from our fellow-creatures,
so long as what we do does not harm them even though they
should think our conduct foolish, perverse, or wrong. Thirdly,
from this liberty of each individual, follows the liberty, within
the same limits, of combination among individuals; freedom to
unite, for any purpose not involving harm to others: the persons
combining being supposed to be of full age, and not forced or
deceived.

No society in which these liberties are not, on the whole, 14
respected, is free, whatever may be its form of government; and
none is completely free in which they do not exist absolute and
unqualified. The only freedom which deserves the name, is that
of pursuing our own good in our own way, so long as we do not
attempt to deprive others of theirs, or impede their efforts to
obtain it. Each is the proper guardian of his own health, whether

bodily, or mental or spiritual. Mankind are greater gainers by suffering each other to live as seems good to themselves, than by compelling each to live as seems good to the rest.

15 Though this doctrine is anything but new, and, to some persons, may have the air of a truism, there is no doctrine which stands more directly opposed to the general tendency of existing opinion and practice. Society has expended fully as much effort in the attempt (according to its lights) to compel people to conform to its notions of personal, as of social excellence. The ancient commonwealths thought themselves entitled to practise, and the ancient philosophers countenanced, the regulation of every part of private conduct by public authority, on the ground that the State had a deep interest in the whole bodily and mental discipline of every one of its citizens, a mode of thinking which may have been admissible in small republics surrounded by powerful enemies, in constant peril of being subverted by foreign attack or internal commotion, and to which even a short interval of relaxed energy and self-command might so easily be fatal, that they could not afford to wait for the salutary permanent effects of freedom. In the modern world, the greater size of political communities, and above all, the separation between the spiritual and temporal authority (which placed the direction of men's consciences in other hands than those which controlled their worldly affairs), prevented so great an interference by law in the details of private life; but the engines of moral repression have been wielded more strenuously against divergence from the reigning opinion in self-regarding, than even in social matters; religion, the most powerful of the elements which have entered into the formation of moral feeling, having almost always been governed either by the ambition of a hierarchy, seeking control over every department of human conduct, or by the spirit of Puritanism. And some of those modern reformers who have placed themselves in strongest opposition to the religions of the past, have been nowhere behind either churches or sects in their assertion of the right of spiritual domination: M. Compte, in particular, whose social system, as unfolded in his *Trait de Politique Positive,* aims at establishing (though by moral more than by legal appliances) a despotism of society over the individual, surpassing anything contemplated in

the political ideal of the most rigid disciplinarian among the ancient philosophers.

Apart from the peculiar tenets of individual thinkers, there is 16 also in the world at large an increasing inclination to stretch unduly the powers of society over the individual, both by the force of opinion and even by that of legislation: and as the tendency of all the changes taking place in the world is to strengthen society, and diminish the power of the individual, this encroachment is not one of the evils which tend spontaneously to disappear, but, on the contrary, to grow more and more formidable. The disposition of mankind, whether as rulers or as fellow-citizens, to impose their own opinions and inclinations as a rule of conduct on others, is so energetically supported by some of the best and by some of the worst feelings incident to human nature, that it is hardly ever kept under restraint by anything but want of power; and as the power is not declining, but growing, unless a strong barrier of moral conviction can be raised against the mischief, we must expect, in the present circumstances of the world, to see it increase.

It will be convenient for the argument, if, instead of at once 17 entering upon the general thesis, we confine ourselves in the first instance to a single branch of it, on which the principle here stated is, if not fully, yet to a certain point, recognized by the current opinions. This one branch is the Liberty of Thought: from which it is impossible to separate the cognate liberty of speaking and of writing. Although these liberties, to some considerable amount, form part of the political morality of all countries which profess religious toleration and free institutions, the grounds, both philosophical and practical, on which they rest, are perhaps not so familiar to the general mind, nor so thoroughly appreciated by many even of the leaders of opinion, as might have been expected. Those grounds, when rightly understood, are of much wider application than to only one division of the subject, and a thorough consideration of this part of the question will be found the best introduction to the remainder. Those to whom nothing which I am about to say will be new, may therefore, I hope, excuse me, if on a subject which for now three centuries has been so often discussed, I venture on one discussion more.

The Declaration of Independence

Thomas Jefferson

In Congress, July 4, 1776
The Unanimous Declaration of the
Thirteen United States of America

1   When in the Course of human events it becomes necessary for one people to dissolve the political bands which have connected them with another, and to assume among the powers of the earth, the separate and equal station to which the Laws of Nature and of Nature's God entitle them, a decent respect to the opinions of mankind requires that they should declare the causes which impel them to the separation.

2   We hold these truths to be self-evident, that all men are created equal, that they are endowed by their Creator with certain unalienable Rights, that among these are Life, Liberty and the pursuit of Happiness. That to secure these rights, Governments are instituted among Men, deriving their just powers from the consent of the governed. That whenever any Form of Government becomes destructive of these ends, it is the Right of the People to alter or to abolish it, and to institute new Government, laying its foundation on such principles and organizing its powers in such form, as to them shall seem most likely to affect their Safety and Happiness. Prudence, indeed, will dictate that Governments long established should not be changed for light and transient causes; and accordingly all experience hath shewn that mankind are more disposed to suffer, while evils are sufferable, than to right themselves by abolishing the forms to which they are accustomed. But when a long train of abuses and usurpations, pursuing invariably the same Object evinces a design to reduce them under absolute Despotism, it is their right, it is their duty, to throw off such Government, and to provide new Guards for their future security. Such has been the patient sufferance of these Colonies; and such is now the necessity which constrains them to alter their former Systems of Government. The history of the present King of Great Britain is a history of repeated injuries and usurpations, all having in direct object the establishment of an absolute

Tyranny over these States. To prove this, let Facts be submitted to a candid world.

He has refused his Assent to Laws, the most wholesome and 3 necessary for the public good.

He has forbidden his Governors to pass laws of immediate 4 and pressing importance, unless suspended in their operation till his Assent should be obtained; and when so suspended, he has utterly neglected to attend to them.

He has refused to pass other Laws for the accommodation of 5 large districts of people, unless those people would relinquish the right of Representation in the Legislature, a right inestimable to them and formidable to tyrants only.

He has called together legislative bodies at places unusual, 6 uncomfortable, and distant from the depository of their Public Records, for the sole purpose of fatiguing them into compliance with his measures.

He has dissolved Representative Houses repeatedly, for oppos- 7 ing with manly firmness his invasions on the rights of the people.

He has refused for a long time, after such dissolutions, to 8 cause others to be elected; whereby the Legislative Powers, inca- pable of Annihilation, have returned to the People at large for their exercise; the State remaining in the mean time exposed to all the dangers of invasion from without, and convulsions within.

He has endeavored to prevent the population of these States; 9 for that purpose obstructing the Laws for Naturalization of For- eigners; refusing to pass others to encourage their migration hither, and raising the conditions of new Appropriations of Lands.

He has obstructed the Administration of Justice, by refusing 10 his Assent to Laws for Establishing Judiciary Powers.

He has made judges dependent on his Will alone, for the tenure 11 of their offices, and the amount and payment of their salaries.

He has erected a multitude of New Offices, and sent hither 12 swarms of Officers to harass our people, and eat out their substance.

He has kept among us, in times of peace, Standing Armies 13 without the Consent of our legislatures.

He has affected to render the Military independent of and 14 superior to the Civil Power.

He has combined with others to subject us to a jurisdiction 15 foreign to our constitution, and unacknowledged by our laws;

giving his Assent to the Acts of pretended Legislation: For quartering large bodies of armed troops among us: For protecting them, by a mock Trial, from punishment for any Murders which they should commit on the Inhabitants of these States: For cutting off our Trade with all parts of the world: For imposing Taxes on us without our Consent: For depriving us in many cases, of the benefits of Trial by Jury: For Transporting us beyond Seas to be tried for pretended offenses: For abolishing the free System of English Laws in a neighboring Province, establishing therein an Arbitrary government, and enlarging its Boundaries so as to render it at once an example and fit instrument for introducing the same absolute rule into these Colonies: For taking away our Charters, abolishing our most valuable Laws and altering fundamentally the Forms of our Governments: For suspending our own Legislatures, and declaring themselves invested with power to legislate for us in all cases whatsoever.

16   He has abdicated Government here, by declaring us out of his Protection and waging War against us.

17   He has plundered our seas, ravaged our Coasts, burnt our towns, and destroyed the lives of our people.

18   He is at this time transporting large Armies of foreign Mercenaries to complete the works of death, desolation and tyranny, already begun with circumstances of Cruelty & Perfidy scarcely paralleled in the most barbarous ages, and totally unworthy the Head of a civilized nation.

19   He has constrained our fellow Citizens taken Captive on the high Seas to bear Arms against their Country, to become the executioners of their friends and Brethren, or to fall themselves by their Hands.

20   He has excited domestic insurrections amongst us, and has endeavored to bring on the inhabitants of our frontiers, the merciless Indian Savages, whose known rule of warfare is an undistinguished destruction of all ages, sexes, and conditions.

21   In every stage of these Oppressions We have Petitioned for Redress in the most humble terms: Our repeated petitions have been answered only by repeated injury. A Prince, whose character is thus marked by every act which may define a Tyrant, is unfit to be the ruler of a free people.

Nor have we been wanting in attention to our British 22 brethren. We have warned them from time to time of attempts by their legislature to extend an unwarrantable jurisdiction over us. We have reminded them of the circumstances of our emigration and settlement here. We have appealed to their native justice and magnanimity, and we have conjured them by the ties of our common kindred to disavow these usurpations, which would inevitably interrupt our connections and correspondence. They too have been deaf to the voice of justice and of consanguinity. We must, therefore, acquiesce in the necessity, which denounces our Separation, and hold them, as we hold the rest of mankind, Enemies in War, in Peace Friends.

We, THEREFORE, the Representatives of the UNITED 23 STATES OF AMERICA, in General Congress, Assembled, appealing to the Supreme Judge of the world for the rectitude of our intentions, do, in the Name, and by Authority of the good People of these Colonies, solemnly publish and declare, That these United Colonies are, and of Right ought to be FREE AND INDEPENDENT STATES: that they are Absolved from all Allegiance to the British Crown, and that all political connection between them and the State of Great Britain, is and ought to be totally dissolved; and that as Free and Independent States; they have full Power to levy War, conclude Peace, contract Alliances, establish Commerce, and to do all the Acts and Things which Independent States may of right do. And for the support of this Declaration, with a firm reliance on the protection of Divine Providence, we mutually pledge to each other our Lives, our Fortunes, and our sacred Honor.

Patriotism: A Menace to Liberty

Emma Goldman

What is patriotism? Is it love of one's birthplace, the place of 1 childhood's recollections and hopes, dreams and aspirations? Is it the place where, in childlike naiveté, we would watch the fleeting clouds, and wonder why we, too, could not run so swiftly? The place where we would count the milliard glittering stars, terror-stricken lest each one "an eye should be," piercing the very depths of our little souls? Is it the place where we would listen to the music of the birds, and long to have wings to fly, even as they, to distant lands? Or the place where we would sit at mother's knee, enraptured by wonderful tales of great deeds and conquests? In short, is it love for the spot, every inch representing dear and precious recollections of a happy, joyous, and playful childhood?

2   If that were patriotism, few American men of today could be called upon to be patriotic, since the place of play has been turned into factory, mill, and mine, while deafening sounds of machinery have replaced the music of the birds. Nor can we longer hear the tales of great deeds, for the stories our mothers tell today are but those of sorrow, tears, and grief.

3   What, then, is patriotism? "Patriotism, sir, is the last resort of scoundrels," said Dr. Johnson. Leo Tolstoy, the greatest anti-patriot of our times, defines patriotism as the principle that will justify the training of wholesale murderers; a trade that requires better equipment for the exercise of man-killing than the making of such necessities of life as shoes, clothing, and houses; a trade that guarantees better returns and greater glory than that of the average workingman.

4   Gustave Hervé, another great anti-patriot, justly calls patriotism a superstition—one far more injurious, brutal, and inhumane than religion. The superstition of religion originated in man's inability to explain natural phenomena. That is, when primitive man heard thunder or saw the lightning, he could not account for either, and therefore concluded that back of them must be a force greater than himself. Similarly he saw a supernatural force in the rain, and in the various other changes in nature. Patriotism, on the other hand, is a superstition artificially created and maintained through a network of lies and falsehoods; a superstition that robs man of his self-respect and dignity, and increases his arrogance and conceit.

5   Indeed, conceit, arrogance, and egotism are the essentials of patriotism. Let me illustrate. Patriotism assumes that our globe is divided into little spots, each one surrounded by an iron gate. Those who have had the fortune of being born on some particular spot, consider themselves better, nobler, grander, more intelligent

than the living beings inhabiting any other spot. It is, therefore, the duty of everyone living on that chosen spot to fight, kill, and die in the attempt to impose his superiority upon all the others.

The inhabitants of the other spots reason in like manner, of 6 course, with the result that, from early infancy, the mind of the child is poisoned with bloodcurdling stories about the Germans, the French, the Italians, Russians, etc. When the child has reached manhood, he is thoroughly saturated with the belief that he is chosen by the Lord himself to defend his country against the attack or invasion of any foreigner. It is for that purpose that we are clamoring for a greater army and navy, more battleships and ammunition. It is for that purpose that America has within a short time spent four hundred million dollars. Just think of it—four hundred million dollars taken from the produce of the people. For surely it is not the rich who contribute to patriotism. They are cosmopolitans, perfectly at home in every land. We in America know well the truth of this. Are not our rich Americans Frenchmen in France, Germans in Germany, or Englishmen in England? And do they not squander with cosmopolitan grace fortunes coined by American factory children and cotton slaves? Yes, theirs is the patriotism that will make it possible to send messages of condolence to a despot like the Russian Tsar, when any mishap befalls him, as President Roosevelt did in the name of his people, when Sergius was punished by the Russian revolutionists.

It is a patriotism that will assist the arch-murderer, Diaz, in 7 destroying thousands of lives in Mexico, or that will even aid in arresting Mexican revolutionists on American soil and keep them incarcerated in American prisons, without the slightest cause or reason.

But, then, patriotism is not for those who represent wealth 8 and power. It is good enough for the people. It reminds one of the historic wisdom of Frederick the Great, the bosom friend of Voltaire, who said: "Religion is a fraud, but it must be maintained for the masses."

That patriotism is rather a costly institution, no one will doubt 9 after considering the following statistics. The progressive increase of the expenditures for the leading armies and navies of the world during the last quarter of a century is a fact of such gravity as to startle every thoughtful student of economic problems. It may be briefly indicated by dividing the time from 1881 to 1905 into five-year periods, and noting the disbursements of several great nations for army and navy purposes during the first and last of those periods. From the first to the last of the periods noted the expenditures of Great Britain increased from $2,101,848,936 to $4,143,226,885, those of France from $3,324,500,000 to $3,455,109,900, those of Germany from $725,000,200 to $2,700,375,600, those of the United States from $1,275,500,750 to $2,650,900,450, those of Russia from $1,900,975,500 to $5,250,445,100, those of Italy from $1,600,975,750 to $1,755,500,100, and those of Japan from $182,900,500 to $700,925,475.

10   It is in connection with this rough estimate of cost per capita that the economic burden of militarism is most appreciable. The irresistible conclusion from available data is that the increase of expenditure for army and navy purposes is rapidly surpassing the growth of population in each of the countries considered in the present calculation. In other words, a continuation of the increased demands of militarism threatens each of those nations with a progressive exhaustion both of men and resources.

11   The awful waste that patriotism necessitates ought to be sufficient to cure the man of even average intelligence from this disease. Yet patriotism demands still more. The people are urged to be patriotic and for that luxury they pay, not only by supporting their "defenders," but even by sacrificing their own children. Patriotism requires allegiance to the flag, which means obedience and readiness to kill father, mother, brother, sister.

12   The usual contention is that we need a standing army to protect the country from foreign invasion. Every intelligent man and woman knows, however, that this is a myth maintained to frighten and coerce the foolish. The governments of the world, knowing each other's interests, do not invade each other. They have learned that they can gain much more by international arbitration of disputes than by war and conquest. Indeed, as Carlyle said, "War is a quarrel between two thieves too cowardly to fight their own battle; therefore they take boys from one village and another village, stick them into uniforms, equip them with guns, and let them loose like wild beasts against each other."

13   It does not require much wisdom to trace every war back to a similar cause. Let us take our own Spanish-American war,

supposedly a great and patriotic event in the history of the United States. How our hearts burned with indignation against the atrocious Spaniards! True, our indignation did not flare up spontaneously. It was nurtured by months of newspaper agitation, and long after Butcher Weyler had killed off many noble Cubans and outraged many Cuban women. Still, in justice to the American Nation be it said, it did grow indignant and was willing to fight, and that it fought bravely. But when the smoke was over, the dead buried, and the cost of the war came back to the people in an increase in the price of commodities and rent—that is, when we sobered up from our patriotic spree it suddenly dawned on us that the cause of the Spanish-American War was the consideration of the price of sugar; or, to be more explicit, that the lives, blood, and money of the American people were used to protect the interests of American capitalists, which were threatened by the Spanish government. That this is not an exaggeration, but is based on absolute facts and figures, is best proven by the attitude of the American government to Cuban labor. When Cuba was firmly in the clutches of the United States, the very soldiers sent to liberate Cuba were ordered to shoot Cuban workingmen during the great cigar-makers' strike, which took place shortly after the war.

Nor do we stand alone in waging war for such causes. The 14 curtain is beginning to be lifted on the motives of the terrible Russo-Japanese War, which cost so much blood and tears. And we see again that back of the fierce Moloch of war stands the still fiercer god of Commercialism. Kuropatkin, the Russian Minister of War during the Russo-Japanese struggle, has revealed the true secret behind the latter. The Tsar and his Grand Dukes, having invested money in Korean concessions, the war was forced for the sole purpose of speedily accumulating large fortunes.

The contention that a standing army and navy is the best 15 security of peace is about as logical as the claim that the most peaceful citizen is he who goes about heavily armed. The experience of every-day life fully proves that the armed individual is invariably anxious to try his strength. The same is historically true of governments. Really peaceful countries do not waste life and energy in war preparations, With the result that peace is maintained.

16   However, the clamor for an increased army and navy is not due to any foreign danger. It is owing to the dread of the growing discontent of the masses and of the international spirit among the workers. It is to meet the internal enemy that the powers of various countries are preparing themselves; an enemy, who, once awakened to consciousness, will prove more dangerous than any foreign invader.

17   The powers that have for centuries been engaged in enslaving the masses have made a thorough study of their psychology. They know that the people at large are like children whose despair, sorrow, and tears can be turned into joy with a little toy. And the more gorgeously the toy is dressed, the louder the colors, the more it will appeal to the million-headed child.

18   An army and navy represents the people's toys. To make them more attractive and acceptable, hundreds and thousands of dollars are being spent for the display of these toys. That was the purpose of the American government in equipping a fleet and sending it along the Pacific coast, that every American citizen should be made to feel the pride and glory of the United States. The city of San Francisco spent one hundred thousand dollars for the entertainment of the fleet; Los Angeles, sixty thousand; Seattle and Tacoma, about one hundred thousand. To entertain the fleet, did I say? To dine and wine a few superior officers, while the "brave boys" had to mutiny to get sufficient food. Yes, two hundred and sixty thousand dollars were spent on fireworks, theatre parties, and revelries, at a time when men, women, and children through the breadth and length of the country were starving in the streets; when thousands of unemployed were ready to sell their labor at any price.

19   Two hundred and sixty thousand dollars! What could not have been accomplished with such an enormous sum? But instead of bread and shelter, the children of those cities were taken to see the fleet, that it may remain, as one of the newspapers said, "a lasting memory for the child."

20   A wonderful thing to remember, is it not? The implements of civilized slaughter. If the mind of the child is to be poisoned with such memories, what hope is there for a true realization of human brotherhood?

We Americans claim to be a peace-loving people. We hate 21
bloodshed; we are opposed to violence. Yet we go into spasms of
joy over the possibility of projecting dynamite bombs from flying
machines upon helpless citizens. We are ready to hang, electro-
cute, or lynch anyone, who, from economic necessity, will risk his
own life in the attempt upon that of some industrial magnate. Yet
our hearts swell with pride at the thought that America is becoming the most powerful nation on earth, and that it will eventually
plant her iron foot on the necks of all other nations.

Such is the logic of patriotism. 22

Considering the evil results that patriotism is fraught with for 23
the average man, it is as nothing compared with the insult and
injury that patriotism heaps upon the soldier himself,—that poor,
deluded victim of superstition and ignorance. He, the savior of his
country, the protector of his nation,—what has patriotism in store
for him? A life of slavish submission, vice, and perversion, during
peace; a life of danger, exposure, and death, during war.

While on a recent lecture tour in San Francisco, I visited the 24
Presidio, the most beautiful spot overlooking the Bay and Golden
Gate Park. Its purpose should have been playgrounds for children, gardens and music for the recreation of the weary. Instead
it is made ugly, dull, and gray by barracks,—barracks wherein the
rich would not allow their dogs to dwell. In these miserable
shanties soldiers are herded like cattle; here they waste their
young days, polishing the boots and brass buttons of their superior officers. Here, too, I saw the distinction of classes: sturdy sons
of a free Republic, drawn up in line like convicts, saluting every
passing shrimp of a lieutenant. American equality, degrading
manhood and elevating the uniform!

Barrack life further tends to develop tendencies of sexual per- 25
version. It is gradually producing along this line results similar to
European military conditions. Havelock Ellis, the noted writer on
sex psychology, has made a thorough study of the subject. I quote:
"Some of the barracks are great centers of male prostitution. . . .
The number of soldiers who prostitute themselves is greater than
we are willing to believe. It is no exaggeration to say that in certain regiments the presumption is in favor of the venality of the
majority of the men. . . . On summer evenings Hyde Park and the

neighborhood of Albert Gate are full of guardsmen and others plying a lively trade, and with little disguise, in uniform or out. . . . In most cases the proceeds form a comfortable addition to Tommy Atkins' pocket money."

26   To what extent this perversion has eaten its way into the army and navy can best be judged from the fact that special houses exist for this form of prostitution. The practice is not limited to England; it is universal. "Soldiers are no less sought after in France than in England or in Germany, and special houses for military prostitution exist both in Paris and the garrison towns."

27   Had Mr. Havelock Ellis included America in his investigation of sex perversion, he would have found that the same conditions prevail in our army and navy as in those of other countries. The growth of the standing army inevitably adds to the spread of sex perversion; the barracks are the incubators.

28   Aside from the sexual effects of barrack life, it also tends to unfit the soldier for useful labor after leaving the army. Men, skilled in a trade, seldom enter the army or navy, but even they, after a military experience, find themselves totally unfitted for their former occupations. Having acquired habits of idleness and a taste for excitement and adventure, no peaceful pursuit can content them. Released from the army, they can turn to no useful work. But it is usually the social riff-raff, discharged prisoners and the like, whom either the struggle for life or their own inclination drives into the ranks. These, their military term over, again turn to their former life of crime, more brutalized and degraded than before. It is a well-known fact that in our prisons there is a goodly number of ex-soldiers; while, on the other hand, the army and navy are to a great extent plied with ex-convicts.

29   Of all the evil results I have just described none seems to me so detrimental to human integrity as the spirit patriotism has produced in the case of Private William Buwalda. Because he foolishly believed that one can be a soldier and exercise his rights as a man at the same time, the military authorities punished him severely. True, he had served his country fifteen years, during which time his record was unimpeachable. According to Gen. Funston, who reduced Buwalda's sentence to three years, "the first duty of an officer or an enlisted man is unquestioned obedience and loyalty to the government, and it makes no difference whether he approves of

that government or not." Thus Funston stamps the true character of allegiance. According to him, entrance into the army abrogates the principles of the Declaration of Independence.

What a strange development of patriotism that turns a think- 30 ing being into a loyal machine!

In justification of this most outrageous sentence of Buwalda, 31 Gen. Funston tells the American people that the soldier's action was "a serious crime equal to treason." Now, what did this "terrible crime" really consist of? Simply in this: William Buwalda was one of fifteen hundred people who attended a public meeting in San Francisco; and, oh, horrors, he shook hands with the speaker, Emma Goldman. A terrible crime, indeed, which the General calls "a great military offense, infinitely worse than desertion."

Can there be a greater indictment against patriotism than that 32 it will thus brand a man a criminal, throw him into prison, and rob him of the results of fifteen years of faithful service?

Buwalda gave to his country the best years of his life and his 33 very manhood. But all that was as nothing. Patriotism is inexorable and, like all insatiable monsters, demands all or nothing. It does not admit that a soldier is also a human being, who has a right to his own feelings and opinions, his own inclinations and ideas. No, patriotism can not admit of that. That is the lesson which Buwalda was made to learn; made to learn at a rather costly, though not at a useless price. When he returned to freedom, he had lost his position in the army, but he regained his self-respect. After all, that is worth three years of imprisonment.

A writer on the military conditions of America, in a recent 34 article, commented on the power of the military man over the civilian in Germany. He said, among other things, that if our Republic had no other meaning than to guarantee all citizens equal rights, it would have just cause for existence. I am convinced that the writer was not in Colorado during the patriotic régime of General Bell. He probably would have changed his mind had he seen how, in the name of patriotism and the Republic, men were thrown into bull-pens, dragged about, driven across the border, and subjected to all kinds of indignities. Nor is that Colorado incident the only one in the growth of military power in the United States. There is hardly a strike where troops and militia do not come to the rescue of those in power, and where they do not act as arrogantly and brutally as do the men wearing the Kaiser's uniform. Then, too, we have the Dick military law. Had the writer forgotten that?

35   A great misfortune with most of our writers is that they are absolutely ignorant on current events, or that, lacking honesty, they will not speak of these matters. And so it has come to pass that the Dick military law was rushed through Congress with little discussion and still less publicity,—a law which gives the President the power to turn a peaceful citizen into a bloodthirsty man-killer, supposedly for the defense of the country, in reality for the protection of the interests of that particular party whose mouth-piece the President happens to be.

36   Our writer claims that militarism can never become such a power in America as abroad, since it is voluntary with us, while compulsory in the Old World. Two very important facts, however, the gentleman forgets to consider. First, that conscription has created in Europe a deep-seated hatred of militarism among all classes of society. Thousands of young recruits enlist under protest and, once in the army, they will use every possible means to desert. Second, that it is the compulsory feature of militarism which has created a tremendous anti-militarist movement, feared by European Powers far more than anything else. After all, the greatest bulwark of capitalism is militarism. The very moment the latter is undermined, capitalism will totter. True, we have no conscription; that is, men are not usually forced to enlist in the army, but we have developed a far more exacting and rigid force—necessity. Is it not a fact that during industrial depressions there is a tremendous increase in the number of enlistments? The trade of militarism may not be either lucrative or honorable, but it is better than tramping the country in search of work, standing in the bread line, or sleeping in municipal lodging houses. After all, it means thirteen dollars per month, three meals a day, and a place to sleep. Yet even necessity is not sufficiently strong a factor to bring into the army an element of character and manhood. No wonder our military authorities complain of the "poor material" enlisting in the army and navy. This admission is a very encouraging sign. It proves that there is still enough of the spirit of independence and love of liberty left in the average American to risk starvation rather than don the uniform.

Thinking men and women the world over are beginning to 37
realize that patriotism is too narrow and limited a conception to
meet the necessities of our time. The centralization of power has
brought into being an international feeling of solidarity among the
oppressed nations of the world; a solidarity which represents a
greater harmony of interests between the workingman of America
and his brothers abroad than between the American miner and
his exploiting compatriot; a solidarity which fears not foreign
invasion, because it is bringing all the workers to the point when
they will say to their masters, "Go and do your own killing. We
have done it long enough for you."

This solidarity is awakening the consciousness of even the sol- 38
diers, they, too, being flesh of the flesh of the great human family. A solidarity that has proven infallible more than once during
past struggles, and which has been the impetus inducing the
Parisian soldiers, during the Commune of 1871, to refuse to obey
when ordered to shoot their brothers. It has given courage to the
men who mutinied on Russian warships during recent years. It
will eventually bring about the uprising of all the oppressed and
downtrodden against their international exploiters.

The proletariat of Europe has realized the great force of that 39
solidarity and has, as a result, inaugurated a war against patriotism and its bloody spectre, militarism. Thousands of men fill the
prisons of France, Germany, Russia, and the Scandinavian countries, because they dared to defy the ancient superstition. Nor is
the movement limited to the working class; it has embraced representatives in all stations of life, its chief exponents being men
and women prominent in art, science, and letters.

America will have to follow suit. The spirit of militarism has 40
already permeated all walks of life. Indeed, I am convinced that
militarism is growing a greater danger here than anywhere else,
because of the many bribes capitalism holds out to those whom
it wishes to destroy.

The beginning has already been made in the schools. Evi- 41
dently the government holds to the Jesuitical conception, "Give
me the child mind, and I will mould the man." Children are
trained in military tactics, the glory of military achievements
extolled in the curriculum, and the youthful minds perverted to
suit the government. Further, the youth of the country is appealed

to in glaring posters to join the army and navy. "A fine chance to see the world!" cries the governmental huckster. Thus innocent boys are morally shanghaied into patriotism, and the military Moloch strides conquering through the Nation.

42   The American workingman has suffered so much at the hands of the soldier, State and Federal, that he is quite justified in his disgust with, and his opposition to, the uniformed parasite. However, mere denunciation will not solve this great problem. What we need is a propaganda of education for the soldier: antipatriotic literature that will enlighten him as to the real horrors of his trade, and that will awaken his consciousness to his true relation to the man to whose labor he owes his very existence. It is precisely this that the authorities fear most. It is already high treason for a soldier to attend a radical meeting. No doubt they will also stamp it high treason for a soldier to read a radical pamphlet. But, then, has not authority from time immemorial stamped every step of progress as treasonable? Those, however, who earnestly strive for social reconstruction can well afford to face all that; for it is probably even more important to carry the truth into the barracks than into the factory. When we have undermined the patriotic lie, we shall have cleared the path for that great structure wherein all nationalities shall be united into a universal brotherhood,—a truly FREE SOCIETY.

The Homeland Security State: How Far Should We Go?

Matthew Brzezinski

1 Until recently, the United States and countries like Israel occupied opposite ends of the security spectrum: one a confident and carefree superpower, seemingly untouchable, the other a tiny garrison state, surrounded by fortifications and barbed wire, fighting for its survival. But the security gap between the U.S. and places like Israel is narrowing. Subways, sewers, shopping centers, food processing and water systems are all now seen as easy prey for terrorists.

There is no clear consensus yet on how to go about protecting 2
ourselves. The federal government recently concluded a 16-month
risk assessment, and last month, the new Department of Homeland
Security was officially born, with an annual budget of $36 billion.
Big money has already been allocated to shore up certain perceived
weaknesses, including the $5.8 billion spent hiring, training and
equipping federal airport screeners and the $3 billion allocated for
"bioterrorism preparedness." All that has been well publicized.
Other measures, like sophisticated radiation sensors and surveillance systems, have been installed in some cities with less fanfare.
Meanwhile, the F.B.I. is carrying out labor-intensive tasks that
would have seemed a ludicrous waste of time 18 months ago, like
assembling dossiers on people who take scuba-diving courses.

This marks only the very beginning. A national conversa- 3
tion is starting about what kind of country we want to live in
and what balance we will tolerate between public safety and
private freedom. The decisions won't come all at once, and we
may be changing our minds a lot, depending on whether there
are more attacks here, what our government tells us and what
we believe. Two weeks ago, Congress decided to sharply cur-
tail the activities of the Total Information Awareness [T.I.A.]
program, a Pentagon project led by Rear Adm. John Poindexter
and invested with power to electronically sift through the private affairs of American citizens. For the time being, it was felt
that the threat of having the government look over our credit-
card statements and medical records was more dangerous than
its promised benefits.

Congress didn't completely shut the door on the T.I.A., 4
though. Agents can still look into the lives of foreigners, and its
functions could be expanded at any time. We could, for instance,
reach the point where we demand the installation of systems, like
the one along the Israeli coastline, to maim or kill intruders in
certain sensitive areas before they have a chance to explain who
they are or why they're there. We may come to think nothing of
American citizens who act suspiciously being held without bail
or denied legal representation for indeterminate periods or tried
in courts whose proceedings are under seal. At shopping malls
and restaurants, we may prefer to encounter heavily armed
guards and be subjected to routine searches at the door. We may

be willing to give up the freedom and ease of movement that has defined American life, if we come to believe our safety depends upon it.

5   For the better part of a generation now, Americans have gone to great lengths to protect their homes—living in gated communities, wiring their property with sophisticated alarms, arming themselves with deadly weapons. Now imagine this kind of intensity turned outward, into the public realm. As a culture, our tolerance for fear is low, and our capacity to do something about it is unrivaled. We could have the highest degree of public safety the world has ever seen. But what would that country look like, and what will it be like to live in it? Perhaps something like this.

ELECTRONIC FRISKING EVERY DAY ON YOUR COMMUTE

6   As a homebound commuter entering Washington's Foggy Bottom subway station swipes his fare card through the turnstile reader, a computer in the bowels of the mass transit authority takes note. A suspicious pattern of movements has triggered the computer's curiosity.

7   The giveaway is a microchip in the new digital fare cards, derived from the electronic ID cards many of us already use to enter our workplaces. It could be in use throughout the U.S. within a couple of years. If embedded with the user's driver's license or national ID number, it would allow transportation authorities to keep tabs on who rides the subway, and on when and where they get on and off.

8   The commuter steps through the turnstile and is scanned by the radiation portal. These would be a natural extension of the hand-held detectors that the police have started using in the New York subways. A cancer patient was actually strip-searched in a New York subway station in 2002 after residue from radiation treatments tripped the meters. But this doesn't happen to our fictitious commuter. The meters barely flicker, registering less than one on a scale of one to nine, the equivalent of a few microroentgens an hour, nowhere near the 3,800 readout that triggers evacuation sirens.

9   Imagine a battery of video cameras following the commuter's progress to the platform, where he reads a newspaper, standing next to an old utility room that contains gas masks. Cops in New

York already have them as part of their standard-issue gear, and a fully secure subway system would need them for everybody, just as every ferryboat must have a life preserver for every passenger. Sensors, which are already used in parts of the New York subway system, would test the air around him for the presence of chemical agents like sarin and mustard gases.

The commuter finishes reading his newspaper, but there is no place to throw it away because all trash cans have been removed, as they were in London when the I.R.A. used them to plant bombs. Cameras show the commuter boarding one of the subway cars, which have been reconfigured to drop oxygen masks from the ceiling in the event of a chemical attack, much like jetliners during decompression. The added security measures have probably pushed fares up throughout the country, maybe as much as 40 percent in some places.

The commuter—now the surveillance subject—gets off at the next stop. As he rides the escalator up, a camera positioned overhead zooms in for a close-up of him. This image, which will be used to confirm his identity, travels through fiber-optic cables to the Joint Operations Command Center at police headquarters. There, a computer scans his facial features, breaks them down into three-dimensional plots and compares them with a databank of criminal mug shots, people on watch lists and anyone who has ever posed for a government-issue ID. The facial-recognition program was originally developed at M.I.T. Used before 9/11 mainly by casinos to ferret out known cardsharps, the system has been tried by airport and law enforcement authorities and costs $75,000 to $100,000 per tower, as the camera stations are called.

"It can be used at A.T.M.'s, car-rental agencies, D.M.V. offices, border crossings," says an executive of Viisage Technology, maker of the Face-Finder recognition system. "These are the sorts of facilities the 19 hijackers used."

Almost instantly, the software verifies the subject's identity and forwards the information to federal authorities. What they do with it depends on the powers of the Total Information Awareness program or whatever its successors will be known as. But let's say that Congress has granted the government authority to note certain suspicious patterns, like when someone buys an airline ticket with cash and leaves the return date open. And let's say the commuter did just that—his credit cards were maxed out, so he had no choice. And he didn't fill in a return date because he wasn't sure when his next consulting assignment was going to start, and he thought he might be able to extend his vacation a few days.

14   On top of that, let's say he was also indiscreet in an e-mail message, making a crude joke to a client about a recent airline crash. Software programs that scan for suspect words are not new. Corporations have long used them to automatically block employee e-mail containing, for instance, multiple references to sex. The National Security Agency's global spy satellites and supercomputers have for years taken the search capability to the next level, processing the content of up to two million calls and e-mail messages per hour around the world.

15   Turning the snooping technology on Americans would not be difficult, if political circumstances made it seem necessary. Right now, there would be fierce resistance to this, but the debate could swing radically to the other side if the government showed that intercepting e-mail could deter terrorists from communicating with one another. Already, says Barry Steinhardt, director of the A.C.L.U. program on technology and liberty, authorities have been demanding records from Internet providers and public libraries about what books people are taking out and what Web sites they're looking at.

16   Once the commuter is on the government's radar screen, it would be hard for him to get off—as anyone who has ever found themselves on a mailing or telemarketers' list can attest. It will be like when you refinance a mortgage—suddenly every financial institution in America sends you a preapproved platinum card. Once a computer detects a pattern, hidden or overt, your identity in the digital world is fixed.

17   Technicians manning the Command Center probably wouldn't know why the subject is on a surveillance list, or whether he should even be on it in the first place. That would be classified, as most aspects of the government's counterterrorist calculations are.

18   Nonetheless, they begin to monitor his movements. Cameras on K Street pick him up as he exits the subway station and hails a waiting taxi. The cab's license plate number, as a matter of routine procedure, is run through another software program—first used in Peru in the 1990's to detect vehicles that have been stolen

or registered to terrorist sympathizers, and most recently introduced in central London to nab motorists who have not paid peak-hour traffic tariffs. Technicians get another positive reading; the cabdriver is also on a watch list. He is a Pakistani immigrant and has traveled back and forth to Karachi twice in the last six months, once when his father died, the other to attend his brother's wedding. These trips seem harmless, but the trackers are trained not to make these sorts of distinctions.

So what they see is the possible beginning of a terrorist 19 conspiracy—one slightly suspicious character has just crossed paths with another slightly suspicious character, and that makes them seriously suspicious. At this moment, the case is forwarded to the new National Counterintelligence Service [N.C.S.], which will pay very close attention to whatever both men do next.

The N.C.S. does not exist yet, but its creation is advocated 20 by the likes of Lt. Gen. William Odom, a former head of the National Security Agency. Whether modeled after Britain's MI5, a domestic spy agency, or Israel's much more proactive and unrestricted Shin Bet, the N.C.S. would most likely require a budget similar to the F.B.I's $4.2 billion and nearly as much personnel as the bureau's 11,400-strong special agent force, mostly for surveillance duties.

N.C.S. surveillance agents dispatched to tail the two subjects 21 in the taxi would have little difficulty following their quarry through Georgetown, up Wisconsin Avenue and into Woodley Park. One tool at their disposal could be a nationwide vehicle tracking system, adapted from the technology used by Singapore's Land Transport Authority to regulate traffic and parking. The system works on the same principle as the E-ZPass toll-road technology, in which scanners at tollbooths read signals from transponders installed on the windshields of passing vehicles to pay tolls automatically. In a future application, electronic readers installed throughout major American metropolitan centers could pinpoint the location of just about any vehicle equipped with mandatory transponders. (American motorists would most likely each have to pay an extra $90 fee, similar to what Singapore charges.)

When the commuter arrives home, N.C.S. agents arrange to 22 put his house under 24-hour aerial surveillance. The same thing happens to the cab-driver when he arrives home. The technology, discreet and effective, is already deployed in Washington. Modified UH-60A Blackhawk helicopters, the kind U.S. Customs uses to intercept drug runners, now patrol the skies over the capital to enforce no-fly zones. The Pentagon deployed its ultrasophisticated RC-7 reconnaissance planes during the sniper siege last fall. The surveillance craft, which have proved their worth along the DMZ in North Korea and against cocaine barons in Colombia, come loaded with long-range night-vision and infrared sensors that permit operators to detect movement and snap photos of virtually anyone's backyard from as far as 20 miles away.

A GOVERNMENT THAT KNOWS WHEN YOU'VE BEEN BAD OR GOOD

23   In the here and now, an aerial photo of my backyard is on file at the Joint Operations Command Center in Washington, which, unlike the N.C.S., already exists. The center looks like NASA, starting with the biometric palm-print scanners on its reinforced doors.

24   The center has not singled me out for any special surveillance. My neighbors' houses are all pictured, too, as are still shots and even three-dimensional images of just about every building, landmark and lot in central D.C.

25   The technology isn't revolutionary. How many times a day is the average American already on camera? There's one in the corner deli where I get my morning coffee and bagel. Another one at the A.T.M. ouside. Yet another one films traffic on Connecticut Avenue when I drive my wife to work. The lobby of her office building has several. So that's at least four, and it's only 9 a.m.

26   There are few legal restraints governing video surveillance. It is perfectly legal for the government to track anyone, anywhere, using cameras except for inside his own home, where a warrant is needed to use thermal imaging that can see all the way into the basement. Backyards or rooftops, however, are fair game.

27   There is a growing network of video cameras positioned throughout the capital that feed into the Joint Operations Command Center, otherwise known as the JOCC, which has been operational since 9/11. The experimental facility is shared by several

government agencies, including the Metropolitan Police Department, the F.B.I., the Secret Service, the State Department and the Defense Intelligence Agency. Agents from different law enforcement bodies man the JOCC's 36 computer terminals, which are arrayed in long rows beneath wall-size projection screens, like the Houston space center. The wall screens simultaneously display live feeds, digital simulations, city maps with the locations of recently released felons and gory crime scene footage.

"From here we can tap into schools, subways, landmarks 28 and main streets," says Chief Charles Ramsey of the D.C. Police, with evident pride. Theoretically, with a few clicks of the mouse the system could also link up with thousands of closed-circuit cameras in shopping malls, department stores and office buildings, and is programmed to handle live feeds from up to six helicopters simultaneously. Ramsey is careful to add that, for now, the majority of the cameras are off-line most of the time, and that the police aren't using them to look into elevators or to spy on individuals.

But they could if they wanted to. I ask for a demonstration of 29 the system's capabilities. A technician punches in a few keystrokes. An aerial photo of the city shot earlier from a surveillance plane flashes on one of the big screens. "Can you zoom in on Dupont Circle?" I ask. The screen flickers, and the thoroughfare's round fountain comes into view. "Go up Connecticut Avenue." The outline of the Hilton Hotel where President Reagan was shot materializes. "Up a few more blocks, and toward Rock Creek Park," I instruct. "There, can you get any closer?" The image blurs and focuses, and I can suddenly see the air-conditioning unit on my roof, my garden furniture and the cypress hedge I recently planted in my yard.

The fact that government officials can, from a remote location, 30 snoop into the backyards of most Washingtonians opens up a whole new level of information they can find out about us almost effortlessly. They could keep track of when you come and go from your house, discovering in the process that you work a second job or that you are carrying on an extramarital affair. Under normal circumstances, there's not much they could do with this information. And for the time being, that is the way most Americans want it. But this is the kind of issue that will come up over the next few years. How many extra tools will we be willing to grant to the police and federal authorities? How much will we allow our notions of privacy to narrow?

31   Because if domestic intelligence agents were able to find out secret details of people's lives, they could get the cooperation of crucial witnesses who might otherwise be inclined to keep quiet. There is more than a whiff of McCarthyism to all this, but perhaps we will be afraid enough to endure it.

THE MALL GUARD WHO CARRIES A MACHINE GUN

32   Imagine a wintry scene: snowdrifts and dirty slush and a long line of people muffled against the cold. This is a line to get into the mall, and it is moving frustratingly slowly. What's the holdup? There is no new blockbuster movie opening that day, or any of those "everything must go" clearance sales that might justify standing outside freezing for 20 minutes. Customers are simply waiting to clear security.

33   Shopping in an environment of total terrorist preparedness promises to be a vastly different experience from anything ever imagined in America. But for millions of people who live in terror-prone places like Israel or the Philippines, tight security at shopping malls has long been a fact of life. "I was shocked when I first came to the States and could go into any shopping plaza without going through security," says Aviv Tene, a 33-year-old Haifa attorney. "It seemed so strange, and risky."

34   It took me just under eight minutes to clear the security checkpoint outside the Dizengoff Center in downtown Tel Aviv. But that was on a rainy weekday morning before the food courts and multiplex theater had opened.

35   The future shopping experience will start at the parking-lot entrance. Booths manned by guards will control access to and from lots to prevent terrorists from emulating the Washington sniper and using parking lots as shooting galleries. Cars entering underground garages will have their trunks searched for explosives, as is the practice in Manila. It has also become common outside New York City hotels. This will guard against car or truck bombs of the type that blew up beneath the World Trade Center in 1993.

No one will be able to drive closer than a hundred yards to 36 mall entrances. Concrete Jersey barriers will stop anyone from crashing a vehicle into the buildings—a favored terrorist tactic for American targets overseas—or into the crowds of customers lining up. Screening will follow the Israeli model: metal barricades will funnel shoppers through checkpoints at all doors. They will be frisked, and both they and their bags will be searched and run through metal detectors. Security would be tightest in winter, says a former senior F.B.I. agent, because AK-47's and grenade belts are easily concealed beneath heavy coats.

What won't be concealed, of course, are the weapons carried 37 by the police at the mall. Major shopping areas will not be patrolled by the docile, paid-by-the-hour guards to whom we're accustomed, but—like airports and New York City tourist attractions—by uniformed cops and soldiers with rifles.

What will it be like to encounter such firearms on a regular 38 basis? I lived for years in Moscow, and after a short time, I rarely noticed the guns. In fact, I tended to feel more uncomfortable when armed guards were *not* around; Israelis traveling in the United States occasionally say the same thing. But despite the powerful presence of guns in popular culture, few Americans have had much contact with the kind of heavy weapons that are now becoming a common sight on city streets. Such prominent displays are meant to convey the notion that the government is doing something to ward off terrorists, but they can have the reverse effect too, of constantly reminding us of imminent danger.

Even more mundane procedures might have the same 39 effect—for example, being asked to produce a national identification card every time you go into a store, much the same way clubgoers have to prove they are of age. The idea of a national identity card, once widely viewed as un-American, is gaining ground in Washington, where some are advocating standardizing driver's licenses throughout the country as a first step in that direction. Though perhaps reminiscent of Big Brother, these cards are not uncommon in the rest of the world, even in Western Europe. In Singapore, the police frequently ask people to produce their papers; it becomes so routine that people cease being bothered by it. How long would it take Americans to become similarly inured?

40 The new ID's, which are advocated by computer industry leaders like Larry Ellison of Oracle, could resemble the digital smart cards that Chinese authorities plan to introduce in Hong Kong by the end of the year. These contain computer chips with room to store biographical, financial and medical histories, and tamperproof algorithms of the cardholder's thumbprint that can be verified by hand-held optical readers. Based on the $394 million Hong Kong has budgeted for smart cards for its 6.8 million residents, a similar program in the U.S. could run as high as $16 billion.

41 Among other things, a national identity card program would make it much harder for people without proper ID to move around and therefore much easier for police and domestic-intelligence agents to track them down. And once found, such people might discover they don't quite have the rights they thought they had. Even now, for instance, U.S. citizens can be declared "enemy combatants" and be detained without counsel. Within a few years, America's counterterrorist agencies could have the kind of sweeping powers of arrest and interrogation that have developed in places like Israel, the Philippines and even France, where the constant threat of terrorism enabled governments to do virtually whatever it takes to prevent terrorism. "As long as you worry too much about making false arrests and don't start taking greater risks," says Offer Einav, a 15-year Shin Bet veteran who now runs a security consulting firm, "you are never going to beat terrorism."

42 In years past, the U.S. has had to rely on other governments to take these risks. For example, the mastermind of the 1993 W.T.C. bombing, Ramzi Yousef, was caught only after Philippine investigators used what official intelligence documents delicately refer to as "tactical interrogation" to elicit a confession from an accomplice arrested in Manila. In U.S. court testimony, the accomplice, Abdul Hakim Murad, later testified that he was beaten to within an inch of his life.

43 In Israel, it is touted that 90 percent of suicide bombers are caught before they get near their targets, a record achieved partly because the Shin Bet can do almost anything it deems necessary to save lives. "They do things we would not be comfortable with in this country," says former Assistant F.B.I. Director Steve Pomerantz, who, along with a growing number of U.S. officials, has traveled to Israel recently for antiterror training seminars.

But the U.S. is moving in the Israeli direction. The U.S.A.   44
Patriot Act, rushed into law six weeks after 9/11, has given government agencies wide latitude to invoke the Foreign Intelligence
Surveillance Act [FISA] and get around judicial restraints on
search, seizure and surveillance of American citizens. FISA, originally intended to hunt international spies, permits the authorities
to wiretap virtually at will and break into people's homes to plant
bugs or copy documents. Last year, surveillance requests by the
federal government under FISA outnumbered for the first time in
U.S. history all of those under domestic law.

New legislative proposals by the Justice Department now seek   45
to take the Patriot Act's antiterror powers several steps further,
including the right to strip terror suspects of their U.S. citizenship.
Under the new bill—titled the Domestic Security Enhancement
Act of 2003—the government would not be required to disclose
the identity of anyone detained in connection with a terror investigation, and the names of those arrested, be they Americans or
foreign nationals, would be exempt from the Freedom of Information Act, according to the Center for Public Integrity, a rights
group in Washington, which has obtained a draft of the bill. An
American citizen suspected of being part of a terrorist conspiracy
could be held by investigators without anyone being notified. He
could simply disappear.

THE FACE-TO-FACE INTERROGATION ON YOUR VACATION

Some aspects of life would, in superficial ways, seem easier,   46
depending on who you are and what sort of specialized ID you
carry. Boarding an international flight, for example, might not
require a passport for frequent fliers. At Schiphol Airport in
Amsterdam, "trusted" travelers—those who have submitted to
background checks—are issued a smart card encoded with the
pattern of their iris. When they want to pass through security, a
scanner checks their eyes and verifies their identities, and they are
off. The whole process takes 20 seconds, according to Dutch officials. At Ben-Gurion in Israel, the same basic function is carried
out by electronic palm readers.

"We start building dossiers the moment someone buys a   47
ticket," says Einav, the Shin Bet veteran who also once served as

head of El Al security. "We have quite a bit of information on our frequent fliers. So we know they are not a security risk."

48   The technology frees up security personnel to focus their efforts on everybody else, who, on my recent trip to Jerusalem, included me. As a holder of a Canadian passport (a favorite of forgers) that has visa stamps from a number of high-risk countries ending in "stan," I was subjected to a 40-minute interrogation. My clothes and belongings were swabbed for explosives residue. Taken to a separate room, I was questioned about every detail of my stay in Israel, often twice to make certain my story stayed consistent. Whom did you meet? Where did you meet? What was the address? Do you have the business cards of the people you met? Can we see them? What did you discuss? Can we see your notes? Do you have any maps with you? Did you take any photographs while you were in Israel? Are you sure? Did you rent a car? Where did you drive to? Do you have a copy of your hotel bill? Why do you have a visa to Pakistan? Why do you live in Washington? Can we see your D.C. driver's license? Where did you live before Washington? Why did you live in Moscow? Are you always this nervous?

49   A Russian speaker was produced to verify that I spoke the language. By the time I was finally cleared, I almost missed my flight. "Sorry for the delay," apologized the young security officer. "Don't take it personally."

50   El Al is a tiny airline that has a fleet of just 30 planes and flies to a small handful of destinations. It is also heavily subsidized by the government. This is what has made El Al and Ben-Gurion safe from terrorists for more than 30 years.

51   Getting the American airline system up to this level would require a great deal more than reinforced cockpit doors and the armed air marshals now aboard domestic and international flights. It would require changing everything, including the cost and frequency of flights. Nothing could be simpler, right now, than flying from New York to Pittsburgh—every day, there are at least a dozen direct flights available from the city's three airports and countless more connecting flights. Bought a week or two in advance, these tickets can be as cheap as $150 round-trip.

52   Making U.S. airlines as security-conscious as El Al would put the U.S. back where the rest of the world is—maybe a flight or two a day from New York to Pittsburgh, at much higher costs,

and no assurance whatsoever you can get on the plane you want. Flights would take longer, and landings might be a little more interesting, because pilots would have to stay away from densely populated areas, where a plane downed by a shoulder-launched Stinger missile could do terrible damage.

EVERY DAY IS SUPER BOWL SUNDAY

But you probably won't be thinking about any of that when you 53 go out to dinner or to the movies or to a ball game. By then, it could all be second nature. The restaurant attendant will go through your purse and wave a metal-detector wand over your jacket, as they do in Tel Aviv. The valet parker will pop open your trunk and look through it before dropping your car off at an underground garage, just as in Manila.

If you take the family to a Dodgers game, you'll be able to 54 tell your kids how, back in the day, they used to have blimps and small planes trailing ad banners over stadiums. The flight restrictions, started at Super Bowl XXXVII in 2002, would not permit any planes within seven miles of any significant sporting events. Fans would have to park at least five miles from the stadium and board shuttle buses to gates. Spectators would be funneled through airport-style metal detectors and watched over by a network of 50 cameras installed throughout the stadium. Air quality would be monitored for pathogens by the type of portable detectors brought in by the Army at last year's Olympics.

Even people with no interest in sports who live in high-rises 55 near stadiums would know whenever game day came round. "Tall buildings near stadiums are also a risk," says Col. Mena Bacharach, a former Israeli secret-service agent who is one of the lead security consultants for the 2004 Summer Olympics in Athens. "They would have to be swept for snipers or R.P.G.'s." *R.P.G.'s?* Those are rocket-propelled grenades, another term that could become an American colloquialism.

It's still too early to tell what all this would mean to ticket 56 prices, but, in a sign of the changing times, the security allocation alone for last month's Super Bowl was $9 million—the equivalent of $134 for every one of the 67,000 fans in attendance.

57   Of course, public awareness programs could help to significantly cut down counterterror costs. In Israel, televised public service announcements similar to antidrug commercials in the U.S. warn viewers to be on the lookout for signs of suspicious activity. The messages are even taught to schoolchildren, along with other important survival tips, like how to assemble gas masks. "I was out with my 7-year-old granddaughter the other day," recalls Joel Feldschuh, a former Israeli brigadier general and president of El Al. "And she sees a bag on the street and starts shouting: 'Granddaddy, granddaddy, look. Quickly call a policeman. It could be left by terrorists.'"

WHAT IS YOUR SECURITY WORTH TO YOU?

58   It is commonly held that a country as big and confident in its freedoms as the United States could never fully protect itself against terrorists. The means available to them are too vast, the potentially deadly targets too plentiful. And there is a strong conviction in many quarters that there is a limit to which Americans will let their daily patterns be disturbed for security precautions. Discussing the possibility that we might all need to be equipped with our own gas masks, as Israelis are, Sergeant McClaskey of Baltimore assured me it would never happen. "If it ever reaches the point where we all need gas masks," McClaskey said, shaking his head with disgust, "then we have lost the war on terror because we are living in fear."

59   What does it really mean, however, to "lose the war on terror"? It's as ephemeral a concept as "winning the war on terror." In what sense will it ever be possible to declare an end of any kind?

60   One thing that makes the decisions of how to protect ourselves so difficult is that the terrorism we face is fundamentally different from what other governments have faced in the past. The Israelis live in tight quarters with an enemy they know well and can readily lay their eyes on. Terror attacks on European countries have always come from colonies or nearby provinces that have generally had specific grievances and demands. Americans don't know exactly who our enemies are or where they are coming from. Two of the recent thwarted terrorists, Richard Reid and Zacarias Moussaoui, were in fact Europeans.

The United States also lacks the national identity that binds 61
Israel and most European countries and helps make the psychic
wounds of terrorism heal faster. In Israel, hours after a bombing, the streets are crowded again—people are determined to
keep going. Immediately after 9/11, that's how many Americans felt, too, but it's not at all clear how long this kind of spirit
will endure.

Nor is it clear how we will absorb the cost. An adviser to 62
President Bush estimates that as much as $100 billion will have
to be spent annually on domestic security over the next 10 years,
if you factor in all the overtime accrued by police departments
every time there is a heightened alert. There are many who
believe, as General Odom does, that the money is "insignificant."
"At the height of the cold war we used to spend 7.2 percent of
G.D.P. on defense and intelligence," he says. "We spend less than
half that now."

Outside of defense and some of the entitlement programs, 63
however, domestic security will dwarf every other kind of federal
spending: education, roads, subsidized housing, environmental
protection. More than that, the decisions we make about how to
protect ourselves—the measures we demand, the ones we resist—
will take over our political discourse and define our ideas about
government in the years to come.

One significant argument against the creation of an American 64
security state, a United States that resembles Israel, is that even
there, in a society rigorously organized around security, the
safety of its citizens is far from guaranteed. But what keeps
Israelis going about their daily lives—and what might help
Americans do the same despite the fear of violence here—is the
conspicuousness of the response and the minor sacrifices that
have to be made every day. The more often we have to have our
bags searched, the better we might feel. Sitting in the kind of traffic jam that would have normally frayed our nerves might seem
almost comforting if it's because all the cars in front of us are
being checked for bombs. We may demand more daily incon-
veniences, more routine abrogations of our rights. These decisions are not only going to change how we go about our days;
they're also going to change our notion of what it means to be
an American. How far do we want to go?

65   "Security is a balancing act," says Einav, the former El Al security chief. "And there are always trade-offs. Give me the resources, and I can guarantee your safety. The question is, What are you willing to pay or put up with to stay safe?"

The Border Patrol State

Leslie Marmon Silko

1 I used to travel the highways of New Mexico and Arizona with a wonderful sensation of absolute freedom as I cruised down the open road and across the vast desert plateaus. On the Laguna Pueblo reservation, where I was raised, the people were patriotic despite the way the U.S. government had treated Native Americans. As proud citizens, we grew up believing the freedom to travel was our inalienable right, a right that some Native Americans had been denied in the early twentieth century. Our cousin, old Bill Pratt, used to ride his horse 300 miles overland from Laguna, New Mexico, to Prescott, Arizona, every summer to work as a fire lookout.

2   In school in the 1950s, we were taught that our right to travel from state to state without special papers or threat of detainment was a right that citizens under communist and totalitarian governments did not possess. That wide open highway told us we were U.S. citizens; we were free. . . .

3   Not so long ago, my companion Gus and I were driving south from Albuquerque, returning to Tucson after a book promotion for the paperback edition of my novel *Almanac of the Dead.* I had settled back and gone to sleep while Gus drove, but I was awakened when I felt the car slowing to a stop. It was nearly midnight on New Mexico State Road 26, a dark, lonely stretch of two-lane highway between Hatch and Deming. When I sat up, I saw the headlights and emergency flashers of six vehicles—Border Patrol cars and a van were blocking both lanes of the highway. Gus stopped the car and rolled down the window to ask what was wrong. But the closest Border Patrolman and his companion did not reply; instead, the first agent ordered us to "step out of the car." Gus asked why, but his question seemed to set them off. Two

more Border Patrol agents immediately approached our car, and one of them snapped, "Are you looking for trouble?" as if he would relish it.

I will never forget that night beside the highway. There was 4 an awful feeling of menace and violence straining to break loose. It was clear that the uniformed men would be only too happy to drag us out of the car if we did not speedily comply with their request (asking a question is tantamount to resistance, it seems). So we stepped out of the car and they motioned for us to stand on the shoulder of the road. The night was very dark, and no other traffic had come down the road since we had been stopped. All I could think about was a book I had read—*Nunca Más*—the official report of a human rights commission that investigated and certified more than 12,000 "disappearances" during Argentina's "dirty war" in the late 1970s.

The weird anger of these Border Patrolmen made me think 5 about descriptions in the report of Argentine police and military officers who became addicted to interrogation, torture and the murder that followed. When the military and police ran out of political suspects to torture and kill, they resorted to the random abduction of citizens off the streets. I thought how easy it would be for the Border Patrol to shoot us and leave our bodies and car beside the highway, like so many bodies found in these parts and ascribed to "drug runners."

Two other Border Patrolmen stood by the white van. The one 6 who had asked if we were looking for trouble ordered his partner to "get the dog," and from the back of the van another patrolman brought a small female German shepherd on a leash. The dog apparently did not heel well enough to suit him, and the handler jerked the leash. They opened the doors of our car and pulled the dog's head into it, but I saw immediately from the expression in her eyes that the dog hated them, and that she would not serve them. When she showed no interest in the inside of our car, they brought her around back to the trunk, near where we were standing. They half-dragged her up into the trunk, but still she did not indicate any stowed-away human beings or illegal drugs.

Their mood got uglier; the officers seemed outraged that the 7 dog could not find any contraband, and they dragged her over to us and commanded her to sniff our legs and feet. To my relief, the strange violence the Border Patrol agents had focused on us now seemed shifted to the dog. I no longer felt so strongly that we would be murdered. We exchanged looks—the dog and I. She was afraid of what they might do, just as I was. The dog's handler jerked the leash sharply as she sniffed us, as if to make her perform better, but the dog refused to accuse us: She had an innate dignity that did not permit her to serve the murderous impulses of those men. I can't forget the expression in the dog's eyes; it was as if she were embarrassed to be associated with them. I had a small amount of medicinal marijuana in my purse that night, but she refused to expose me. I am not partial to dogs, but I will always remember the small German shepherd that night.

8   Unfortunately, what happened to me is an everyday occurrence here now. Since the 1980s, on top of greatly expanding border checkpoints, the Immigration and Naturalization Service and the Border Patrol have implemented policies that interfere with the rights of U.S. citizens to travel freely within our borders. I.N.S. agents now patrol all interstate highways and roads that lead to or from the U.S.-Mexico Border in Texas, New Mexico, Arizona and California. Now, when you drive east from Tucson on Interstate 10 toward El Paso, you encounter an I.N.S. check station outside Las Cruces, New Mexico. When you drive north from Las Cruces up Interstate 25, two miles north of the town of Truth or Consequences, the highway is blocked with orange emergency barriers, and all traffic is diverted into a two-lane Border Patrol checkpoint—ninety-five miles north of the U.S.-Mexico border.

9   I was detained once at Truth or Consequences, despite my and my companion's Arizona driver's licenses. Two men, both Chicanos, were detained at the same time, despite the fact that they too presented ID and spoke English without the thick Texas accents of the Border Patrol agents. While we were stopped, we watched as other vehicles—whose occupants were white—were waved through the checkpoint. White people traveling with brown people, however, can expect to be stopped on suspicion they work with the sanctuary movement, which shelters refugees. White people who appear to be clergy, those who

wear ethnic clothing or jewelry and women with very long hair or very short hair (they could be nuns) are also frequently detained; white men with beards or men with long hair are likely to be detained, too, because Border Patrol agents have "profiles" of "those sorts" of white people who may help political refugees. (Most of the political refugees from Guatemala and El Salvador are Native American or mestizo [of mixed Indian and European heritage] because the indigenous people of the Americas have continued to resist efforts by invaders to displace them from their ancestral lands.) Alleged increase in illegal immigration by people of Asian ancestry means that the Border Patrol now routinely detains anyone who appears to be Asian or part Asian, as well.

Once your car is diverted from the Interstate Highway into 10 the checkpoint area, you are under the control of the Border Patrol, which in practical terms exercises a power that no highway patrol or city patrolman possesses: They are willing to detain anyone, for no apparent reason. Other law-enforcement officers need a shred of probable cause in order to detain anyone. On the books, so does the Border Patrol; but on the road, it's another matter. They'll order you to stop your car and step out; then they'll ask you to open the trunk. If you ask why or request a search warrant, you'll be told that they'll have to have a dog sniff the car before they can request a search warrant, and the dog might not get there for two or three hours. The search warrant might require an hour or two past that. They make it clear that if you force them to obtain a search warrant for the car, they will make you submit to a strip search as well.

Traveling in the open, though, the sense of violation can be 11 even worse. Never mind high-profile cases like that of former Border Patrol agent Michael Elmer, acquitted of murder by claiming self-defense, despite admitting that as an officer he shot an "illegal" immigrant in the back and then hid the body, which remained undiscovered until another Border Patrolman reported the event. (Last month, Elmer was convicted of reckless endangerment in a separate incident, for shooting at least ten rounds from his M-16 too close to a group of immigrants as they were crossing illegally into Nogales in March 1992.) Or that in El Paso, a high school football coach driving a vanload of his players in full uniform was pulled over on the freeway and a Border Patrol agent put a cocked revolver to his head. (The football coach was Mexican-American, as were most of the players in his van; the incident eventually caused a federal judge to issue a restraining order against the Border Patrol.) We've a mountain of personal experiences like that which never make the newspapers. A history professor at U.C.L.A. told me she had been traveling by train from Los Angeles to Albuquerque twice a month doing research. On each of her trips, she had noticed that the Border Patrol agents were at the station in Albuquerque scrutinizing the passengers. Since she is six feet tall and of Irish and German ancestry, she was not particularly concerned. Then one day when she stepped off the train in Albuquerque, two Border Patrolmen accosted her, wanting to know what she was doing, and why she was traveling between Los Angeles and Albuquerque twice a month. She presented identification and an explanation deemed "suitable" by the agents, and was allowed to go about her business.

12   Just the other day, I mentioned to a friend that I was writing this article and he told me about his 73-year-old father, who is half Chinese and had set out alone by car from Tucson to Albuquerque the week before. His father had become confused by road construction and missed a turnoff from Interstate 10 to Interstate 25; when he turned around and circled back, he missed the turnoff a second time. But when he looped back for yet another try, Border Patrol agents stopped him and forced him to open his trunk. After they satisfied themselves that he was not smuggling Chinese immigrants, they sent him on his way. He was so rattled by the event that he had to be driven home by his daughter.

13   This is the police state that has developed in the southwestern United States since the 1980s. No person, no citizen, is free to travel without the scrutiny of the Border Patrol. In the city of South Tucson, where 80 percent of the respondents were Chicano or Mexicano, a joint research project by the University of Wisconsin and the University of Arizona recently concluded that one out of every five people there had been detained, mistreated verbally or nonverbally, or questioned by I.N.S. agents in the past two years.

Manifest Destiny may lack its old grandeur of theft and 14
blood—"lock the door" is what it means now, with racism a
trump card to be played again and again, shamelessly, by both
major political parties. "Immigration," like "street crime" and
"welfare fraud," is a political euphemism that refers to people
of color. Politicians and media people talk about "illegal aliens"
to dehumanize and demonize undocumented immigrants, who
are for the most part people of color. Even in the days of Spanish
and Mexican rule, no attempts were made to interfere with the
flow of people and goods from south to north and north to
south. It is the U.S. government that has continually attempted
to sever contact between the tribal people north of the border
and those to the south.*

Now that the "Iron Curtain" is gone, it is ironic that the U.S. 15
government and its Border Patrol are constructing a steel wall ten
feet high to span sections of the border with Mexico. While politicians and multinational corporations extol the virtues of NAFTA
[the North American Free Trade Agreement] and "free trade" (in
goods, not flesh), the ominous curtain is already up in a six-mile
section of the border crossing at Mexicali; two miles are being
erected but are not yet finished at Naco; and at Nogales, sixty
miles south of Tucson, the steel wall has been all rubber-stamped
and awaits construction. Like the pathetic multimillion-dollar
"antidrug" border surveillance balloons that were continually
deflated by high winds and made only a couple of meager inter-
ceptions before they blew away, the fence along the border is a
theatrical prop, a bit of pork for contractors. Border entrepreneurs
have already used blowtorches to cut passageways through the
fence to collect "tolls" and are doing a brisk business. Back in
Washington, the I.N.S. announces a $300 million computer con-
tract to modernize its record-keeping and Congress passes a crime
bill that shunts $255 million to the I.N.S. for 1995, $181 million
earmarked for border control, which is to include 700 new partners for the men who stopped Gus and me in our travels, and the

---

*The Treaty of Guadalupe Hidalgo, signed in 1848, recognizes the right of the
Tobano O'Odom (Papago) people to move freely across the U.S.-Mexico border
without documents. A treaty with Canada guarantees similar rights to those of
the Iroquois nation in traversing the U.S.-Canada border.

history professor, and my friends' father, and as many as they could from South Tucson.

16   It is no use; borders haven't worked, and they won't work, not now, as the indigenous people of the Americas reassert their kinship and solidarity with one another. A mass migration is already under way; its roots are not simply economic. The Uto-Aztecan languages are spoken as far north as Taos Pueblo near the Colorado border, all the way south to Mexico City. Before the arrival of the Europeans, the indigenous communities throughout this region not only conducted commerce, the people shared cosmologies, and oral narratives about the Maize Mother, the Twin Brothers and their Grandmother, Spider Woman, as well as Quetzalcoatl the benevolent snake. The great human migration within the Americas cannot be stopped; human beings are natural forces of the Earth, just as rivers and winds are natural forces.

17   Deep down the issue is simple: The so-called "Indian Wars" from the days of Sitting Bull and Red Cloud have never really ended in the Americas. The Indian people of southern Mexico, of Guatemala and those left in El Salvador, too, are still fighting for their lives and for their land against the "cavalry" patrols sent out by the government of those lands. The Americas are Indian country, and the "Indian problem" is not about to go away.

18   One evening at sundown, we were stopped in traffic at a railroad crossing in downtown Tucson while a freight train passed us, slowly gaining speed as it headed north to Phoenix. In the twilight I saw the most amazing sight: Dozens of human beings, mostly young men, were riding the train; everywhere, on flat cars, inside open boxcars, perched on top of boxcars, hanging off ladders on tank cars and between boxcars. I couldn't count fast enough, but I saw fifty or sixty people headed north. They were dark young men, Indian and mestizo; they were smiling and a few of them waved at us in our cars. I was reminded of the ancient story of Aztlán, told by the Aztecs but known in other Uto-Aztecan communities as well. Aztlán is the beautiful land to the north, the origin place of the Aztec people. I don't remember how or why the people left Aztlán to journey farther south, but the old story says that one day, they will return.

Stripped of More than My Clothes

Daria MonDesire

The most comforting part of a trip abroad used to be the part that 1
brought me home.

There were only so many Yucatan pyramids to descend 2
dizzily or Moorish castles to sigh over before not-to-be-denied
nesting instincts kicked in and I missed the chaotic confusion of
home. Souvenir mugs would get packed away, wet bathing suits
tossed into carry-ons and unmailed postcards readied for repen-
tant hand delivery.

Once aloft, I'd settle into a window seat, savor being above 3
the clouds and think about the noisy welcome that awaited me.

Then came the day I found myself in a gray, windowless room 4
in San Juan's airport politely being strip-searched by U.S. Customs agents.

There have, in my life, been two occasions when underwear 5
was removed against my will. The first occurred at the hands of
a rapist. The second time was at the hands of my government.

The agents told me they'd picked me out because I was 6
dressed in bulky clothes: a backless sundress, a light cotton shirt
and sandals. They told me that if they'd failed to stop me, their
boss would have wanted to know why. They told me, after they'd
made me remove my underwear and prove to their satisfaction
the sanitary pad was there for its intended purpose, that I should
consider working undercover as a drug agent.

Then they let me go. 7

Drugs have taken a numbing toll on this country. Lives have 8
been lost, minds wasted. Heroin and cocaine should not be
allowed to flow onto our shores unchallenged and unabated. Yet
there's something chilling about a federal policy where law-abiding
American citizens are forced to disrobe, detained without counsel, subjected to intrusive body cavity searches and at times held
for as long as it takes laxatives to empty their stomachs.

Last year, 50,892 international airline passengers went 9
through the rigors of some type of body search courtesy of the
U.S. Customs Service—most of them "pat-downs" that fall short
of the service's definition of a strip-search. One would surmise,

given the professionalism of U.S. Customs officers, that drugs and maybe a mango or two would turn up on at least half the passengers subjected to such scrutiny.

10   Guess again. According to the Customs Service, 96% of them were found to be carrying nothing more than memories of a Caribbean honeymoon, gaudy sombreros destined to collect dust on a family room wall or mildewed laundry in need of a washer. Even three out of four of the 2,797 travelers subjected to partial or full strip searches, X-ray exams or cavity searches turned out not to be carrying drugs or contraband.

11   Those strip-searched were everyday people going about their everyday lives, until a federal agent labeled them with two loaded words: "potential courier." Had a municipal police department or a state police force attempted to do what U.S. Customs zealously did, constitutional safeguards against unreasonable search and seizure would bring the attempts to a screeching halt.

12   I can't say with absolute certainty why I, the one African-American on my flight, also was the one passenger on my flight singled out for that search several years ago. The official Customs line is that it focuses on high-risk flights from high-risk countries. Perhaps Grenada is famous for more than nutmeg and American intervention. Perhaps I should have taken care of those unpaid parking tickets. Perhaps I was a victim of a vast, right-wing conspiracy. It's all so wearying to think that, in addition to everything else being black in America entails, it may signal prima facie grounds for agents of my government to strip me.

13   This much is clear: Minorities bear the brunt of the examinations. Of the total number of airline passengers who were searched in some manner in 1998 and on whom Customs kept race-identifying statistics, two-thirds were black, Latino or Asian.

14   Customs officials, noting that three times as many whites as blacks were strip-searched, say they don't discriminate against blacks.

15   This official position, however, does not include the opinion of Cathy Harris, a Customs inspector in Atlanta who has filed complaints alleging discrimination against black travelers. Nor is it supported by about four dozen black women who launched a class-action lawsuit in Chicago against the Customs Service

alleging they were targeted for strip-searches because of their race. According to their attorney, Edward M. Fox, they include a 15-year-old searched while traveling with her white mother and aunt, who were not searched, a mentally retarded woman and a travel agent who has been repeatedly searched. Fox says he's now heard from more than 90 women from across the country.

The low number of body searches leading to drug seizures, the lawsuits and the complaints have convinced the Customs Service that things are not going swimmingly. A new commissioner, Raymond W. Kelly, has a consultant examining the agency's policies. Customs officers are taking classes in cultural diversity. Some targeted passengers are being given the option of having machines scan their bodies.   16

Here's my proposal. Let's level the probing field and make it, indeed, a war against drugs.   17

Strip-search everyone who travels out of the country.   18

Strip-search Martha Stewart the second she steps off the Concorde. Strip-search Al Gore, members of Congress, all nine Supreme Court justices and every last one of the Daughters of the American Revolution. Strip-search Barbara Walters, Ivana Trump and ditto for The Donald. Strip search the Toujours Provence tourists, the Tuscany villa vacationers and the Hollywood-St. Barts brigade. Strip-search everyone who heretofore labored under the privileged assumption they could return to this country with some shred of dignity.   19

And then let the chips fall where they may.   20

We Should Relinquish Some Liberty in Exchange for Security

Mona Charen

It will be interesting to see how the debate over civil liberties and the war on terror plays out now that the electorate has given President George W. Bush such a vote of confidence. Since September 11, the left has pitched fits about military commissions, alleged   1 attorney–client privilege infringements, telephone taps, surveillance of suspected terrorists, fingerprinting and photographing of some foreign visitors, and particularly round-ups of visa violators. Each of these measures has been met with loud objections from liberals who are convinced that the Bush administration is on the verge of creating a police state.

2   Others see the world differently. Instead of an out-of-control government behemoth spying on you and me in complete disregard for civil liberties, they see our domestic and foreign intelligence services as toothless watchdogs, powerless to detect or stop terrorism after decades of liberal "reforms."

3   No one, least of all a conservative concerned about government power, should take civil liberties protection lightly. But the liberal reforms of the past generation have gone way beyond protecting the privacy rights of American citizens—they've protected the ability of international terrorists to function in this country virtually unimpeded. Everyone now knows that FBI agent Colleen Rowley pleaded with her superiors for permission to inspect the computer of Zacharias Moussaoui, only to be told that she lacked "probable cause." If investigators had searched that laptop, they would have found the name and phone number of one the ringleaders of the September 11 plot.

4   This bit of recent history is raised to imply that the FBI screwed up in August 2001. Yet when the suggestion is made that perhaps the "probable cause" standard be brought down a notch, say to "reasonable suspicion," the civil-liberties types go ballistic. When the Justice Department interviewed several thousand men from Arab nations, *The New York Times* decried the "vast roundup" and the American Civil Liberties Union shrilled that this "dragnet approach . . . is likely to magnify concerns of racial and ethnic profiling." In fact, as Professor Robert Turner of the University of Virginia Law School relates, interviewees were treated politely and asked, among other things, whether they had encountered any acts of bigotry.

5   Before September 11, and thanks to a process of emasculation stretching back to the Church committee hearings of the 1970s, the FBI and CIA were forbidden to share information. Even within the FBI, thanks to "the wall" inaugurated under Attorney General Janet Reno, a counter-terrorism agent examining a terror cell in

Buffalo could not walk down the hall and chat with a criminal investigator who was looking into money laundering by the same people. The FBI was forbidden to conduct general Internet searches, or to visit public places open to all.

Seventy-five percent of the American people told the Gallup 6 organization that the Bush administration has not gone too far in restricting civil liberties. Fifty percent thought they'd gone far enough, but 25 percent thought they should have been tougher. Only 11 percent thought the administration had gone too far.

What liberals are urging is that suspected terrorists, here or 7 abroad, be accorded the full panoply of rights we give to ordinary criminal defendants. But this judicializes war. President Bill Clinton adhered to this model and accordingly turned down an opportunity to capture Osama bin Laden because he feared we might not have proper evidence for a criminal indictment.

But the war powers of the presidency, long respected by the 8 courts, permit special action in the case of war. Even before September 11, bin Laden had declared war on the United States and was clearly ineligible for a criminal trial. He was morally and legally an enemy combatant. Similarly, though, President Bush has not taken any action since September 11 that was not also approved overwhelmingly by the Congress.

But the key point is this: If we err on the side of civil liber- 9 ties instead of on the side of security, hundreds of thousands or millions of Americans could die. If we err on the side of security, many people will be inconvenienced and a few individuals may be wrongly imprisoned for some time. In which direction would you lean?

Chapter

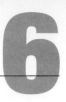

The Law and the Individual: How Should Society Enforce Its Rules?

From *Crito*

Plato

1 *SOCRATES:* . . . Ought a man to do what he admits to be right, or ought he to betray the right?

2 *CRITO:* He ought to do what he thinks right.

3 *SOCRATES:* But if this is true, what is the application? In leaving the prison against the will of the Athenians, do I wrong any? Or rather do I not wrong those whom I ought least to wrong? Do I not desert the principles which are acknowledged by us to be just—what do you say?

4 *CRITO:* I cannot tell, Socrates; for I do not know.

5 *SOCRATES:* Then consider the matter in this way:—Imagine that I am about to play truant (you may call the proceeding by any name which you like), and the laws of the government come and interrogate me: "Tell us, Socrates," they say: "what are you about? Are you not going by an act of yours to overturn us—the laws, and the whole state, as far as in you lies? Do you imagine that a state can subsist and not be overthrown, in which the decisions of law have no power, but are set aside and trampled upon by individuals?" What will be our answer, Crito, to these and the like words? Any one, and especially a rhetorician, will have a good deal to say on behalf of the law which requires a sentence to be carried out. He will

argue that this law should not be set aside; and shall we reply, "Yes, but the state has injured us and given an unjust sentence." Suppose I say that?

CRITO: Very good, Socrates.   6

SOCRATES: "And was that our agreement with you?" the law 7 would answer; "or were you to abide by the sentence of the state?" And if I were to express my astonishment at their words, the law would probably add: "Answer, Socrates, instead of opening your eyes—you are in the habit of asking and answering questions. Tell us,—What complaint have you to make against us which justifies you in attempting to destroy us and the state? In the first place did we not bring you into existence? Your father married your mother by our aid and begat you. Say whether you have any objection to urge against those of us who regulate marriage?" None, I should reply. "Or against those of us who after birth regulate the nurture and education of children, in which you also were trained? Were not the laws, which have the charge of education, right in commanding your father to train you in music and gymnastics?" Right, I should reply. "Well then, since you were brought into the world and nurtured and educated by us, can you deny in the first place that you are our child and slave, as your fathers were before you? And if this is true you are not on equal terms with us; nor can you think that you have a right to do to us what we are doing to you. Would you have any right to strike or revile or do any other evil to your father or your master, if you had one, because you have been struck or reviled by him, or received some other evil at his hands?—you would not say this? And because we think right to destroy you, do you think that you have any right to destroy us in return, and your country as far as in you lies? Will you, O professor of true virtue, pretend that you are justified in this? Has a philosopher like you failed to discover that our country is more to be valued and higher and holier far than mother or father or any ancestor, and more to be regarded in the eyes of the gods and of men of understanding? Also to be soothed, and gently and reverently entreated when angry, even more than a father, and either to be persuaded, or if not persuaded, to be obeyed? And when we are punished by her, whether with imprisonment or stripes, the punishment is to be endured in silence, and if she leads us to wounds or death in battle, thither we follow as is right; neither may any one yield or retreat or leave his rank, but whether in battle or in a court of law, or in any other place, he must do what his city and his country order him; or he must change their view of what is just: and if he may do no violence to his father or mother, much less may he do violence to his country." What answer shall we make to this, Crito? Do the laws speak truly, or do they not?

8 *CRITO:* I think that they do.

9 *SOCRATES:* Then the laws will say, "Consider, Socrates, if we are speaking truly that in your present attempt you are going to do us an injury. For, having brought you into the world, and nurtured and educated you, and given you and every other citizen a share in every good which we had to give, we further proclaim to any Athenian by the liberty which we allow him, that if he does not like us when he has become of age and has seen the ways of the city, and made our acquaintance, he may go where he pleases and take his goods with him. None of us laws will forbid him or interfere with him. Any one who does not like us and the city, and who wants to emigrate to a colony or to any other city, may go where he likes, retaining his property. But he who has experience of the manner in which we order justice and administer the state, and still remains, has entered into an implied contract that he will do as we command him. And he who disobeys us is, as we maintain, thrice wrong; first, because in disobeying us he is disobeying his parents; secondly, because we are the authors of his education; thirdly, because he has made an agreement with us that he will duly obey our commands; and he neither obeys them nor convinces us that our commands are unjust; and we do not rudely impose them, but give him the alternative of obeying or convincing us;—that is what we offer, and he does neither.

10   "These are the sort of accusations to which, as we were saying, you, Socrates, will be exposed if you accomplish your intentions; you, above all other Athenians." Suppose now I

ask, why I rather than anybody else? They will justly retort
upon me that I above all other men have acknowledged the
agreement. "There is clear proof," they will say, "Socrates, that
we and the city were not displeasing to you. Of all Athenians you have been the most constant resident in the city,
which, as you never leave, you may be supposed to love. For
you never went out of the city either to see the games, except
once when you went to the Isthmus, or to any other place
unless when you were on military service; nor did you travel
as other men do. Nor had you any curiosity to know other
states or their laws: your affections did not go beyond us and
our state; we were your special favorites, and you acquiesced
in our government of you; and here in this city you begat your
children, which is a proof of your satisfaction. Moreover, you
might in the course of the trial, if you had liked, have fixed
the penalty at banishment; the state which refuses to let you
go now would have let you go then. But you pretended that
you preferred death to exile, and that you were not unwilling to die. And now you have forgotten these fine sentiments,
and pay no respect to us the laws, of whom you are the
destroyer; and are doing what only a miserable slave would
do, running away and turning your back upon the compacts
and agreements which you made as a citizen. And first of all
answer this very question: Are we right in saying that you
agreed to be governed according to us in deed, and not in
word only? Is that true or not?" How shall we answer, Crito?
Must we not assent?

CRITO: We cannot help it, Socrates.   11

SOCRATES: Then will they not say: "You, Socrates, are breaking   12
the covenants and agreements which you made with us at
your leisure, not in any haste or under any compulsion or
deception, but after you have had seventy years to think of
them, during which time you were at liberty to leave the
city, if we were not to your mind, or if our covenants
appeared to you to be unfair. You had your choice, and
might have gone either to Lacedaemon or Crete, both which
states are often praised by you for their good government,
or to some other Hellenic or foreign state. Whereas you,
above all our Athenians, seemed to be so fond of the state,

or, in other words, of us her laws (and who would care about a state which has no laws?), that you never stirred out of her; the halt, the blind, the maimed were not more stationary in her than you were. And now you run away and forsake your agreements. Not so, Socrates, if you will take our advice; do not make yourself ridiculous by escaping out of the city.

13   "For just consider, if you transgress and err in this sort of way, what good will you do either to yourself or to your friends? That your friends will be driven into exile and deprived of citizenship, or will lose their property, is tolerably certain; and you yourself, if you fly to one of the neighboring cities, as, for example, Thebes or Megara, both of which are well governed, will come to them as an enemy, Socrates, and their government will be against you, and all patriotic citizens will cast an evil eye upon you as a subverter of the laws, and you will confirm in the minds of the judges the justice of their own condemnation of you. For he who is a corrupter of the laws is more than likely to be a corrupter of the young and foolish portion of mankind. Will you then flee from well-ordered citizens and virtuous men? And is existence worth having on these terms? Or will you go to them without shame, and talk to them, Socrates? And what will you say to them? What you say here about virtue and justice and institutions and laws being the best things among men? Would that be decent of you? Surely not. But if you go away from well-governed states to Crito's friends in Thessaly, where there is a great disorder and licence, they will be charmed to hear the tale of your escape from prison, set off with ludicrous particulars of the manner in which you were wrapped in a goatskin or some other disguise, and metamorphosed as the manner is of runaways; but will there be no one to remind you that in your old age you were ashamed to violate the most sacred laws from a miserable desire of a little more life? Perhaps not, if you keep them in a good temper; but if they are out of temper you will hear many degrading things; you will live, but how?—as the flatterer of all men, and the servant of all men; and doing what?—eating and drinking in Thessaly, having gone

abroad in order that you may get a dinner. And where will
be your fine sentiments about justice and virtue? Say that
you wish to live for the sake of your children—you want to
bring them up and educate them—will you take them into
Thessaly and deprive them of Athenian citizenship? Is this
the benefit which you will confer upon them? Or are you
under the impression that they will be better cared for and
educated here if you are still alive, although absent from
them; for your friends will take care of them? Do you fancy
that if you are an inhabitant of Thessaly they will take care
of them, and if you are an inhabitant of the other world that
they will not take care of them? Nay: but if they who call
themselves friends are good for anything, they will—to be
sure they will.

"Listen, then, Socrates, to us who have brought you up. 14
Think not of life and children first, and of justice afterwards,
but of justice first, that you may be justified before the
princes of the world below. For neither will you nor any that
belong to you be happier or holier or juster in this life, or
happier in another, if you do as Crito bids. Now you depart
in innocence, a sufferer and not a doer of evil; a victim, not
of the laws of men. But if you go forth, returning evil for
evil, and injury for injury, breaking the covenants and agreements which you have made with us, and wronging those
whom you ought least of all to wrong, that is to say, yourself, your friends, your country, and us, we shall be angry
with you while you live, and our brethren, the laws in the
world below, will receive you as an enemy; for they will
know that you have done your best to destroy us. Listen,
then, to us and not to Crito."

This, dear Crito, is the voice which I seem to hear mur- 15
muring in my ears, like the sound of the flute in the ears of
the mystic; that voice, I say, is humming in my ears, and prevents me from hearing any other. And I know that anything
more which you may say will be vain. Yet speak, if you have
anything to say.

CRITO: I have nothing to say, Socrates.   16

SOCRATES: Leave me then, Crito, to fulfill the will of God, and to 17
follow whither he leads.

Civil Disobedience

Henry David Thoreau

1   I heartily accept the motto—"That government is best which governs least;" and I should like to see it acted up to more rapidly and systematically. Carried out, it finally amounts to this, which also I believe,—"That government is best which governs not at all;" and when men are prepared for it, that will be the kind of government which they will have. Government is at best but an expedient; but most governments are usually, and all governments are sometimes, inexpedient. The objections which have been brought against a standing army, and they are many and weighty, and deserve to prevail, may also at last be brought against a standing government. The standing army is only an arm of the standing government. The government itself, which is only the mode which the people have chosen to execute their will, is equally liable to be abused and perverted before the people can act through it. Witness the present Mexican war, the work of comparatively a few individuals using the standing government as their tool; for, in the outset, the people would not have consented to this measure.

2   This American government,—what is it but a tradition, though a recent one, endeavoring to transmit itself unimpaired to posterity, but each instant losing some of its integrity? It has not the vitality and force of a single living man; for a single man can bend it to his will. It is a sort of wooden gun to the people themselves; and, if ever they should use it in earnest as a real one against each other, it will surely split. But it is not the less necessary for this; for the people must have some complicated machinery or other, and hear its din, to satisfy that idea of government which they have. Governments show thus how successfully men can be imposed on, even impose on themselves, for their own advantage. It is excellent, we must all allow; yet this government never of itself furthered any enterprise, but by the alacrity with which it got out of its way. *It* does not keep the country free. *It* does not settle the West. It does not educate. The character inherent in the American people has done all that has been accomplished; and it would have done somewhat more, if the government had not sometimes got in its way. For government is

an expedient by which men would fain succeed in letting one another alone; and, as has been said, when it is most expedient, the governed are most let alone by it. Trade and commerce, if they were not made of India rubber, would never manage to bounce over the obstacles which legislators are continually putting in their way; and, if one were to judge these men wholly by the effects of their actions, and not partly by their intentions, they would deserve to be classed and punished with those mischievous persons who put obstructions on the railroads.

But, to speak practically and as a citizen, unlike those who call themselves no-government men, I ask for, not at once no government, but *at once* a better government. Let every man make known what kind of government would command his respect, and that will be one step toward obtaining it. 3

After all, the practical reason why, when the power is once in the hands of the people, a majority are permitted, and for a long period continue, to rule, is not because they are most likely to be in the right, nor because this seems fairest to the minority, but because they are physically the strongest. But a government in which the majority rule in all cases cannot be based on justice, even as far as men understand it. Can there not be a government in which majorities do not virtually decide right and wrong, but conscience?—in which majorities decide only those questions to which the rule of expediency is applicable? Must the citizen ever for a moment, or in the least degree, resign his conscience to the legislator? Why has every man a conscience, then? I think that we should be men first, and subjects afterward. It is not desirable to cultivate a respect for the law, so much as for the right. The only obligation which I have a right to assume, is to do at any time what I think right. It is truly enough said, that a corporation has no conscience; but a corporation of conscientious men is a corporation *with* a conscience. Law never made men a whit more just; and, by means of their respect for it, even the well-disposed are daily made the agents of injustice. A common and natural result of an undue respect for law is, that you may see a file of soldiers, colonel, captain, corporal, privates, powder-monkeys and all, marching in admirable order over hill and dale to the wars, against their wills, aye, against their common sense and consciences, which makes it very steep marching indeed, and produces a palpitation 4 of the heart. They have no doubt that it is a damnable business in which they are concerned; they are all peaceably inclined. Now, what are they? Men at all? or small moveable forts and magazines, at the service of some unscrupulous man in power? Visit the Navy Yard, and behold a marine, such a man as an American government can make, or such as it can make a man with its black arts, a mere shadow and reminiscence of humanity, a man laid out alive and standing, and already, as one may say, buried under arms with funeral accompaniments, though it may be

> "Not a drum was heard, nor a funeral note,
> As his corse to the ramparts we hurried;
> Not a soldier discharged his farewell shot
> O'er the grave where our hero we buried."

5   The mass of men serve the State thus, not as men mainly, but as machines, with their bodies. They are the standing army, and the militia, jailers, constables, *posse comitatus,* &c. In most cases there is no free exercise whatever of the judgment or of the moral sense; but they put themselves on a level with wood and earth and stones; and wooden men can perhaps be manufactured that will serve the purpose as well. Such command no more respect than men of straw, or a lump of dirt. They have the same sort of worth only as horses and dogs. Yet such as these even are commonly esteemed good citizens. Others, as most legislators, politicians, lawyers, ministers, and office-holders, serve the State chiefly with their heads; and, as they rarely make any moral distinctions, they are as likely to serve the devil, without intending it, as God. A very few, as heroes, patriots, martyrs, reformers in the great sense, and *men,* serve the State with their consciences also, and so necessarily resist it for the most part; and they are commonly treated by it as enemies. A wise man will only be useful as a man, and will not submit to be "clay," and "stop a hole to keep the wind away," but leave that office to his dust at least:—

> "I am too high-born to be propertied,
> To be a secondary at control,
> Or useful serving-man and instrument
> To any sovereign state throughout the world."

He who gives himself entirely to his fellow-men appears to   6
them useless and selfish; but he who gives himself partially to
them is pronounced a benefactor and philanthropist.

How does it become a man to behave toward this American   7
government to-day? I answer that he cannot without disgrace be
associated with it. I cannot for an instant recognize that political
organization as *my* government which is the *slave's* government also.

All men recognize the right of revolution; that is, the right to   8
refuse allegiance to and to resist the government, when its
tyranny or its inefficiency are great and unendurable. But almost
all say that such is not the case now. But such was the case, they
think, in the Revolution of '75. If one were to tell me that this was
a bad government because it taxed certain foreign commodities
brought to its ports, it is most probable that I should not make an
ado about it, for I can do without them: all machines have their
friction; and possibly this does enough good to counterbalance the
evil. At any rate, it is a great evil to make a stir about it. But when
the friction comes to have its machine, and oppression and robbery are organized, I say, let us not have such a machine any
longer. In other words, when a sixth of the population of a nation
which has undertaken to be the refuge of liberty are slaves, and
a whole country is unjustly overrun and conquered by a foreign
army, and subjected to military law, I think that it is not too soon
for honest men to rebel and revolutionize. What makes this duty
the more urgent is the fact, that the country so overrun is not our
own, but ours is the invading army.

Paley, a common authority with many on moral questions, in   9
his chapter on the "Duty of Submission to Civil Government,"
resolves all civil obligation into expediency; and he proceeds to
say, "that so long as the interest of the whole society requires it,
that is, so long as the established government cannot be resisted
or changed without public inconveniency, it is the will of God that
the established government be obeyed, and no longer."—"This
principle being admitted, the justice of every particular case of
resistance is reduced to a computation of the quantity of the danger and grievance on the one side, and of the probability and
expense of redressing it on the other." Of this, he says, every man
shall judge for himself. But Paley appears never to have contemplated those cases to which the rule of expediency does not apply,

in which a people, as well as an individual, must do justice, cost
what it may. If I have unjustly wrested a plank from a drowning
man, I must restore it to him though I drown myself. This, according to Paley, would be inconvenient. But he that would save his life,
in such a case, shall lose it. This people must cease to hold slaves,
and to make war on Mexico, though it cost them their existence
as a people.

10   In their practice, nations agree with Paley; but does any one
think that Massachusetts does exactly what is right at the present crisis?

> "A drab of state, a cloth-o'-silver slut,
> To have her train borne up, and her soul trail
>   in the dirt."

Practically speaking, the opponents to a reform in Massachusetts are not a hundred thousand politicians at the South, but a
hundred thousand merchants and farmers here, who are more
interested in commerce and agriculture than they are in humanity,
and are not prepared to do justice to the slave and to Mexico, *cost
what it may.* I quarrel not with far-off foes, but with those who, near
at home, co-operate with, and do the bidding of those far away,
and without whom the latter would be harmless. We are accustomed to say, that the mass of men are unprepared; but improvement is slow, because the few are not materially wiser or better
than the many. It is not so important that many should be as good
as you, as that there be some absolute goodness somewhere; for
that will leaven the whole lump. There are thousands who are *in
opinion* opposed to slavery and to the war, who yet in effect do
nothing to put an end to them; who, esteeming themselves children of Washington and Franklin, sit down with their hands in
their pockets, and say that they know not what to do, and do nothing; who even postpone the question of freedom to the question
of free-trade, and quietly read the prices-current along with the latest advices from Mexico, after dinner, and, it may be, fall asleep
over them both. What is the price-current of an honest man and
patriot to-day? They hesitate, and they regret, and sometimes they
petition; but they do nothing in earnest and with effect. They will
wait, well disposed, for others to remedy the evil, that they may

no longer have it to regret. At most, they give only a cheap vote, and a feeble countenance and God-speed, to the right, as it goes by them. There are nine hundred and ninety-nine patrons of virtue to one virtuous man; but it is easier to deal with the real possessor of a thing than with the temporary guardian of it.

All voting is a sort of gaming, like chequers or backgammon, 11 with a slight moral tinge to it, a playing with right and wrong, with moral questions; and betting naturally accompanies it. The character of the voters is not staked. I cast my vote, perchance, as I think right; but I am not vitally concerned that that right should prevail. I am willing to leave it to the majority. Its obligation, therefore, never exceeds that of expediency. Even voting *for the right* is *doing* nothing for it. It is only expressing to men feebly your desire that it should prevail. A wise man will not leave the right to the mercy of chance, nor wish it to prevail through the power of the majority. There is but little virtue in the action of masses of men. When the majority shall at length vote for the abolition of slavery, it will be because they are indifferent to slavery, or because there is but little slavery left to be abolished by their vote. *They* will then be the only slaves. Only *his* vote can hasten the abolition of slavery who asserts his own freedom by his vote.

I hear of a convention to be held at Baltimore, or elsewhere, 12 for the selection of a candidate for the Presidency, made up chiefly of editors, and men who are politicians by profession; but I think, what is it to any independent, intelligent, and respectable man what decision they may come to, shall we not have the advantage of his wisdom and honesty, nevertheless? Can we not count upon some independent votes? Are there not many individuals in the country who do not attend conventions? But no: I find that the respectable man, so called, has immediately drifted from his position, and despairs of his country, when his country has more reason to despair of him. He forthwith adopts one of the candidates thus selected as the only *available* one, thus proving that he is himself *available* for any purposes of the demagogue. His vote is of no more worth than that of any unprincipled foreigner or hireling native, who may have been bought. Oh for a man who is a *man*, and, as my neighbor says, has a bone in his back which you cannot pass your hand through! Our statistics are at fault: the population has been returned too large. How many *men* are there to a square thousand miles in this country? Hardly one. Does not America offer any inducement for men to settle here? The American has dwindled into an Odd Fellow,—one who may be known by the development of his organ of gregarious-ness, and a manifest lack of intellect and cheerful self-reliance; whose first and chief concern, on coming into the world, is to see that the alms-houses are in good repair; and, before yet he has lawfully donned the virile garb, to collect a fund for the support of the widows and orphans that may be; who, in short, ventures to live only by the aid of the mutual insurance company, which has promised to bury him decently.

13   It is not a man's duty, as a matter of course, to devote himself to the eradication of any, even the most enormous wrong; he may still properly have other concerns to engage him; but it is his duty, at least, to wash his hands of it, and, if he gives it no thought longer, not to give it practically his support. If I devote myself to other pursuits and contemplations, I must first see, at least, that I do not pursue them sitting upon another man's shoulders. I must get off him first, that he may pursue his contemplations too. See what gross inconsistency is tolerated. I have heard some of my townsmen say, "I should like to have them order me out to help put down an insurrection of the slaves, or to march to Mexico,—see if I would go;" and yet these very men have each, directly by their allegiance, and so indirectly, at least, by their money, furnished a substitute. The soldier is applauded who refuses to serve in an unjust war by those who do not refuse to sustain the unjust gov-ernment which makes the war; is applauded by those whose own act and authority he disregards and sets at nought; as if the State were penitent to that degree that it hired one to scourge it while it sinned, but not to that degree that it left off sinning for a moment. Thus, under the name of order and civil government, we are all made at last to pay homage to and support our own meanness. After the first blush of sin, comes its indifference; and from immoral it becomes, as it were, *un*moral, and not quite unnecessary to that life which we have made.

14   The broadest and most prevalent error requires the most dis-interested virtue to sustain it. The slight reproach to which the virtue of patriotism is commonly liable, the noble are most likely to incur. Those who, while they disapprove of the character and

measures of a government, yield to it their allegiance and support, are undoubtedly its most conscientious supporters, and so frequently the most serious obstacles to reform. Some are petitioning the State to dissolve the Union, to disregard the requisitions of the President. Why do they not dissolve it themselves—the union between themselves and the State,—and refuse to pay their quota into its treasury? Do not they stand in the same relation to the State, that the State does to the Union? And have not the same reasons prevented the State from resisting the Union, which have prevented them from resisting the State?

How can a man be satisfied to entertain an opinion merely, and enjoy *it*? Is there any enjoyment in it, if his opinion is that he is aggrieved? If you are cheated out of a single dollar by your neighbor, you do not rest satisfied with knowing that you are cheated, or with saying that you are cheated, or even with petitioning him to pay you your due; but you take effectual steps at once to obtain the full amount, and see that you are never cheated again. Action from principle,—the perception and the performance of right,— changes things and relations; it is essentially revolutionary, and does not consist wholly with any thing which was. It not only divides states and churches, it divides families; aye, it divides the *individual*, separating the diabolical in him from the divine. 15

Unjust laws exist: shall we be content to obey them, or shall we endeavor to amend them, and obey them until we have succeeded, or shall we transgress them at once? Men generally, under such a government as this, think that they ought to wait until they have persuaded the majority to alter them. They think that, if they should resist, the remedy would be worse than the evil. But it is the fault of the government itself that the remedy is worse than the evil. *It* makes it worse. Why is it not more apt to anticipate and provide for reform? Why does it not cherish its wise minority? Why does it cry and resist before it is hurt? Why does it not encourage its citizens to be on the alert to point out its faults, and *do* better than it would have them? Why does it always crucify Christ, and excommunicate Copernicus and Luther, and pronounce Washington and Franklin rebels? 16

One would think, that a deliberate and practical denial of its authority was the only offence never contemplated by government; else, why has it not assigned its definite, its suitable and 17 proportionate penalty? If a man who has no property refuses but once to earn nine shillings for the State, he is put in prison for a period unlimited by any law that I know, and determined only by the discretion of those who placed him there; but if he should steal ninety times nine shillings from the State, he is soon permitted to go at large again.

18   If the injustice is part of the necessary friction of the machine of government, let it go, let it go: perchance it will wear smooth,— certainly the machine will wear out. If the injustice has a spring, or a pulley, or a rope, or a crank, exclusively for itself, then perhaps you may consider whether the remedy will not be worse than the evil; but if it is of such a nature that it requires you to be the agent of injustice to another, then, I say, break the law. Let your life be a counter friction to stop the machine. What I have to do is to see, at any rate, that I do not lend myself to the wrong which I condemn.

19   As for adopting the ways which the State has provided for remedying the evil, I know not of such ways. They take too much time, and a man's life will be gone. I have other affairs to attend to. I came into this world, not chiefly to make this a good place to live in, but to live in it, be it good or bad. A man has not every thing to do, but something; and because he cannot do *every thing*, it is not necessary that he should do *something* wrong. It is not my business to be petitioning the governor or the legislature any more than it is theirs to petition me; and, if they should not hear my petition, what should I do then? But in this case the State has provided no way: its very Constitution is the evil. This may seem to be harsh and stubborn and unconciliatory; but it is to treat with the utmost kindness and consideration the only spirit that can appreciate or deserves it. So is all change for the better, like birth and death which convulse the body.

20   I do not hesitate to say, that those who call themselves abolitionists should at once effectually withdraw their support, both in person and property, from the government of Massachusetts, and not wait till they constitute a majority of one, before they suffer the right to prevail through them. I think that it is enough if they have God on their side, without waiting for that other one. Moreover, any man more right than his neighbors, constitutes a majority of one already.

I meet this American government, or its representative the   21
State government, directly, and face to face, once a year, no more,
in the person of its tax-gatherer; this is the only mode in which a
man situated as I am necessarily meets it; and it then says distinctly,
Recognize me; and the simplest, the most effectual, and, in the
present posture of affairs, the indispensablest mode of treating
with it on this head, of expressing your little satisfaction with and
love for it, is to deny it then. My civil neighbor, the tax-gatherer,
is the very man I have to deal with,—for it is, after all, with men
and not with parchment that I quarrel,—and he has voluntarily
chosen to be an agent of the government. How shall he ever know
well what he is and does as an officer of the government, or as a
man, until he is obliged to consider whether he shall treat me,
his neighbor, for whom he has respect, as a neighbor and well-
disposed man, or as a maniac and disturber of the peace, and see
if he can get over this obstruction to his neighborliness without a
ruder and more impetuous thought or speech corresponding with
his action? I know this well, that if one thousand, if one hundred,
if ten men whom I could name,—if ten *honest* men only,—aye, if
one Honest man, in this State of Massachusetts, *ceasing to hold
slaves,* were actually to withdraw from this copartnership, and be
locked up in the county jail therefor, it would be the abolition of
slavery in America. For it matters not how small the beginning
may seem to be: what is once well done is done for ever. But we
love better to talk about it: that we say is our mission. Reform
keeps many scores of newspapers in its service, but not one man.
If my esteemed neighbor, the State's ambassador, who will devote
his days to the settlement of the question of human rights in the
Council Chamber, instead of being threatened with the prisons of
Carolina, were to sit down the prisoner of Massachusetts, that
State which is so anxious to foist the sin of slavery upon her
sister,—though at present she can discover only an act of inhos-
pitality to be the ground of a quarrel with her,—the Legislature
would not wholly waive the subject the following winter.

Under a government which imprisons any unjustly, the true   22
place for a just man is also a prison. The proper place to-day, the
only place which Massachusetts has provided for her freer and
less desponding spirits, is in her prisons, to be put out and
locked out of the State by her own act, as they have already put

themselves out by their principles. It is there that the fugitive slave, and the Mexican prisoner on parole, and the Indian come to plead the wrongs of his race, should find them; on that separate, but more free and honorable ground, where the State places those who are not *with* her but *against* her,—the only house in a slave-state in which a free man can abide with honor. If any think that their influence would be lost there, and their voices no longer afflict the ear of the State, that they would not be as an enemy within its walls, they do not know by how much truth is stronger than error, nor how much more eloquently and effectively he can combat injustice who has experienced a little in his own person. Cast your whole vote, not a strip of paper merely, but your whole influence. A minority is powerless while it conforms to the majority; it is not even a minority then; but it is irresistible when it clogs by its whole weight. If the alternative is to keep all just men in prison, or give up war and slavery, the State will not hesitate which to choose. If a thousand men were not to pay their tax-bills this year, that would not be a violent and bloody measure, as it would be to pay them, and enable the State to commit violence and shed innocent blood. This is, in fact, the definition of a peaceable revolution, if any such is possible. If the tax-gatherer, or any other public officer, asks me, as one has done, "But what shall I do?" my answer is, "If you really wish to do any thing, resign your office." When the subject has refused allegiance, and the officer has resigned his office, then the revolution is accomplished. But even suppose blood should flow. Is there not a sort of blood shed when the conscience is wounded? Through this wound a man's real manhood and immortality flow out, and he bleeds to an everlasting death. I see this blood flowing now.

23   I have contemplated the imprisonment of the offender, rather than the seizure of his goods,—though both will serve the same purpose,—because they who assert the purest right, and consequently are most dangerous to a corrupt State, commonly have not spent much time in accumulating property. To such the State renders comparatively small service, and a slight tax is wont to appear exorbitant, particularly if they are obliged to earn it by special labor with their hands. If there were one who lived wholly without the use of money, the State itself would hesitate to demand it of him. But the rich man—not to make any invidious

comparison—is always sold to the institution which makes him rich. Absolutely speaking, the more money, the less virtue; for money comes between a man and his objects, and obtains them for him; and it was certainly no great virtue to obtain it. It puts to rest many questions which he would otherwise be taxed to answer; while the only new question which it puts is the hard but superfluous one, how to spend it. Thus his moral ground is taken from under his feet. The opportunities of living are diminished in proportion as what are called the "means" are increased. The best thing a man can do for his culture when he is rich is to endeavour to carry out those schemes which he entertained when he was poor. Christ answered the Herodians according to their condition. "Show me the tribute-money," said he;—and one took a penny out of his pocket;—If you use money which has the image of Caesar on it, and which he has made current and valuable, that is, *if you are men of the State,* and gladly enjoy the advantages of Caesar's government, then pay him back some of his own when he demands it; "Render therefore to Caesar that which is Caesar's, and to God those things which are God's,"—leaving them no wiser than before as to which was which; for they did not wish to know.

When I converse with the freest of my neighbors, I perceive 24 that, whatever they may say about the magnitude and seriousness of the question, and their regard for the public tranquility, the long and the short of the matter is, that they cannot spare the protection of the existing government, and they dread the consequences of disobedience to it to their property and families. For my own part, I should not like to think that I ever rely on the protection of the State. But, if I deny the authority of the State when it presents its tax-bill, it will soon take and waste all my property, and so harass me and my children without end. This is hard. This makes it impossible for a man to live honestly and at the same time comfortably in outward respects. It will not be worth the while to accumulate property; that would be sure to go again. You must hire or squat somewhere, and raise but a small crop, and eat that soon. You must live within yourself, and depend upon yourself, always tucked up and ready for a start, and not have many affairs. A man may grow rich in Turkey even, if he will be in all respects a good subject of the Turkish government.

Confucius said,—"If a State is governed by the principles of reason, poverty and misery are subjects of shame; if a State is not governed by the principles of reason, riches and honors are the subjects of shame." No: until I want the protection of Massachusetts to be extended to me in some distant southern port, where my liberty is endangered, or until I am bent solely on building up an estate at home by peaceful enterprise, I can afford to refuse allegiance to Massachusetts, and her right to my property and life. It costs me less in every sense to incur the penalty of disobedience to the State, than it would to obey. I should feel as if I were worth less in that case.

25   Some years ago, the State met me in behalf of the church, and commanded me to pay a certain sum toward the support of a clergyman whose preaching my father attended, but never I myself. "Pay it," it said, "or be locked up in the jail." I declined to pay. But, unfortunately, another man saw fit to pay it. I did not see why the schoolmaster should be taxed to support the priest, and not the priest the schoolmaster; for I was not the State's schoolmaster, but I supported myself by voluntary subscription. I did not see why the lyceum should not present its tax-bill, and have the State to back its demand, as well as the church. However, at the request of the selectmen, I condescended to make some such statement as this in writing:—"Know all men by these presents, that I, Henry Thoreau, do not wish to be regarded as a member of any incorporated society which I have not joined." This I gave to the town-clerk; and he has it. The State, having thus learned that I did not wish to be regarded as a member of that church, has never made a like demand on me since; though it said that it must adhere to its original presumption that time. If I had known how to name them, I should then have signed off in detail from all the societies which I never signed on to; but I did not know where to find a complete list.

26   I have paid no poll-tax for six years. I was put into a jail once on this account, for one night; and, as I stood considering the walls of solid stone, two or three feet thick, the door of wood and iron, a foot thick, and the iron grating which strained the light, I could not help being struck with the foolishness of that institution which treated me as if I were mere flesh and blood and bones, to be locked up. I wondered that it should have concluded at length

that this was the best use it could put me to, and had never thought to avail itself of my services in some way. I saw that, if there was a wall of stone between me and my towns-men, there was a still more difficult one to climb or break through, before they could get to be as free as I was. I did not for a moment feel confined, and the walls seemed a great waste of stone and mortar. I felt as if I alone of all my townsmen had paid my tax. They plainly did not know how to treat me, but behaved like persons who are underbred. In every threat and in every compliment there was a blunder; for they thought that my chief desire was to stand the other side of that stone wall. I could not but smile to see how industriously they locked the door on my meditations, which followed them out again without let or hinderance, and *they* were really all that was dangerous. As they could not reach me, they had resolved to punish my body; just as boys, if they cannot come at some person against whom they have a spite, will abuse his dog. I saw that the State was half-witted, that it was timid as a lone woman with her silver spoons, and that it did not know its friends from its foes, and I lost all my remaining respect for it, and pitied it.

Thus the State never intentionally confronts a man's sense, intellectual or moral, but only his body, his senses. It is not armed with superior wit or honesty, but with superior physical strength. I was not born to be forced. I will breathe after my own fashion. Let us see who is the strongest. What force has a multitude? They only can force me who obey a higher law than I. They force me to become like themselves. I do not hear of *men* being *forced* to live this way or that by masses of men. What sort of life were that to live? When I meet a government which says to me, "Your money or your life," why should I be in haste to give it my money? It may be in a great strait, and not know what to do: I cannot help that. It must help itself; do as I do. It is not worth the while to snivel about it. I am not responsible for the successful working of the machinery of society. I am not the son of the engineer. I perceive that, when an acorn and a chestnut fall side by side, the one does not remain inert to make way for the other, but both obey their own laws, and spring and grow and flourish as best they can, till one, perchance, overshadows and destroys the other. If a plant cannot live according to its nature, it dies; and so a man.

28   The night in prison was novel and interesting enough. The prisoners in their shirtsleeves were enjoying a chat and the evening air in the door-way, when I entered. But the jailer said, "Come, boys, it is time to lock up;" and so they dispersed, and I heard the sound of their steps returning into the hollow apartments. My room-mate was introduced to me by the jailer, as "a first-rate fellow and a clever man." When the door was locked, he showed me where to hang my hat, and how he managed matters there. The rooms were whitewashed once a month; and this one, at least, was the whitest, most simply furnished, and probably the neatest apartment in the town. He naturally wanted to know where I came from, and what brought me there; and, when I had told him, I asked him in my turn how he came there, presuming him to be an honest man, of course; and, as the world goes, I believe he was. "Why," said he, "they accuse me of burning a barn; but I never did it." As near as I could discover, he had probably gone to bed in a barn when drunk, and smoked his pipe there; and so a barn was burnt. He had the reputation of being a clever man, had been there some three months waiting for his trial to come on, and would have to wait as much longer; but he was quite domesticated and contented, since he got his board for nothing, and thought that he was well treated.

29   He occupied one window, and I the other; and I saw, that if one stayed there long, his principal business would be to look out the window. I had soon read all the tracts that were left there, and examined where former prisoners had broken out, and where a grate had been sawed off, and heard the history of the various occupants of that room; for I found that even here there was a history and a gossip which never circulated beyond the walls of the jail. Probably this is the only house in the town where verses are composed, which are afterward printed in a circular form, but not published. I was shown quite a long list of verses which were composed by some young men who had been detected in an attempt to escape, who avenged themselves by singing them.

30   I pumped my fellow-prisoner as dry as I could, for fear I should never see him again; but at length he showed me which was my bed, and left me to blow out the lamp.

31   It was like travelling into a far country, such as I had never expected to behold, to lie there for one night. It seemed to me that

I never had heard the town-clock strike before, nor the evening sounds of the village; for we slept with the windows open, which were inside the grating. It was to see my native village in the light of the middle ages, and our Concord was turned into a Rhine stream, and visions of knights and castles passed before me. They were the voices of old burghers that I heard in the streets. I was an involuntary spectator and auditor of whatever was done and said in the kitchen of the adjacent village-inn,—a wholly new and rare experience to me. It was a closer view of my native town. I was fairly inside of it. I never had seen its institutions before. This is one of its peculiar institutions; for it is a shire town. I began to comprehend what its inhabitants were about.

In the morning, our breakfasts were put through the hole in 32 the door, in small oblong-square tin pans, made to fit, and holding a pint of chocolate, with brown bread, and an iron spoon. When they called for the vessels again, I was green enough to return what bread I had left; but my comrade seized it, and said that I should lay that up for lunch or dinner. Soon after, he was let out to work at haying in a neighboring field, whither he went every day, and would not be back till noon; so he bade me good-day, saying that he doubted if he should see me again.

When I came out of prison,—for some one interfered, and 33 paid the tax,—I did not perceive that great changes had taken place on the common, such as he observed who went in a youth, and emerged a tottering and gray-headed man; and yet a change had to my eyes come over the scene,—the town, and State, and country,—greater than any that mere time could effect. I saw yet more distinctly the State in which I lived. I saw to what extent the people among whom I lived could be trusted as good neighbors and friends; that their friendship was for summer weather only; that they did not greatly purpose to do right; that they were a distinct race from me by their prejudices and superstitions, as the Chinamen and Malays are; that, in their sacrifices to humanity, they ran no risks, not even to their property; that, after all, they were not so noble but they treated the thief as he had treated them, and hoped, by a certain outward observance and a few prayers, and by walking in a particular straight though useless path from time to time, to save their souls. This may be to judge my neighbors harshly; for I believe that most of them are not aware that they have such an institution as the jail in their village.

34   It was formerly the custom in our village, when a poor debtor came out of jail, for his acquaintances to salute him, looking through their fingers, which were crossed to represent the grating of a jail window, "How do ye do?" My neighbors did not thus salute me, but first looked at me, and then at one another, as if I had returned from a long journey. I was put into jail as I was going to the shoemaker's to get a shoe which was mended. When I was let out the next morning, I proceeded to finish my errand, and, having put on my mended shoe, joined a huckleberry party, who were impatient to put themselves under my conduct; and in half an hour,—for the horse was soon tackled,—was in the midst of a huckleberry field, on one of our highest hills, two miles off; and then the State was nowhere to be seen.

35   This is the whole history of "My Prisons."

36   I have never declined paying the highway tax, because I am as desirous of being a good neighbor as I am of being a bad subject; and, as for supporting schools, I am doing my part to educate my fellow-countrymen now. It is for no particular item in the tax-bill that I refuse to pay it. I simply wish to refuse allegiance to the State, to withdraw and stand aloof from it effectually. I do not care to trace the course of my dollar, if I could, till it buys a man, or a musket to shoot one with,—the dollar is innocent,—but I am concerned to trace the effects of my allegiance. In fact, I quietly declare war with the State, after my fashion, though I will still make what use and get what advantage of her I can, as is usual in such cases.

37   If others pay the tax which is demanded of me, from a sympathy with the State, they do but what they have already done in their own case, or rather they abet injustice to a greater extent than the State requires. If they pay the tax from a mistaken interest in the individual taxed, to save his property or prevent his going to jail, it is because they have not considered wisely how far they let their private feelings interfere with the public good.

38   This, then, is my position at present. But one cannot be too much on his guard in such a case, lest his action be biassed by obstinacy, or an undue regard for the opinions of men. Let him see that he does only what belongs to himself and to the hour.

I think sometimes, Why, this people mean well; they are only 39
ignorant; they would do better if they knew how: why give your
neighbors this pain to treat you as they are not inclined to? But I
think, again, this is no reason why I should do as they do, or
permit others to suffer much greater pain of a different kind.
Again, I sometimes say to myself, When many millions of men,
without heat, without ill-will, without personal feeling of any
kind, demand of you a few shillings only, without the possibility,
such is their constitution, of retracting or altering their present
demand, and without the possibility, on your side, of appeal to
any other millions, why expose yourself to this overwhelming
brute force? You do not resist cold and hunger, the winds and the
waves, thus obstinately; you quietly submit to a thousand similar
necessities. You do not put your head into the fire. But just in
proportion as I regard this as not wholly a brute force, but partly
a human force, and consider that I have relations to those millions
as to so many millions of men, and not of mere brute or inanimate things, I see that appeal is possible, first and instantaneously,
from them to the Maker of them, and, secondly, from them to
themselves. But, if I put my head deliberately into the fire, there
is no appeal to fire or to the Maker of fire, and I have only
myself to blame. If I could convince myself that I have any right
to be satisfied with men as they are, and to treat them accordingly, and not according, in some respects, to my requisitions
and expectations of what they and I ought to be, then, like a good
Mussulman and fatalist, I should endeavor to be satisfied with
things as they are, and say it is the will of God. And, above all,
there is this difference between resisting this and a purely brute
or natural force, that I can resist this with some effect; but I cannot
expect, like Orpheus, to change the nature of the rocks and trees
and beasts.

I do not wish to quarrel with any man or nation. I do not 40
wish to split hairs, to make fine distinctions, or set myself up as
better than my neighbors. I seek rather, I may say, even an excuse
for conforming to the laws of the land. I am but too ready to
conform to them. Indeed I have reason to suspect myself on this
head; and each year, as the tax-gatherer comes round, I find
myself disposed to review the acts and position of the general
and state governments, and the spirit of the people, to discover

a pretext for conformity. I believe that the State will soon be able to take all my work of this sort out of my hands, and then I shall be no better a patriot than my fellow-countrymen. Seen from a lower point of view, the Constitution, with all its faults, is very good; the law and the courts are very respectable; even this State and this American government are, in many respects, very admirable and rare things, to be thankful for, such as a great many have described them; but seen from a point of view a little higher, they are what I have described them; seen from a higher still, and the highest, who shall say what they are, or that they are worth looking at or thinking of at all?

41   However, the government does not concern me much, and I shall bestow the fewest possible thoughts on it. It is not many moments that I live under a government, even in this world. If a man is thought-free, fancy-free, imagination-free, that which is *not* never for a long time appearing *to be* to him, unwise rulers or reformers cannot fatally interrupt him.

42   I know that most men think differently from myself; but those whose lives are by profession devoted to the study of these or kindred subjects, content me as little as any. Statesmen and legislators, standing so completely within the institution, never distinctly and nakedly behold it. They speak of moving society, but have no resting-place without it. They may be men of a certain experience and discrimination, and have no doubt invented ingenious and even useful systems, for which we sincerely thank them; but all their wit and usefulness lie within certain not very wide limits. They are wont to forget that the world is not governed by policy and expediency. Webster never goes behind government, and so cannot speak with authority about it. His words are wisdom to those legislators who contemplate no essential reform in the existing government; but for thinkers, and those who legislate for all time, he never once glances at the subject. I know of those whose serene and wise speculations on this theme would soon reveal the limits of his mind's range and hospitality. Yet, compared with the cheap professions of most reformers, and the still cheaper wisdom and eloquence of politicians in general, his are almost the only sensible and valuable words, and we thank Heaven for him. Comparatively, he is always strong, original, and, above all,

practical. Still his quality is not wisdom, but prudence. The lawyer's truth is not Truth, but consistency, or a consistent expediency. Truth is always in harmony with herself, and is not concerned chiefly to reveal the justice that may consist with wrong-doing. He well deserves to be called, as he has been called, the Defender of the Constitution. There are really no blows to be given by him but defensive ones. He is not a leader, but a follower. His leaders are the men of '87. "I have never made an effort," he says, "and never propose to make an effort; I have never countenanced an effort, and never mean to countenance an effort, to disturb the arrangement as originally made, by which the various States came into the Union." Still thinking of the sanction which the Constitution gives to slavery, he says, "Because it was a part of the original compact,—let it stand." Notwithstanding his special acuteness and ability, he is unable to take a fact out of its merely political relations, and behold it as it lies absolutely to be disposed of by the intellect,—what, for instance, it behoves a man to do here in America to-day with regard to slavery, but ventures, or is driven, to make some such desperate answer as the following, while professing to speak absolutely, and as a private man,—from which what new and singular code of social duties might be inferred?—"The manner," says he, "in which the government of those States where slavery exists are to regulate it, is for their own consideration, under their responsibility to their constituents, to the general laws of propriety, humanity, and justice, and to God. Associations formed elsewhere, springing from a feeling of humanity, or any other cause, have nothing whatever to do with it. They have never received any encouragement from me, and they never will."

They who know of no purer sources of truth, who have traced   43
up its stream no higher, stand, and wisely stand, by the Bible and the Constitution, and drink at it there with reverence and humility; but they who behold where it comes trickling into this lake or that pool, gird up their loins once more, and continue their pilgrimage toward its fountain-head.

No man with a genius for legislation has appeared in   44
America. They are rare in the history of the world. There are orators, politicians, and eloquent men, by the thousand; but the speaker has not yet opened his mouth to speak, who is capable

of settling the much-vexed questions of the day. We love eloquence for its own sake, and not for any truth which it may utter, or any heroism it may inspire. Our legislators have not yet learned the comparative value of free-trade and of freedom, of union, and of rectitude, to a nation. They have no genius or talent for comparatively humble questions of taxation and finance, commerce and manufactures and agriculture. If we were left solely to the wordy wit of legislators in Congress for our guidance, uncorrected by the seasonable experience and the effectual complaints of the people, America would not long retain her rank among the nations. For eighteen hundred years, though perchance I have no right to say it, the New Testament, has been written; yet where is the legislator who has wisdom and practical talent enough to avail himself of the light which it sheds on the science of legislation?

45   The authority of government, even such as I am willing to submit to,—for I will cheerfully obey those who know and can do better than I, and in many things even those who neither know nor can do so well,—is still an impure one: to be strictly just, it must have the sanction and consent of the governed. It can have no pure right over my person and property but what I concede to it. The progress from an absolute to a limited monarchy, from a limited monarchy to a democracy, is a progress toward a true respect for the individual. Is a democracy, such as we know it, the last improvement possible in government? Is it not possible to take a step further towards recognizing and organizing the rights of man? There will never be a really free and enlightened State, until the State comes to recognize the individual as a higher and independent power, from which all its own power and authority are derived, and treats him accordingly. I please myself with imagining a State at last which can afford to be just to all men, and to treat the individual with respect as a neighbor; which even would not think it inconsistent with its own repose, if a few were to live aloof from it, not meddling with it, nor embraced by it, who fulfilled all the duties of neighbors and fellow-men. A State which bore this kind of fruit, and suffered it to drop off as fast as it ripened, would prepare the way for a still more perfect and glorious State, which also I have imagined, but not yet anywhere seen.

Letter from Birmingham Jail

Martin Luther King, Jr.

My dear Fellow Clergymen,

While confined here in the Birmingham city jail, I came across 1
your recent statement calling our present activities "unwise and
untimely." Seldom, if ever, do I pause to answer criticism of my
work and ideas. If I sought to answer all of the criticisms that
cross my desk, my secretaries would be engaged in little else in
the course of the day, and I would have no time for constructive
work. But since I feel that you are men of genuine good will and
your criticisms are sincerely set forth, I would like to answer your
statement in what I hope will be patient and reasonable terms.

I think I should give the reason for my being in Birmingham, 2
since you have been influenced by the argument of "outsiders
coming in." I have the honor of serving as president of the Southern Christian Leadership Conference, an organization operating in
every southern state, with headquarters in Atlanta, Georgia. We
have some eighty-five affiliate organizations all across the South—
one being the Alabama Christian Movement for Human Rights.
Whenever necessary and possible we share staff, educational and
financial resources with our affiliates. Several months ago our
local affiliate here in Birmingham invited us to be on call to
engage in a nonviolent direct-action program if such were deemed
necessary. We readily consented and when the hour came we
lived up to our promises. So I am here, along with several
members of my staff, because we were invited here. I am here
because I have basic organizational ties here.

Beyond this, I am in Birmingham because injustice is here. Just 3
as the eighth century prophets left their little villages and carried
their "thus saith the Lord" far beyond the boundaries of their
hometowns; and just as the Apostle Paul left his little village of
Tarsus and carried the gospel of Jesus Christ to practically every
hamlet and city of the Graeco-Roman world, I too am compelled
to carry the gospel of freedom beyond my particular hometown.
Like Paul, I must constantly respond to the Macedonian call for aid.

Moreover, I am cognizant of the interrelatedness of all 4
communities and states. I cannot sit idly by in Atlanta and not be

concerned about what happens in Birmingham. Injustice anywhere is a threat to justice everywhere. We are caught in an
inescapable network of mutuality, tied in a single garment of
destiny. Whatever affects one directly affects all indirectly. Never
again can we afford to live with the narrow, provincial "outside
agitator" idea. Anyone who lives in the United States can never
be considered an outsider anywhere in this country.

5   You deplore the demonstrations that are presently taking
place in Birmingham. But I am sorry that your statement did not
express a similar concern for the conditions that brought the
demonstrations into being. I am sure that each of you would want
to go beyond the superficial social analyst who looks merely at
effects, and does not grapple with underlying causes. I would not
hesitate to say that it is unfortunate that so-called demonstrations
are taking place in Birmingham at this time, but I would say in
more emphatic terms that it is even more unfortunate that the
white power structure of this city left the Negro community with
no other alternative.

6   In any nonviolent campaign there are four basic steps: (1) collection of the facts to determine whether injustices are alive,
(2) negotiation, (3) self-purification, and (4) direct action. We have
gone through all of these steps in Birmingham. There can be no
gainsaying of the fact that racial injustice engulfs this community.

7   Birmingham is probably the most thoroughly segregated city
in the United States. Its ugly record of police brutality is known
in every section of this country. Its injust treatment of Negroes in
the courts is a notorious reality. There have been more unsolved
bombings of Negro homes and churches in Birmingham than any
city in this nation. These are the hard, brutal and unbelievable
facts. On the basis of these conditions Negro leaders sought to
negotiate with the city fathers. But the political leaders consistently refused to engage in good faith negotiation.

8   Then came the opportunity last September to talk with some
of the leaders of the economic community. In these negotiating
sessions certain promises were made by the merchants—such as
the promise to remove the humiliating racial signs from the
stores. On the basis of these promises Rev. Shuttlesworth and the
leaders of the Alabama Christian Movement for Human Rights
agreed to call a moratorium on any type of demonstrations. As

the weeks and months unfolded we realized that we were the victims of a broken promise. The signs remained. Like so many experiences of the past we were confronted with blasted hopes, and the dark shadow of a deep disappointment settled upon us. So we had no alternative except that of preparing for direct action, whereby we would present our very bodies as a means of laying our case before the conscience of the local and national community. We were not unmindful of the difficulties involved. So we decided to go through a process of self-purification. We started having workshops on nonviolence and repeatedly asked ourselves the questions, "Are you able to accept blows without retaliating?" "Are you able to endure the ordeals of jail?" We decided to set our direct-action program around the Easter season, realizing that with the exception of Christmas, this was the largest shopping period of the year. Knowing that a strong economic withdrawal program would be the by-product of direct action, we felt that this was the best time to bring pressure on the merchants for the needed changes. Then it occurred to us that the March election was ahead and so we speedily decided to postpone action until after election day. When we discovered that Mr. Connor was in the run-off, we decided again to postpone action so that the demonstrations could not be used to cloud the issues. At this time we agreed to begin our nonviolent witness the day after the run-off.

This reveals that we did not move irresponsibly into direct 9 action. We too wanted to see Mr. Connor defeated; so we went through postponement after postponement to aid in this community need. After this we felt that direct action could be delayed no longer.

You may well ask, "Why direct action? Why sit-ins, marches, 10 etc.? Isn't negotiation a better path?" You are exactly right in your call for negotiation. Indeed, this is the purpose of direct action. Nonviolent direct action seeks to create such a crisis and establish such creative tension that a community that has constantly refused to negotiate is forced to confront the issue. It seeks so to dramatize the issue that it can no longer be ignored. I just referred to the creation of tension as a part of the work of the nonviolent resister. This may sound rather shocking. But I must confess that I am not afraid of the word tension. I have earnestly worked and preached against violent tension, but there is a type of constructive nonviolent tension that is necessary for growth. Just as Socrates felt that it was necessary to create a tension in the mind so that individuals could rise from the bondage of myths and half-truths to the unfettered realm of creative analysis and objective appraisal, we must see the need of having nonviolent gadflies to create the kind of tension in society that will help men to rise from the dark depths of prejudice and racism to the majestic heights of understanding and brotherhood. So the purpose of the direct action is to create a situation so crisis-packed that it will inevitably open the door to negotiation. We, therefore, concur with you in your call for negotiation. Too long has our beloved Southland been bogged down in the tragic attempt to live in monologue rather than dialogue.

11   One of the basic points in your statement is that our acts are untimely. Some have asked, "Why didn't you give the new administration time to act?" The only answer that I can give to this inquiry is that the new administration must be prodded about as much as the outgoing one before it acts. We will be sadly mistaken if we feel that the election of Mr. Boutwell will bring the millennium to Birmingham. While Mr. Boutwell is much more articulate and gentle than Mr. Connor, they are both segregationists, dedicated to the task of maintaining the status quo. The hope I see in Mr. Boutwell is that he will be reasonable enough to see the futility of massive resistance to desegregation. But he will not see this without pressure from the devotees of civil rights. My friends, I must say to you that we have not made a single gain in civil rights without determined legal and nonviolent pressure. History is the long and tragic story of the fact that privileged groups seldom give up their privileges voluntarily. Individuals may see the moral light and voluntarily give up their unjust posture; but as Reinhold Niebuhr has reminded us, groups are more immoral than individuals.

12   We know through painful experience that freedom is never voluntarily given by the oppressor; it must be demanded by the oppressed. Frankly, I have never yet engaged in a direct action movement that was "well-timed," according to the timetable of those who have not suffered unduly from the disease of segregation. For years now I have heard the words "Wait!" It rings in the

ear of every Negro with a piercing familiarity. This "Wait" has almost always meant "Never." It has been a tranquilizing thalidomide, relieving the emotional stress for a moment, only to give birth to an ill-formed infant of frustration. We must come to see with the distinguished jurist of yesterday that "justice too long delayed is justice denied." We have waited for more than 340 years for our constitutional and God-given rights. The nations of Asia and Africa are moving with jetlike speed toward the goal of political independence, and we still creep at horse and buggy pace toward the gaining of a cup of coffee at a lunch counter. I guess it is easy for those who have never felt the stinging darts of segregation to say, "Wait." But when you have seen vicious mobs lynch your mothers and fathers at will and drown your sisters and brothers at whim; when you have seen hate-filled policemen curse, kick, brutalize and even kill your black brothers and sisters with impunity; when you see the vast majority of your twenty million Negro brothers smothering in an airtight cage of poverty in the midst of an affluent society; when you suddenly find your tongue twisted and your speech stammering as you seek to explain to your six-year-old daughter why she can't go to the public amusement park that has just been advertised on television, and see tears welling up in her little eyes when she is told that Funtown is closed to colored children, and see the depressing clouds of inferiority begin to form in her little mental sky, and see her begin to distort her little personality by unconsciously developing a bitterness toward white people; when you have to concoct an answer for a five-year-old son asking in agonizing pathos: "Daddy, why do white people treat colored people so mean?"; when you take a cross-country drive and find it necessary to sleep night after night in the uncomfortable corners of your automobile because no motel will accept you; when you are humiliated day in and day out by nagging signs reading "white" and "colored"; when your first name becomes "nigger" and your middle name becomes "boy" (however old you are) and your last name becomes "John," and when your wife and mother are never given the respected title "Mrs."; when you are harried by day and haunted by night by the fact that you are a Negro, living constantly at tiptoe stance never quite knowing what to expect next, and plagued with inner fears and outer resentments; when you are forever fighting a degenerating sense of "nobodiness"; then you will understand why we find it difficult to wait. There comes a time when the cup of endurance runs over, and men are no longer willing to be plunged into an abyss of injustice where they experience the blackness of corroding despair. I hope, sirs, you can understand our legitimate and unavoidable impatience.

13   You express a great deal of anxiety over our willingness to break laws. This is certainly a legitimate concern. Since we so diligently urge people to obey the Supreme Court's decision of 1954 outlawing segregation in the public schools, it is rather strange and paradoxical to find us consciously breaking laws. One may well ask, "How can you advocate breaking some laws and obeying others?" The answer is found in the fact that there are two types of laws: there are *just* and there are *unjust* laws. I would agree with Saint Augustine that "An unjust law is no law at all."

14   Now what is the difference between the two? How does one determine when a law is just or unjust? A just law is a man-made code that squares with the moral law or the law of God. An unjust law is a code that is out of harmony with the moral law. To put it in the terms of Saint Thomas Aquinas, an unjust law is a human law that is not rooted in eternal and natural law. Any law that uplifts human personality is just. Any law that degrades human personality is unjust. All segregation statutes are unjust because segregation distorts the soul and damages the personality. It gives the segregator a false sense of superiority, and the segregated a false sense of inferiority. To use the words of Martin Buber, the great Jewish philosopher, segregation substitutes an "I–it" relationship for the "I–thou" relationship, and ends up relegating persons to the status of things. So segregation is not only politically, economically and sociologically unsound, but it is morally wrong and sinful. Paul Tillich has said that sin is separation. Isn't segregation an existential expression of man's tragic separation, an expression of his awful estrangement, his terrible sinfulness? So I can urge men to disobey segregation ordinances because they are morally wrong.

15   Let us turn to a more concrete example of just and unjust laws. An unjust law is a code that a majority inflicts on a minority that is not binding on itself. This is difference made legal. On the other hand a just law is a code that a majority compels a

minority to follow that it is willing to follow itself. This is sameness made legal.

Let me give another explanation. An unjust law is a code 16 inflicted upon a minority which that minority had no part in enacting or creating because they did not have the unhampered right to vote. Who can say that the legislature of Alabama which set up the segregation laws was democratically elected? Throughout the state of Alabama all types of conniving methods are used to prevent Negroes from becoming registered voters and there are some counties without a single Negro registered to vote despite the fact that the Negro constitutes a majority of the population. Can any law set up in such a state be considered democratically structured?

These are just a few examples of unjust and just laws. There 17 are some instances when a law is just on its face and unjust in its application. For instance, I was arrested Friday on a charge of parading without a permit. Now there is nothing wrong with an ordinance which requires a permit for a parade, but when the ordinance is used to preserve segregation and to deny citizens the First Amendment privilege of peaceful assembly and peaceful protest, then it becomes unjust.

I hope you can see the distinction I am trying to point out. In 18 no sense do I advocate evading or defying the law as the rabid segregationist would do. This would lead to anarchy. One who breaks an unjust law must do it *openly, lovingly* (not hatefully as the white mothers did in New Orleans when they were seen on television screaming, "nigger, nigger, nigger"), and with a willingness to accept the penalty. I submit that an individual who breaks a law that conscience tells him is unjust, and willingly accepts the penalty by staying in jail to arouse the conscience of the community over its injustice, is in reality expressing the very highest respect for law.

Of course, there is nothing new about this kind of civil dis- 19 obedience. It was seen sublimely in the refusal of Shadrach, Meshach and Abednego to obey the laws of Nebuchadnezzar because a higher moral law was involved. It was practiced superbly by the early Christians who were willing to face hungry lions and the excruciating pain of chopping blocks, before submitting to certain unjust laws of the Roman Empire. To a degree academic freedom is a reality today because Socrates practiced civil disobedience.

20   We can never forget that everything Hitler did in Germany was "legal" and everything the Hungarian freedom fighters did in Hungary was "illegal." It was "illegal" to aid and comfort a Jew in Hitler's Germany. But I am sure that if I had lived in Germany during that time I would have aided and comforted my Jewish brothers even though it was illegal. If I lived in a Communist country today where certain principles dear to the Christian faith are suppressed, I believe I would openly advocate disobeying these anti-religious laws. I must make two honest confessions to you, my Christian and Jewish brothers. First, I must confess that over the last few years I have been gravely disappointed with the white moderate. I have almost reached the regrettable conclusion that the Negro's great stumbling block in the stride toward freedom is not the White Citizen's Counciler or the Ku Klux Klanner, but the white moderate who is more devoted to "order" than to justice; who prefers a negative peace which is the absence of tension to a positive peace which is the presence of justice; who constantly says, "I agree with you in the goal you seek, but I can't agree with your methods of direct action"; who paternalistically feels that he can set the timetable for another man's freedom; who lives by the myth of time and who constantly advised the Negro to wait until a "more convenient season." Shallow understanding from people of good will is more frustrating than absolute misunderstanding from people of ill will. Lukewarm acceptance is much more bewildering than outright rejection.

21   I had hoped that the white moderate would understand that law and order exist for the purpose of establishing justice, and that when they fail to do this they become dangerously structured dams that block the flow of social progress. I had hoped that the white moderate would understand that the present tension of the South is merely a necessary phase of the transition from an obnoxious negative peace, where the Negro passively accepted his unjust plight, to a substance-filled positive peace, where all men will respect the dignity and worth of human personality. Actually, we who engage in nonviolent direct action are not the creators of tension. We merely bring to the surface the hidden tension that is

already alive. We bring it out in the open where it can be seen and dealt with. Like a boil that can never be cured as long as it is covered up but must be opened with all its pus-flowing ugliness to the natural medicines of air and light, injustice must likewise be exposed, with all of the tension its exposing creates, to the light of human conscience and the air of national opinion before it can be cured.

In your statement you asserted that our actions, even though peaceful, must be condemned because they precipitate violence. But can this assertion be logically made? Isn't this like condemning the robbed man because his possession of money precipitated the evil act of robbery? Isn't this like condemning Socrates because his unswerving commitment to truth and his philosophical delvings precipitated the misguided popular mind to make him drink the hemlock? Isn't this like condemning Jesus because His unique God-consciousness and never-ceasing devotion to His will precipitated the evil act of crucifixion? We must come to see, as federal courts have consistently affirmed, that it is immoral to urge an individual to withdraw his efforts to gain his basic constitutional rights because the quest precipitates violence. Society must protect the robbed and punish the robber.

I had also hoped that the white moderate would reject the myth of time. I received a letter this morning from a white brother in Texas which said: "All Christians know that the colored people will receive equal rights eventually, but it is possible that you are in too great of a religious hurry. It has taken Christianity almost two thousand years to accomplish what it has. The teachings of Christ take time to come to earth." All that is said here grows out of a tragic misconception of time. It is the strangely irrational notion that there is something in the very flow of time that will inevitably cure all ills. Actually time is neutral. It can be used either destructively or constructively. I am coming to feel that the people of ill will have used time much more effectively than the people of good will. We will have to repent in this generation not merely for the vitriolic words and actions of the bad people, but for the appalling silence of the good people. We must come to see that human progress never rolls in on wheels of inevitability. It comes through the tireless efforts and persistent work of men willing to be co-workers with God, and without this hard work time itself becomes an ally of the forces of social stagnation. We must use time creatively, and forever realize that the time is always ripe to do right. Now is the time to make real the promise of democracy, and transform our pending national elegy into a creative psalm of brotherhood. Now is the time to lift our national policy from the quicksand of racial injustice to the solid rock of human dignity.

24   You spoke of our activity in Birmingham as extreme. At first I was rather disappointed that fellow clergymen would see my nonviolent efforts as those of the extremist. I started thinking about the fact that I stand in the middle of two opposing forces in the Negro community. One is a force of complacency made up of Negroes who, as a result of long years of oppression, have been so completely drained of self-respect and a sense of "somebodiness" that they have adjusted to segregation, and, of a few Negroes in the middle class who, because of a degree of academic and economic security, and because at points they profit by segregation, have unconsciously become insensitive to the problems of the masses. The other force is one of bitterness and hatred, and comes perilously close to advocating violence. It is expressed in the various black nationalist groups that are springing up over the nation, the largest and best known being Elijah Muhammad's Muslim movement. This movement is nourished by the contemporary frustration over the continued existence of racial discrimination. It is made up of people who have lost faith in America, who have absolutely repudiated Christianity, and who have concluded that the white man is an incurable "devil." I have tried to stand between these two forces, saying that we need not follow the "do-nothingism" of the complacent or the hatred and despair of the black nationalist. There is the more excellent way of love and nonviolent protest. I'm grateful to God that, through the Negro church, the dimension of nonviolence entered our struggle. If this philosophy had not emerged, I am convinced that by now many streets of the South would be flowing with floods of blood. And I am further convinced that if our white brothers dismiss us as "rabble-rousers" and "outside agitators" those of us who are working through the channels of nonviolent direct action and refuse to support our nonviolent efforts, millions of Negroes, out of frustration and despair, will seek solace and security in black

nationalist ideologies, a development that will lead inevitably to a frightening racial nightmare.

Oppressed people cannot remain oppressed forever. The urge for freedom will eventually come. This is what happened to the American Negro. Something within has reminded him of his birthright of freedom; something without has reminded him that he can gain it. Consciously and unconsciously, he has been swept in by what the Germans call the *Zeitgeist,* and with his black brothers of Africa, and his brown and yellow brothers of Asia, South America and the Caribbean, he is moving with a sense of cosmic urgency toward the promised land of racial justice. Recognizing this vital urge that has engulfed the Negro community, one should readily understand public demonstrations. The Negro has many pent-up resentments and latent frustrations. He has to get them out. So let him march sometime; let him have his prayer pilgrimages to the city hall; understand why he must have sit-ins and freedom rides. If his repressed emotions do not come out in these nonviolent ways, they will come out in ominous expressions of violence. This is not a threat; it is a fact of history. So I have not said to my people "get rid of your discontent." But I have tried to say that this normal and healthy discontent can be channelized through the creative outlet of nonviolent direct action. Now this approach is being dismissed as extremist. I must admit that I was initially disappointed in being so categorized.

But as I continued to think about the matter I gradually gained a bit of satisfaction from being considered an extremist. Was not Jesus an extremist in love—"Love your enemies, bless them that curse you, pray for them that despitefully use you." Was not Amos an extremist for justice—"Let justice roll down like waters and righteousness like a mighty stream." Was not Paul an extremist for the gospel of Jesus Christ—"I bear in my body the marks of the Lord Jesus." Was not Martin Luther an extremist— "Here I stand; I can do none other so help me God." Was not John Bunyan an extremist—"I will stay in jail to the end of my days before I make a butchery of my conscience." Was not Abraham Lincoln an extremist—"This nation cannot survive half slave and half free." Was not Thomas Jefferson an extremist—"We hold these truths to be self-evident, that all men are created equal." So the question is not whether we will be extremist but what kind of extremist will we be. Will we be extremists for hate or will we be extremists for love? Will we be extremists for the preservation of injustice—or will we be extremists for the cause of justice? In that dramatic scene on Calvary's hill, three men were crucified. We must not forget that all three were crucified for the same crime—the crime of extremism. Two were extremists for immorality, and thusly fell below their environment. The other, Jesus Christ, was an extremist for love, truth and goodness, and thereby rose above his environment. So, after all, maybe the South, the nation and the world are in dire need of creative extremists.

27   I had hoped that the white moderate would see this. Maybe I was too optimistic. Maybe I expected too much. I guess I should have realized that few members of a race that has oppressed another race can understand or appreciate the deep groans and passionate yearnings of those that have been oppressed and still fewer have the vision to see that injustice must be rooted out by strong, persistent and determined action. I am thankful, however, that some of our white brothers have grasped the meaning of this social revolution and committed themselves to it. They are still all too small in quantity, but they are big in quality. Some like Ralph McGill, Lillian Smith, Harry Golden and James Dabbs have written about our struggle in eloquent, prophetic and understanding terms. Others have marched with us down nameless streets of the South. They have languished in filthy roach-infested jails, suffering the abuse and brutality of angry policemen who see them as "dirty nigger-lovers." They, unlike so many of their moderate brothers and sisters, have recognized the urgency of the moment and sensed the need for powerful "action" antidotes to combat the disease of segregation.

28   Let me rush on to mention my other disappointment. I have been so greatly disappointed with the white church and its leadership. Of course, there are some notable exceptions. I am not unmindful of the fact that each of you has taken some significant stands on this issue. I commend you, Rev. Stallings, for your Christian stance on this past Sunday, in welcoming Negroes to your worship service on a non-segregated basis. I commend the Catholic leaders of this state for integrating Springhill College several years ago.

29   But despite these notable exceptions I must honestly reiterate that I have been disappointed with the church. I do not say that

as one of the negative critics who can always find something wrong with the church. I say it as a minister of the gospel, who loves the church; who was nurtured in its bosom; who has been sustained by its spiritual blessings and who will remain true to it as long as the cord of life shall lengthen.

I had the strange feeling when I was suddenly catapulted into the leadership of the bus protest in Montgomery several years ago that we would have the support of the white church. I felt that the white ministers, priests and rabbis of the South would be some of our strongest allies. Instead, some have been outright opponents, refusing to understand the freedom movement and misrepresenting its leaders; all too many others have been more cautious than courageous and have remained silent behind the anesthetizing security of the stained-glass windows.

In spite of my shattered dreams of the past, I came to Birmingham with the hope that the white religious leadership of this community would see the justice of our cause, and with, deep moral concern, serve as the channel through which our just grievances would get to the power structure. I had hoped that each of you would understand. But again I have been disappointed. I have heard numerous religious leaders of the South call upon their worshippers to comply with a desegregation decision because it is the *law*, but I have longed to hear white ministers say, "Follow this decree because integration is morally *right* and the Negro is your brother." In the midst of blatant injustices inflicted upon the Negro, I have watched white churches stand on the sideline and merely mouth pious irrelevancies and sanctimonious trivialities. In the midst of a mighty struggle to rid our nation of racial and economic injustice, I have heard so many ministers say, "Those are social issues with which the gospel has no real concern," and I have watched so many churches commit themselves to a completely otherwordly religion which made a strange distinction between body and soul, the sacred and the secular.

So here we are moving toward the exit of the twentieth century with a religious community largely adjusted to the status quo, standing as a taillight behind other community agencies rather than a headlight leading men to higher levels of justice.

I have traveled the length and breadth of Alabama, Mississippi and all the other southern states. On sweltering summer days and crisp autumn mornings I have looked at her beautiful churches with their lofty spires pointing heavenward. I have beheld the impressive outlay of her massive religious education buildings. Over and over again I have found myself asking: "What kind of people worship here? Who is their God? Where were their voices when the lips of Governor Barnett dripped with words of interposition and nullification? Where were they when Governor Wallace gave the clarion call for defiance and hatred? Where were their voices of support when tired, bruised and weary Negro men and women decided to rise from the dark dungeons of complacency to the bright hills of creative protest?"

34   Yes, these questions are still in my mind. In deep disappointment, I have wept over the laxity of the church. But be assured that my tears have been tears of love. There can be no deep disappointment where there is not deep love. Yes, I love the church; I love her sacred walls. How could I do otherwise? I am in the rather unique position of being the son, the grandson and the great-grandson of preachers. Yes, I see the church as the body of Christ. But, oh! How we have blemished and scarred that body through social neglect and fear of being nonconformists.

35   There was a time when the church was very powerful. It was during that period when the early Christians rejoiced when they were deemed worthy to suffer for what they believed. In those days the church was not merely a thermometer that recorded the ideas and principles of popular opinion; it was a thermostat that transformed the mores of society. Wherever the early Christians entered a town the power structure got disturbed and immediately sought to convict them for being "disturbers of the peace" and "outside agitators." But they went on with the conviction that they were "a colony of heaven," and had to obey God rather than man. They were small in number but big in commitment. They were too God-intoxicated to be "astronomically intimidated." They brought an end to such ancient evils as infanticide and gladiatorial contest.

36   Things are different now. The contemporary church is often a weak, ineffectual voice with an uncertain sound. It is so often the arch-supporter of the status quo. Far from being disturbed by the presence of the church, the power structure of the average community is consoled by the church's silent and often vocal sanction of things as they are.

But the judgment of God is upon the church as never before. If ₃₇ the church of today does not recapture the sacrificial spirit of the early church, it will lose its authentic ring, forfeit the loyalty of millions, and be dismissed as an irrelevant social club with no meaning for the twentieth century. I am meeting young people every day whose disappointment with the church has risen to outright disgust.

Maybe again, I have been too optimistic. Is organized religion ₃₈ too inextricably bound to the status quo to save our nation and the world? Maybe I must turn my faith to the inner spiritual church, the church within the church, as the true *ecclesia* and the hope of the world. But again I am thankful to God that some noble souls from the ranks of organized religion have broken loose from the paralyzing chains of conformity and joined us as active partners in the struggle for freedom. They have left their secure congregations and walked the streets of Albany, Georgia, with us. They have gone through the highways of the South on tortuous rides for freedom. Yes, they have gone to jail with us. Some have been kicked out of their churches, and lost support of their bishops and fellow ministers. But they have gone with the faith that right defeated is stronger than evil triumphant. These men have been the leaven in the lump of the race. Their witness has been the spiritual salt that has preserved the true meaning of the gospel in these troubled times. They have carved a tunnel of hope through the dark mountain of disappointment.

I hope the church as a whole will meet the challenge of this deci- ₃₉ sive hour. But even if the church does not come to the aid of justice, I have no despair about the future. I have no fear about the outcome of our struggle in Birmingham, even if our motives are presently misunderstood. We will reach the goal of freedom in Birmingham and all over the nation, because the goal of America is freedom. Abused and scorned though we may be, our destiny is tied up with the destiny of America. Before the Pilgrims landed at Plymouth we were here. Before the pen of Jefferson etched across the pages of history the majestic words of the Declaration of Independence, we were here. For more than two centuries our foreparents labored in this country without wages; they made cotton king; and they built the homes of their masters in the midst of brutal injustice and shameful humiliation—and yet out of a bottomless vitality they continued to thrive and develop. If the inexpressible cruelties of slavery could not stop us, the opposition we now face will surely fail. We will win our freedom because the sacred heritage of our nation and the eternal will of God are embodied in our echoing demands.

40   I must close now. But before closing I am impelled to mention one other point in your statement that troubled me profoundly. You warmly commended the Birmingham police force for keeping "order" and "preventing violence." I don't believe you would have so warmly commended the police force if you had seen its angry violent dogs literally biting six unarmed, nonviolent Negroes. I don't believe you would so quickly commend the policemen if you would observe their ugly and inhuman treatment of Negroes here in the city jail; if you would watch them push and curse old Negro women and young Negro girls; if you would see them slap and kick old Negro men and young boys; if you will observe them, as they did on two occasions, refuse to give us food because we wanted to sing our grace together. I'm sorry that I can't join you in your praise for the police department.

41   It is true that they have been rather disciplined in their public handling of the demonstrators. In this sense they have been rather publicly "nonviolent." But for what purpose? To preserve the evil system of segregation. Over the last few years I have consistently preached that nonviolence demands that the means we use must be as pure as the ends we seek. So I have tried to make it clear that it is wrong to use immoral means to attain moral ends. But now I must affirm that it is just as wrong, or even more so, to use moral means to preserve immoral ends. Maybe Mr. Connor and his policemen have been rather publicly nonviolent, as Chief Pritchett was in Albany, Georgia, but they have used the moral means of nonviolence to maintain the immoral end of flagrant racial injustice. T. S. Eliot has said that there is no greater treason than to do the right deed for the wrong reason.

42   I wish you had commended the Negro sit-inners and demonstrators of Birmingham for their sublime courage, their willingness to suffer and their amazing discipline in the midst of the most inhuman provocation. One day the South will recognize its real heroes. They will be the James Merediths, courageously and with a majestic sense of purpose facing jeering and hostile mobs and the agonizing loneliness that characterizes the life of the pioneer. They will be old, oppressed, battered Negro women, symbolized

in a seventy-two-year-old woman of Montgomery, Alabama, who rose up with a sense of dignity and with her people decided not to ride the segregated buses, and responded to one who inquired about her tiredness with ungrammatical profundity: "My feet is tired, but my soul is rested." They will be the young high school and college students, young ministers of the gospel and a host of their elders courageously and nonviolently sitting-in at lunch counters and willingly going to jail for conscience's sake. One day the South will know that when these disinherited children of God sat down at lunch counters they were in reality standing up for the best in the American dream and the most sacred values in our Judeo-Christian heritage, and thusly, carrying our whole nation back to those great wells of democracy which were dug deep by the Founding Fathers in the formulation of the Constitution and the Declaration of Independence.

Never before have I written a letter this long (or should I say 43 a book?). I'm afraid that it is much too long to take your precious time. I can assure you that it would have been much shorter if I had been writing from a comfortable desk, but what else is there to do when you are alone for days in the dull monotony of a narrow jail cell other than write long letters, think strange thoughts, and pray long prayers?

If I have said anything in this letter that is an overstatement 44 of the truth and is indicative of an unreasonable impatience, I beg you to forgive me. If I have said anything in this letter that is an understatement of the truth and is indicative of my having a patience that makes me patient with anything less than brotherhood, I beg God to forgive me.

I hope this letter finds you strong in the faith. I also hope that 45 circumstances will soon make it possible for me to meet each of you, not as an integrationist or a civil rights leader, but as a fellow clergyman and a Christian brother. Let us all hope that the dark clouds of racial prejudice will soon pass away and the deep fog of misunderstanding will be lifted from our fear-drenched communities and in some not too distant tomorrow the radiant stars of love and brotherhood will shine over our great nation with all of their scintillating beauty.

Yours for the cause of Peace and Brotherhood,

Martin Luther King, Jr.

Executions Are Too Costly—Morally

Helen Prejean

1   I think of the running debate I engage in with "church" people about the death penalty. "Proof texts" from the Bible usually punctuate these discussions without regard for the cultural context or literary genre of the passages invoked. (Will D. Campbell, a Southern Baptist minister and writer, calls this use of scriptural quotations "biblical quarterbacking.")

2   It is abundantly clear that the Bible depicts murder as a crime for which death is considered the appropriate punishment, and one is hard-pressed to find a biblical "proof text" in either the Hebrew Testament or the New Testament which unequivocally refutes this. Even Jesus' admonition "Let him without sin cast the first stone," when he was asked the appropriate punishment for an adulteress (John 8:7)—the Mosaic law prescribed death—should be read in its proper context. This passage is an "entrapment" story, which sought to show Jesus' wisdom in besting his adversaries. It is not an ethical pronouncement about capital punishment.

3   Similarly, the "eye for eye" passage from Exodus, which pro-death penalty advocates are fond of quoting, is rarely cited in its original context, in which it is clearly meant to limit revenge.

4   The passage, including verse 22, which sets the context reads:

> If, when men come to blows, they hurt a woman who is pregnant and she suffers a miscarriage, though she does not die of it, the man responsible must pay the compensation demanded of him by the woman's master; he shall hand it over after arbitration. But should she die, you shall give life for life, eye for eye, tooth for tooth, hand for hand, foot for foot, burn for burn, wound for wound, stroke for stroke. (Exodus 21:22–25)

5   In the example given (patently patriarchal: the woman is considered the negotiable property of her male master), it is clear that punishment is to be measured out according to the seriousness of the offense. If the child is lost but not the mother, the punishment is less grave than if both mother and child are lost. *Only* an eye for an eye, *only* a life for a life is the intent of the passage. Restraint was badly needed. It was not uncommon for an offended family

or clan to slaughter entire communities in retaliation for an offense against one of their members.

Even granting the call for restraint in this passage, it is nonethe- 6 less clear—here and in numerous other instances throughout the Hebrew Bible—that the punishment for murder was death.

But we must remember that such prescriptions of the Mosaic 7 Law were promulgated in a seminomadic culture in which the preservation of a fragile society—without benefit of prisons and other institutions—demanded quick, effective, harsh punishment of offenders. And we should note the numerous other crimes for which the Bible prescribes death as punishment:

contempt of parents (Exodus 21:15, 17; Leviticus 24:17);

trespass upon sacred ground (Exodus 19:12–13; Numbers 1:51; 18:7);

sorcery (Exodus 22:18; Leviticus 20:27);

bestiality (Exodus 22:19; Leviticus 20:15–16);

sacrifice to foreign gods (Exodus 22:20; Deuteronomy 13:1–9);

profaning the sabbath (Exodus 31:14);

adultery (Leviticus 20:10; Deuteronomy 22:22–24);

incest (Leviticus 20:11–13);

homosexuality (Leviticus 20:13);

and prostitution (Leviticus 21:19; Deuteronomy 22:13–21).

And this is by no means a complete list. 8

But no person with common sense would dream of appro- 9 priating such a moral code today, and it is curious that those who so readily invoke the "eye for an eye, life for life" passage are quick to shun other biblical prescriptions which also call for death, arguing that modern societies have evolved over the three thousand or so years since biblical times and no longer consider such exaggerated and archaic punishments appropriate.

Such nuances are lost, of course, in "biblical quarterbacking," 10 and more and more I find myself steering away from such futile discussions. Instead, I try to articulate what I personally believe about Jesus and the ethical thrust he gave to humankind: an impetus toward compassion, a preference for disarming enemies without humiliating and destroying them, and a solidarity with poor and suffering people.

11   So, what happened to the impetus of love and compassion Jesus set blazing into history?

12   The first Christians adhered closely to the way of life Jesus had taught. They died in amphitheaters rather than offer homage to worldly emperors. They refused to fight in emperors' wars. But then a tragic diversion happened, which Elaine Pagels has deftly explored in her book *Adam, Eve, and the Serpent:* in 313 C.E. the Emperor Constantine entered the Christian church.

13   Pagels says, "Christian bishops, once targets for arrest, torture, and execution, now received tax exemptions, gifts from the imperial treasury, prestige, and even influence at court; the churches gained new wealth, power and prominence."

14   Unfortunately, the exercise of power practiced by Christians in alliance with the Roman Empire—with its unabashed allegiance to the sword—soon bore no resemblance to the purely moral persuasion that Jesus had taught.

15   In the fifth century, Pagels points out, Augustine provided the theological rationale the church needed to justify the use of violence by church and state governments. Augustine persuaded church authorities that "original sin" so damaged every person's ability to make moral choices that external control by church and state authorities over people's lives was necessary and justified. The "wicked" might be "coerced by the sword" to "protect the innocent," Augustine taught. And thus was legitimated for Christians the authority of secular government to "control" its subjects by coercive and violent means—even punishment by death.

16   In the latter part of the twentieth century, however, two flares of hope—Mohandas K. Gandhi and Martin Luther King—have demonstrated that Jesus' counsel to practice compassion and tolerance even toward one's enemies can effect social change. Susan Jacoby, analyzing the moral power that Gandhi and King unleashed in their campaigns for social justice, finds a unique form of aggression:

17   " 'If everyone took an eye for an eye,' Gandhi said, 'the whole world would be blind.' But Gandhi did not want to take anyone's eye; he wanted to force the British out of India. . . ."

> Nonviolence and nonaggression are generally regarded as interchangeable concepts—King and Gandhi frequently used

them that way—but nonviolence, as employed by Gandhi in India and by King in the American South, might reasonably be viewed as a highly disciplined form of aggression. If one defines aggression in the primary dictionary sense of "attack," nonviolent resistance proved to be the most powerful attack imaginable on the powers King and Gandhi were trying to overturn. The writings of both men are filled with references to love as a powerful force against oppression, and while the two leaders were not using the term "force" in the military sense, they certainly regarded nonviolence as a tactical weapon as well as an expression of high moral principle. The root meaning of Gandhi's concept of *satyagraha* . . . is "holding on to truth" . . . Gandhi also called *satyagraha* the "love force" or "soul force" and explained that he had discovered "in the earliest stages that pursuit of truth did not permit violence being inflicted on one's opponent, but that he must be weaned from error by patience and sympathy. . . . And patience means self-suffering." So the doctrine came to mean vindication of truth, not by the infliction of suffering on the opponent, but on one's self.

King was even more explicit on this point: the purpose of civil disobedience, he explained many times, was to force the defenders of segregation to commit brutal acts in public and thus arouse the conscience of the world on behalf of those wronged by racism. King and Gandhi did not succeed because they changed the hearts and minds of southern sheriffs and British colonial administrators (although they did, in fact, change some minds) but because they *made the price of maintaining control too high for their opponents* [emphasis mine].

That, I believe, is what it's going to take to abolish the death 18 penalty in this country: we must persuade the American people that government killings are too costly for us, not only financially, but—more important—morally.

The death penalty *costs* too much. Allowing our government to 19 kill citizens compromises the deepest moral values upon which this country was conceived: the inviolable dignity of human persons.

I have no doubt that we will one day abolish the death penalty 20 in America. It will come sooner if people like me who know the truth about executions do our work well and educate the public. It will come slowly if we do not. Because, finally, I know that it is not a question of malice or ill will or meanness of spirit that prompts our citizens to support executions. It is, quite simply, that people don't know the truth of what is going on. That is not by accident. The secrecy surrounding executions makes it possible for executions to continue. I am convinced that if executions were made public, the torture and violence would be unmasked, and we would be shamed into abolishing executions. We would be embarrassed at the brutalization of the crowds that would gather to watch a man or woman be killed. And we would be humiliated to know that visitors from other countries—Japan, Russia, Latin America, Europe—were watching us kill our own citizens—we, who take pride in being the flagship of democracy in the world.

Unsung Heroes: Juries Offer True Justice

Alan Dershowitz

1 The American jury, one of the great bastions of liberty, is under increasing attack. Many lawyers regard it as, at best, a necessary evil. It slows the process of adjudication. Its outcomes are unpredictable. It is inexpert at deciding complex issues. It is subject to emotional, even bigoted, appeals. Its verdicts lack consistency, since different juries arrive at different conclusions in cases with similar facts. It seems anachronistic in our age of efficiency and specialization.

2 In England, where the jury originated, it has been all but abolished in civil cases. In the United States, where our Constitution forbids its abolition in most cases, it has been limited wherever possible. Moreover, the traditional size of juries has been reduced from twelve to six in many cases, and the requirement of unanimity has been changed in many states to a two-thirds majority.

3 At an even more fundamental level, the cumbersomeness of juries has resulted in relatively few cases actually being tried: The vast majority are settled before trial, in criminal cases by a plea bargain and in civil cases by a financial compromise. The expense and unpredictability of jury trials have also driven many institutional litigants such as stock brokerage firms to demand that their

customers waive trial by jury and accept the more streamlined mechanism of arbitration.

In sum, it's fair to say that if our Constitution did not man- 4 date the right to trial by jury in most criminal and civil cases, the jury would be in danger of becoming an endangered species of adjudication.

It's ironic, though not at all surprising, that as we Americans 5 unappreciatively chip away at the right to trial by jury, reformers in several Eastern European nations are calling for its transplantation onto their foreign soil. Having experienced totalitarian judicial and political systems, they are searching for mechanisms that promise some popular checks on the abuse of governmental power.

They have seen enough of Communist efficiency, predictabil- 6 ity, expertise, and objectivity. They understand, as some Americans seem not to, that making the judicial "trains run on time" is not the sole criterion by which to judge a legal system. For a trial to be fair, the adjudicator must be *independent* of the powers that be, willing and able to stand up to pressures to do the government's bidding.

The American jury has passed that difficult test with flying 7 colors, from the colonial period when it acquitted John Peter Zenger of politically inspired charges of libel to recent juries that have ruled in favor of such unpopular defendants as John Hinkley, Peggy McMartin Buckey, Imelda Marcos, and John DeLorean.

Juries, unlike judges, do not become routinized: Every case is 8 their first and only case. It is their opportunity to do justice, and most jurors take their role quite seriously.

Many judges, especially some who have been on the bench 9 for years, regard criminal defendants as presumptively guilty, since most who have come before them have pleaded guilty or been convicted. Juries, on the other hand, really seem to believe in the presumption of innocence and require the prosecution to prove each case beyond a reasonable doubt.

Nor can anyone *whisper* to a jury. Everything said to them is 10 said openly and on the record. They hear only the evidence that is properly admissible. They do not learn that the prosecutor believes that the defendant is a bad or dangerous man—unless there is admissible evidence to support these assertions. The jurors are umpires, not fans.

11   The very independence and unaccountability of juries also make them a potentially dangerous institution in some settings. Racist juries in the pre–civil rights South routinely acquitted white killers of African Americans. Some contemporary jurors, who regard themselves as foot soldiers in the war against drugs, seem willing to convict anyone with a Colombian passport of drug charges.

12   But the jury is simply one part of our system of checks and balances. It, too, must be kept in check by other institutions of government, such as trial and appellate judges.

13   In addition to recent efforts at limiting the role of juries, there is another serious danger on the horizon. Sophisticated social scientists are becoming increasingly involved on behalf of wealthy litigants in trying to select jurors who will favor their side. Since the average litigant cannot afford this expensive luxury—he can barely scrape up the money for exorbitant legal fees—only the most powerful plaintiffs or defendants will be able to manipulate jury selection to their advantage. These "designer juries" threaten to skew the randomness of the jury and destroy its objectivity.

14   In the end, the jury system, like democracy itself, is the worst mechanism for achieving justice, "except," as Winston Churchill said about democracy, "for all the others." Even with its imperfections, the American jury serves as a powerful check on the abuses of governmental power.

15   Our system of checks and balances may not be the most efficient mechanism for governing. But it is the envy of all who treasure liberty and believe in government by the people. American jurors are the people administering justice.

Adult Crime, Adult Time

Linda J. Collier

1 When prosecutor Brent Davis said he wasn't sure if he could charge 11-year-old Andrew Golden and 13-year-old Mitchell Johnson as adults after Tuesday afternoon's slaughter in Jonesboro, Arkansas, I cringed. But not for the reasons you might think.

I knew he was formulating a judgment based on laws that ₂
have not had a major overhaul for more than 100 years. I knew
his hands were tied by the longstanding creed that juvenile
offenders, generally defined as those under the age of 18, are
to be treated rather than punished. I knew he would have to do
legal cartwheels to get the case out of the juvenile system.
But most of all, I cringed because today's juvenile suspects—
even those who are accused of committing the most violent
crimes—are still regarded by the law as children first and
criminals second.

As astonishing as the Jonesboro events were, this is hardly the ₃
first time that children with access to guns and other weapons have
brought tragedy to a school. Only weeks before the Jonesboro
shootings, three girls in Paducah, Kentucky, were killed in their
school lobby when a 14-year-old classmate allegedly opened fire on
them. Authorities said he had several guns with him, and the
alleged murder weapon was one of seven stolen from a neighbor's
garage. And the day after the Jonesboro shootings, a 14-year-old in
Daly City, California, was charged as a juvenile after he allegedly
fired at his middle-school principal with a semiautomatic handgun.

It's not a new or unusual phenomenon for children to com- ₄
mit violent crimes at younger and younger ages, but it often takes
a shocking incident to draw our attention to a trend already in
progress. According to the U.S. Department of Justice, crimes
committed by juveniles have increased by 60 percent since 1984.
Where juvenile delinquency was once limited to truancy or van-
dalism, juveniles now are more likely to be the perpetrators of
serious and deadly crimes such as arson, aggravated assault, rape
and murder. And these violent offenders increasingly include
those as young as the Jonesboro suspects. Since 1965, the number
of 12-year-olds arrested for violent crimes has doubled and the
number of 13- and 14-year-olds has tripled, according to government statistics.

Those statistics are a major reason why we need to revamp ₅
our antiquated juvenile justice system. Nearly every state, including Arkansas, has laws that send most youthful violent offenders
to the juvenile courts, where they can only be found "delinquent"
and confined in a juvenile facility (typically not past age 21). In
recent years, many states have enacted changes in their juvenile

crime laws, and some have lowered the age at which a juvenile can be tried as an adult for certain violent crimes. Virginia, for example, has reduced its minimum age to 14, and suspects accused of murder and aggravated malicious wounding are automatically waived to adult court. Illinois is now sending some 13-year-olds to adult court after a hearing in juvenile court. In Kansas, a 1996 law allows juveniles as young as 10 to be prosecuted as adults in some cases. These are steps in the right direction, but too many states still treat violent offenders under 16 as juveniles who belong in the juvenile system.

6   My views are not those of a frustrated prosecutor. I have represented children as a court-appointed guardian *ad litem,* or temporary guardian, in the Philadelphia juvenile justice system. Loosely defined, a guardian *ad litem* is responsible for looking after the best interest of a neglected or rebellious child who has come into the juvenile courts. It is often a humbling experience as I try to help children whose lives have gone awry, sometimes because of circumstances beyond their control.

7   My experience has made me believe that the system is doing a poor job at treatment as well as punishment. One of my "girls," a chronic truant, was a foster child who longed to be adopted. She often talked of how she wanted a pink room, a frilly bunk bed and sisters with whom she could share her dreams. She languished in foster care from ages 2 to 13 because her drug-ravaged mother would not relinquish her parental rights. Initially, the girl refused to tolerate the half-life that the state had maintained was in her best interest. But as it became clear that we would never convince her mother to give up her rights, the girl became a frequent runaway. Eventually she ended up pregnant, wandering from place to place and committing adult crimes to survive. No longer a child, not quite a woman, she is the kind of teenager offender for whom the juvenile system has little or nothing to offer.

8   A brief history: Proceedings in juvenile justice began in 1890 in Chicago, where the original mandate was to save wayward children and protect them from the ravages of society. The system called for children to be processed through an appendage of the family court. By design, juveniles were to be kept away from the court's criminal side, the district attorney and adult correctional institutions.

Typically, initial procedures are informal, non-threatening 9 and not open to public scrutiny. A juvenile suspect is interviewed by an "intake" officer who determines the child's fate. The intake officer may issue a warning, lecture and release; he may detain the suspect; or, he may decide to file a petition, subjecting the child to juvenile "adjudication" proceedings. If the law allows, the intake officer may make a recommendation that the juvenile be transferred to adult criminal court.

An adjudication is similar to a hearing, rather than a trial, 10 although the juvenile may be represented by counsel and a juvenile prosecutor will represent the interests of the community. It is important to note that throughout the proceedings, no matter which side of the fence the parties are on, the operating principle is that everyone is working in the best interests of the child. Juvenile court judges do not issue findings of guilt, but decide whether a child is delinquent. If delinquency is found, the judge must decide the child's fate. Should the child be sent the child back to the family—assuming there is one? Declare him or her "in need of supervision," which brings in the intense help of social services? Remove the child from the family and place him or her in foster care? Confine the child to a state institution for juvenile offenders?

This system was developed with truants, vandals and petty 11 thieves in mind. But this model is not appropriate for the violent juvenile offender of today. Detaining a rapist or murderer in a juvenile facility until the age of 18 or 21 isn't even a slap on the hand. If a juvenile is accused of murdering, raping or assaulting someone with a deadly weapon, the suspect should automatically be sent to adult criminal court. What's to ponder?

With violent crime becoming more prevalent among the jun- 12 ior set, it's a mystery why there hasn't been a major overhaul of juvenile justice laws long before now. Will the Jonesboro shootings be the incident that makes us take a hard look at the current system? When it became evident that the early release of Jesse Timmendequas—whose murder of 7-year-old Megan Kanka in New Jersey sparked national outrage—had caused unwarranted tragedy, legislative action was swift. Now New Jersey has Megan's Law, which requires the advance notification of a sexual predator's release into a neighborhood. Other states have followed suit.

13   It is unequivocally clear that the same type of mandate is needed to establish a uniform minimum age for trying juveniles as adults. As it stands now, there is no consistency in state laws governing waivers to adult court. One reason for this lack of uniformity is the absence of direction from the federal government or Congress. The Bureau of Justice Statistics reports that adjacent states such as New York and Pennsylvania respond differently to 16-year-old criminals, with New York tending to treat offenders of that age as adults and Pennsylvania handling them in the juvenile justice system.

14   Federal prosecution of juveniles is not totally unheard of, but it is uncommon. The Bureau of Justice Statistics estimates that during 1994, at least 65 juveniles were referred to the attorney general for transfer to adult status. In such cases, the U.S. attorney's office must certify a substantial federal interest in the case and show that one of the following is true: The state does not have jurisdiction; the state refuses to assume jurisdiction or the state does not have adequate services for juvenile offenders; the offense is a violent felony, drug trafficking or firearm offense as defined by the U.S. Code.

15   Exacting hurdles, but not insurmountable. In the Jonesboro case, prosecutor Davis has been exploring ways to enlist the federal court's jurisdiction. Whatever happens, federal prosecutions of young offenders are clearly not the long-term answer. The states must act. So as far as I can see, the next step is clear: Children who knowingly engage in adult conduct and adult crimes should automatically be subject to adult rules and adult prison time.

One Big Happy Prison

Michael Moore

1   It was a few minutes after 10:00 p.m. on October 4, 2000, one month before the presidential election. The previous night, the first of three debates between Al Gore and George W. Bush had taken place.

On this balmy October evening in Lebanon, Tennessee, John ₂
Adams, sixty-four, had just sat down in his favorite tan recliner
to watch the evening news. His cane, the result of a stroke a few
years earlier, rested beside him. A well-respected member of
Lebanon's African-American community, Adams was now on disability after working for years at the Precision Rubber plant.

The anchors on TV were dishing out their postmortems on the ₃
debate. Adams and his wife, Lorine, were discussing their intention to vote for Al Gore when there was a knock at the door.

Mrs. Adams left the room, came to the door, and asked who ₄
was there. Two men demanded that she open the door and let
them in. She asked again who they were, but they refused to identify themselves. She again refused to open the door.

At that moment, two unidentified officers from the Lebanon ₅
Police Department's drug task force broke down the door,
grabbed Mrs. Adams, and immediately handcuffed her. Seven
other officers burst into the house. Two of them ran around the
corner into the back room, guns drawn, and pumped several bullets into John Adams. Three hours later, he was pronounced dead
at Vanderbilt University Medical Center.

The raid on the Adams house had been ordered after an ₆
undercover informant purchased drugs in the house at 1120
Joseph Street. Lebanon's narcotics unit, funded along with thousands of others around the country as part of the Clinton administration's "War on Drugs," obtained warrants from a local judge
to arrest the occupants of the house.

The only problem: the Adamses live at 70 Joseph Street. The ₇
drug-war police had the wrong house.

A few miles down the road in Nashville, as John Adams was ₈
being accidentally executed, scores of paid and volunteer staff bus-
tled about inside Al Gore's national campaign headquarters. Their
main concern that night was damage control, as they tried to distract voters from the spectacle of their candidate sighing through
Bush's responses the previous night. Phones were lighting up,
shipments of bumper stickers and yard signs were being rerouted,
strategists were huddling to plan the next day's campaign stops.
On the table sat copies of Gore's anticrime proposals, including
more funding for additional police and more money to fight the
Drug War. None of them knew that their out-of-control efforts to

eradicate drugs had just cost them a potential vote, that of an elderly black man across town.

9   Killing off your voters is no way to win an election.

10   This was just one of too many incidents in recent years where innocent people have been shot by local or federal drug police who thought they "had their man."

11   Worse still is the way so many citizens have been locked up in the past decade thanks to Clinton/Gore policies. At the beginning of the nineties, there were about a million people in prison in the United States. By the end of the Clinton/Gore years, that number had grown to TWO MILLION. The bulk of this increase was the result of new laws being enforced against drug users, not pushers. Eighty percent of those who go to prison for drugs are in there for possession, not dealing. The penalties for crack use are three times as high as those for cocaine use.

12   It doesn't take much to figure out why the drug of choice in the white community is treated with so much more leniency than the drug that constitutes the only affordable high in the poor black and Hispanic community. For eight years there was an intense, aggressive move to lock up as many of these minority citizens as possible. Instead of providing the treatment their condition demands, we dealt with the problem by sending them to rot inside a prison cell.

13   But forget for a moment about helping the less fortunate. Who was the genius in the Clinton/Gore administration who said, "Hey, I've got an idea—why don't we go after the black and Hispanic community—plenty of drug users there! Lock 'em up in record numbers, decimating the voting power of a group that votes for our side nine to one!"

14   It doesn't make sense, does it? What kind of campaign would purposely destroy its own voting base? You don't see Republicans sitting around trying to plot ways to incarcerate corporate executives and NRA members. Trust me, you won't see Karl Rove convening a White House meeting to figure out a way to lock up and strip the voting rights from a million members of the Christian Coalition.

15   In fact, just the opposite. The Bush people are committed to seeing that none of their supporters ever enjoys the hospitality of a prison shower room. Much was made after Clinton left office of the pardons he granted to dubious fat cats like Marc Rich. The

entire country was up in arms over the absolution given to a fugitive who got away without paying his taxes. A rich person who got away without paying taxes! We were shocked SHOCKED!

And yet no attention at all was paid to the "pardons" of David Lamp, Vincent Mietlicki, John Wadsworth, or James Weathers Jr. And no one called for a congressional investigation of why criminal charges were dropped against Koch Industries, the largest privately held oil company in America, whose CEO and vice president are the brothers Charles and David Koch. Why was this? 16

Because those "pardons" came during the reign of George W. Bush. 17

In September 2000, the federal government brought a 97 count indictment against Koch Industries and its four employees—Lamp, Mietlicki, Wadsworth, and Weathers, who were Koch's environmental and plant managers—for knowingly releasing 91 metric tons of benzene, a cancer-causing agent, into the air and water, and for covering up the deadly release from federal regulators. 18

This wasn't Koch's first run-in with the law; it wasn't even their first that year. Earlier in 2000, Koch had been fined $35 million for illegal pollution in six states. 19

But with the George W. Bush's election "decided," Koch's fortunes suddenly changed. Koch executives had just contributed some $800,000 to Bush's presidential campaign and other Republican candidates and causes. In January, as John Ashcroft waited in the wings, the government dropped the charges first from 97 to 11 and then to a mere nine. 20

Koch Industries, however, still faced fines totaling $352 million. Bush's new administration, now firmly in place, quickly fixed that. In March, they dropped two more charges. Then, two days before the case was to go to court, Ashcroft's Justice Department settled the case. 21

Koch Industries pled guilty to a new charge of falsifying documents, and the government dropped all environmental charges against the company, including all felony counts against their four employees. 22

Following hard on the heels of their generosity, the Koch executives facing possible prison terms were freed from any prosecution. The company itself had all 90 of the serious counts against 23 it dismissed and in the end paid a fine that wiped out the 7 remaining counts. According to the *Houston Chronicle*, "Koch executives celebrated the conclusion of the case," company spokesman Jay Rosser crowing about how the dropping of charges was proof of Koch's "vindication."

24   I won't defend the actions of Marc Rich, but correct me if I'm wrong: I believe the willful spewing into the air and water of a deadly chemical that causes cancer (and will surely contribute to who knows how many people's deaths) is a little more serious than skipping out on Rudy Giuliani to go on an eighteen-year ski trip to Switzerland. Yet I'm sure none of you have heard of the pardons granted to Charles and David Koch and their oil company and its executives. Why should you? It was just business as usual, under a national press that's thoroughly asleep at the wheel.

25   It's too bad that Anthony Lemar Taylor forgot to send in his contribution to the Bush campaign. Taylor was another repeat offender—a petty thief who decided one day in 1999 to pretend he was golf superstar Tiger Woods.

26   Though Taylor looked nothing at all like Woods (but, hey, they all look alike, don't they?), he was able to use a fake driver's license and credit cards identifying him as Tiger Woods to purchase a 70-inch TV, a few stereos, and a used luxury car.

27   Then somebody finally figured out he wasn't Tiger Woods, and he was arrested and tried for theft and perjury.

28   His sentence? TWO HUNDRED YEARS TO LIFE!

29   You read it right. Two hundred years to life, thanks to California's "three-strikes" law, which says that upon a third criminal conviction, you're put away for life. To date, no corporate executive has been sent away for life after being caught three times polluting a river or ripping off its customers. In America, we reserve that special treatment for those who happen to be poor or African-American or fail to contribute to one of our fine political parties.

30   Of course, sometimes the justice system, ever the steamroller, is so hell-bent on punishing the havenots it doesn't care who it locks up, guilty or not.

31   Kerry Sanders, the youngest child of nine, suffered from paranoid schizophrenia. By the age of twenty-seven he had fought the demons in his mind for over seven years and had been in and out

of mental institutions for much of that time. Sometimes, when he went off his medication, he would end up on the streets of Los Angeles, as he did one day in October 1993.

While sleeping on a bench outside the USC Medical Center,   32 Kerry was arrested for trespassing. But Kerry's luck turned worse when a routine warrant check showed that one Robert Sanders, a career criminal, had escaped five weeks earlier from a New York State prison, where he was serving time for attempting to kill a man over cocaine in 1990.

Of course, Kerry Sanders of California wasn't Robert Sanders   33 of New York. But I guess "Kerry" and "Robert" are close enough, and California and New York . . .

well, um, they're both BIG STATES, after all. . . .   34

Unfortunately for Kerry, what he did share with Robert was   35 a birthday.

That was enough for the L.A. cop, even though the same com-   36 puterized warrant search showed that Kerry Sanders had been stopped for jaywalking on a Los Angeles street in July 1993— while Robert Sanders was still in his New York prison.

No matter: Kerry Sanders was sent to New York to serve out   37 Robert Sanders's sentence. He remained in the New York penitentiary for two years, while his mother searched all over Los Angeles for him. Somehow the L.A. cops failed to compare the two records—which would have revealed that their guy had the wrong fingerprints.

Kerry had only one person in the whole process who was sup-   38 posed to help him—the public defender appointed to protect his interests. But this thirty-year veteran PD encouraged him not to fight extradition. The PD explained to Kerry that fighting back would only prolong his stay in the L.A. county jail before being returned to New York anyway. Apparently the PD didn't even notice that Kerry was "slow," much less suffering from severe mental illness. Or would it have even mattered?

The PD failed to ask basic questions. He failed to spend more   39 than a brief few minutes with a helpless client. He never looked into whether Kerry had any family who might be contacted to assist in his defense.

The PD also failed to check the system for any pending cases,   40 or a prior record, or his client's financial status. He didn't even take the time to match the description on the warrant with Kerry, much less demand a fingerprint or booking photo comparison. So what, you say? After all, both men were black; they were both the same age—they even shared a birthdate! Isn't that good enough?

41   It gets worse. During the hearing to waive Kerry Sanders' right to fight the New York extradition, he was asked to sign a form. The form read: "I, Robert Sanders, do hereby freely and voluntarily state that I am the identical Robert Sanders"—and then Kerry signed it "Kerry Sanders."

42   He also drew doodles all over one copy of the waiver.

43   No bells? No red flags? Not for this public defender!

44   Finally given his chance to appear before a judge, Kerry was asked if he had read the document he had signed. He said he had not. The judge stopped the extradition proceeding.

45   "Did you sign it?" asked the judge.

46   "Yeah," Kerry replied.

47   "Why did you sign it?"

48   "Because they told me to sign it," Kerry Sanders answered.

49   Kerry's public defender was ordered by the judge to review the form again with his client. Within minutes the judge was satisfied, and both the court and the public defender moved on to the next case.

50   After Kerry Sanders was sold down the river by his L.A. public defender, he was shipped across the country to spend the next two years in Green Haven maximum-security prison, sixty miles north of New York City, where he was sexually assaulted by other inmates.

51   In October 1995, after federal agents in Cleveland arrested the real Robert Sanders, Kerry Sanders was reunited with his mother, Mary Sanders Lee. Had it not been for the chance arrest of Robert Sanders, Kerry Sanders would still be in prison today.

52   Kerry was sent home from Green Haven with $48.13, a plastic bag with some medicine, a soda, and a pack of cigarettes. He told his sister, Roberta: "They took me to New York. It was so cold there. They put me in this little room."

53   This is not a rare case of the system making a horrible mistake. In a sense, it is not even a mistake. It is the natural result of a society that recklessly locks up anyone who may be a criminal, even if they aren't a criminal, because it's better to be safe than right. Our

courts are nothing but a haphazard assembly line for the poor to be routed away from us, out of sight—out of my damn way!

Well, this is America, and I guess if it's good enough to 54 remove thousands of innocent black men from the voting rolls in Florida, it should be good enough to railroad an innocent black man in Los Angeles.

In this assembly-line system of justice, the one thing that 55 mucks up the wholesale delivery of the accused to jail is the jury trial. Why? Because jury trials are shit-disturbers. They force everyone to do their job. The judges, prosecutors, and public defenders do everything in their power to coerce the defendant into accepting a guilty plea to AVOID THE BRUTAL PRISON SENTENCE WE WILL GIVE YOU IF YOU DEMAND A JURY TRIAL. If they can get the defendant not only to plead guilty but also to sign a waiver of his right to appeal, then they've hit a home run—and everyone can laugh about it later at the country club.

My sister, Anne, was a public defender in California. She 56 insisted on defending her clients, and getting them a jury trial if that's what they wanted. For that, she was subjected to incredible harassment from the other PDs in the office. In 1998 the public defender's office in her county allowed only one felony client out of almost nine hundred defendants to have a jury trial.

Obviously, that didn't mean every single one of the other 899 57 accused were guilty. They were just coerced into pleading that way, with many of them ending up in prison, perhaps for crimes they didn't commit. But we'll never know, because their Sixth Amendment right to a trial by a jury of their peers was taken from them.

With this standardized railroading of the poor going on daily 58 in every city in America, our justice system has nothing to do with justice. Our judges and lawyers are more like glorified garbage men, rounding up and disposing of society's refuse—ethnic cleansing, American style.

What happens when this fast-track chute sends innocent peo- 59 ple to their death? It took only one college class full of kids at Northwestern University in Evanston, Illinois, to uncover and prove that five individuals on Illinois's death row were, in fact, innocent. Those students and their professor saved the lives of five people.

60   If one college class could do that, how many other hundreds of innocent people on death rows across the country are also sitting there awaiting their permanent disposal?

61   Thirty-eight states have the death penalty. So does the federal government and the U.S. military. Twelve states, plus the District of Columbia (that little piece of swampland with a majority of African-Americans and those offensive license plates), do not.

62   Since 1976, there have been over seven hundred executions in the United States.

63   The top execution-happy states are:

Texas (248 executions—nearly one-third of all U.S. executions since 1976)

Virginia (82)

Florida (51)

Missouri (50)

Oklahoma (43)

Louisiana (26)

South Carolina (25)

Arkansas (24)

Alabama (23)

Arizona (22)

North Carolina (17)

Delaware (13)

Illinois (12)

California (9)

Nevada (9)

Indiana (8)

Utah (6)

64   A shocking recent death penalty study of 4,578 cases in a twenty-three-year period (1973–1995) concluded that the courts found serious, reversible error in nearly 7 of every 10 capital sentence cases that were fully reviewed during the period. It also found that death sentences were being overturned in 2 out of 3 appeals. The overall prejudicial review error rate was 68 percent.

Since 1973, some ninety-five death row inmates have been 65
fully exonerated by the courts—that is, found innocent of the
crimes for which they were sentenced to die. Ninety-six persons
have been released as a result of DNA testing.

And what were the most common errors? 66

1. Egregiously incompetent defense lawyers who didn't even 67
   look for, or missed important evidence that would have
   proved innocence or demonstrated that their client didn't
   deserve to die.
2. Police or prosecutors who did discover that kind of evidence 68
   but suppressed it, actively derailing the judicial process.

In half the years studied, including the most recent one, the 69
error rate was over 60 percent. High error rates exist across
the country. In 85 percent of death penalty cases the error rates
are 60 percent or higher. Three-fifths have error rates of 70 percent
or higher.

Catching these errors takes time—a national average of nine 70
years from death sentence to execution. In most cases, death row
inmates wait years for the lengthy review procedures needed to
uncover all these errors—whereupon their death sentences are
very often reversed. This imposes a terrible cost on taxpayers, victims' families, the judicial system, and the wrongly condemned.

Among the inmates involved in the study who had their 71
death verdicts overturned, nearly all were given a sentence less
than death (82 percent), and many were found innocent on retrial
(7 percent).

The number of errors has risen since 1996, when President 72
Clinton made it tougher for death row inmates to prove their
innocence by signing into law a one-year limit on the time inmates
have to appeal to federal courts after exhausting their appeals in
state courts. In light of the study that proved how many of these
inmates are either innocent or not legally deserving of the death
penalty, this attempt to curb their appeals was simply outrageous.

We are one of the few countries in the world that puts to death 73
both the mentally retarded and juvenile offenders. The United
States is among only six countries that impose the death penalty
on juveniles. The others are Iran, Nigeria, Pakistan, Saudi Arabia,
and Yemen.

74   The United States is also the only country besides Somalia that has not signed the United Nations Convention on the Rights of the Child. Why? Because it contains a provision prohibiting the execution of children under eighteen, and we want to remain free to execute our children.

75   *No other industrialized nation executes its children.*

76   Even China prohibits the death penalty for those under eighteen—this from a country that has shown an intolerable lack of respect for human rights.

77   Currently the total number of death row inmates in the United States tops 3,700. Seventy of those death row inmates are minors (or were when they committed their crime).

78   But our Supreme Court doesn't find it cruel and unusual punishment (in the terms of the Eighth Amendment to the U.S. Constitution) to execute those who were sixteen years old when they committed a capital crime. This despite the fact that same court has ruled that sixteen-year-olds do not have "the maturity or judgment" to sign contracts.

79   Odd, isn't it, that a child's diminished capacity for signing contracts is viewed as a legal barrier to enforcing a contract, but when it comes to the right to be executed, a child's capacity is equal to that of an adult?

80   Eighteen states allow juvenile offenders as young as sixteen to be executed. Five others allow the execution of those who were seventeen or older when they committed their crime. In 1999 Oklahoma executed Sean Sellers, who was sixteen at the time of the murders he was found guilty of committing. Sellers's multiple personality disorder wasn't revealed to the jury that convicted him. A federal appeals court found that Sellers might have been "factually innocent" because of his mental disorder, but that "innocence alone is not sufficient to grant federal relief." Unbelievable.

81   The American public is not stupid, and now that the truth has been coming out about the innocent people who have been sent to death row, they are at least responding with a sense of shame. Just a few years ago public opinion polls showed that upwards of 80 percent of the American people supported the death penalty. But now, with the truth out, a recent *Washington Post*/ABC News poll found that public approval of capital

punishment has declined, while the proportion of Americans who favor replacing the death penalty with life in prison has increased. Fifty-one percent favored halting all executions until a commission is established to determine whether the death penalty is being administered fairly.

Sixty-eight percent said the death penalty is unfair because 82 innocent people are sometimes executed. Recent Gallup Polls have shown that support for the death penalty is at a nineteen year low. Sixty-five percent agreed that a poor person is more likely than a person of average or above-average income to receive the death penalty for the same crime. Fifty percent agreed that a black person is more likely than a white person to receive the death penalty for the same crime. Even in the killing machine known as the state of Texas, the *Houston Chronicle* reported that 59 percent of Texans surveyed believed that their state has executed an innocent person!, while 72 percent favor changing state law to include the sentencing option of life without parole, and 60 percent are now opposed to the state executing an inmate who is mentally retarded.

What we have done, in this great country, is to wage a war 83 not on crime but on the poor we feel comfortable blaming for it. Somewhere along the way we forgot about people's rights, because we didn't want to spend the money.

We live in a society that rewards and honors corporate 84 gangsters—corporate leaders who directly and indirectly plunder the earth's resources and look out for the shareholders' profits above all else—while subjecting the poor to a random and brutal system of "justice."

But the public is starting to realize this is wrong.   85

We need to reorder society so that every person within it is 86 seen as precious, sacred, and valuable, and that NO man is above the law, no matter how many candidates he buys off. Until this changes, we can utter the words "with liberty and justice for all" only with shame.

7

Marriage and Divorce: How Should You Take This Person to Be Your Spouse?

I Want a Wife

Judy Brady

1   I belong to that classification of people known as wives. I am A Wife. And, not altogether incidentally, I am a mother.

2   Not too long ago a male friend of mine appeared on the scene fresh from a recent divorce. He had one child, who is, of course, with his ex-wife. He is looking for another wife. As I thought about him while I was ironing one evening, it suddenly occurred to me that I, too, would like to have a wife. Why do I want a wife?

3   I would like to go back to school so that I can become economically independent, support myself, and if need be, support those dependent upon me. I want a wife who will work and send me to school. And while I am going to school I want a wife to take care of my children. I want a wife to keep track of the children's doctor and dentist appointments. And to keep track of mine, too. I want a wife to make sure my children eat properly and are kept clean. I want a wife who will wash the children's clothes and keep them mended. I want a wife who is a good nurturing attendant to my children, who arranges for their schooling, makes sure that they have an adequate social life with their peers,

takes them to the park, the zoo, etc. I want a wife who takes care of the children when they are sick, a wife who arranges to be around when the children need special care, because, of course, I cannot miss classes at school. My wife must arrange to lose time at work and not lose the job. It may mean a small cut in my wife's income from time to time, but I guess I can tolerate that. Needless to say, my wife will arrange and pay for the care of the children while my wife is working.

I want a wife who will take care of *my* physical needs. I want a wife who will keep my house clean. A wife who will pick up after my children, a wife who will pick up after me. I want a wife who will keep my clothes clean, ironed, mended, replaced when need be, and who will see to it that my personal things are kept in their proper place so that I can find what I need the minute I need it. I want a wife who cooks the meals, a wife who is a *good* cook. I want a wife who will plan the menus, do the necessary grocery shopping, prepare the meals, serve them pleasantly, and then do the cleaning up while I do my studying. I want a wife who will care for me when I am sick and sympathize with my pain and loss of time from school. I want a wife to go along when our family takes a vacation so that someone can continue to care for me and my children when I need a rest and change of scene.

I want a wife who will not bother me with rambling complaints about a wife's duties. But I want a wife who will listen to me when I feel the need to explain a rather difficult point I have come across in my course of studies. And I want a wife who will type my papers for me when I have written them.

I want a wife who will take care of the details of my social life. When my wife and I are invited out by my friends, I want a wife who will take care of the baby-sitting arrangements. When I meet people at school that I like and want to entertain, I want a wife who will have the house clean, will prepare a special meal, serve it to me and my friends, and not interrupt when I talk about things that interest me and my friends. I want a wife who will have arranged that the children are fed and ready for bed before my guests arrive so that the children do not bother us. I want a wife who takes care of the needs of my guests so that they feel comfortable, who makes sure that they have an ashtray, that they are passed the hors d'oeuvres, that they are offered a second helping of the food, that their wine glasses are replenished when necessary, that their coffee is served to them as they like it. And I want a wife who knows that sometimes I need a night out by myself.

7   I want a wife who is sensitive to my sexual needs, a wife who makes love passionately and eagerly when I feel like it, a wife who makes sure that I am satisfied. And, of course, I want a wife who will not demand sexual attention when I am not in the mood for it. I want a wife who assumes the complete responsibility for birth control, because I do not want more children. I want a wife who will remain sexually faithful to me so that I do not have to clutter up my intellectual life with jealousies. And I want a wife who understands that *my* sexual needs may entail more than strict adherence to monogamy. I must, after all, be able to relate to people as fully as possible.

8   If, by chance, I find another person more suitable as a wife than the wife I already have, I want the liberty to replace my present wife with another one. Naturally, I will expect a fresh, new life; my wife will take the children and be solely responsible for them so that I am left free.

9   When I am through with school and have a job, I want my wife to quit working and remain at home so that my wife can more fully and completely take care of a wife's duties.

10   My God, who *wouldn't* want a wife?

Declaration of Sentiments

Elizabeth Cady Stanton

1 When, in the course of human events, it becomes necessary for one portion of the family of man to assume among the people of the earth a position different from that which they have hitherto occupied, but one to which the laws of nature and of nature's God entitle them, a decent respect to the opinions of mankind requires that they should declare the causes that impel them to such a course.

2   We hold these truths to be self-evident: that all men and women are created equal; that they are endowed by their Creator

with certain inalienable rights; that among these are life, liberty, and the pursuit of happiness; that to secure these rights governments are instituted, deriving their just powers from the consent of the governed. Whenever any form of government becomes destructive of these ends, it is the right of those who suffer from it to refuse allegiance to it, and to insist upon the institution of a new government, laying its foundation on such principles, and organizing its powers in such form, as to them shall seem most likely to effect their safety and happiness. Prudence, indeed, will dictate that governments long established should not be changed for light and transient causes; and accordingly all experience hath shown that mankind are more disposed to suffer, while evils are sufferable, than to right themselves by abolishing the forms to which they were accustomed. But when a long train of abuses and usurpations, pursuing invariably the same object evinces a design to reduce them under absolute despotism, it is their duty to throw off such government, and to provide new guards for their future security. Such has been the patient sufferance of the women under this government, and such is now the necessity which constrains them to demand the equal station to which they are entitled.

The history of mankind is a history of repeated injuries and 3 usurpations on the part of man toward woman, having in direct object the establishment of an absolute tyranny over her. To prove this, let facts be submitted to a candid world.

He has never permitted her to exercise her inalienable right 4 to the elective franchise.

He has compelled her to submit to laws, in the formation of 5 which she had no voice.

He has withheld from her rights which are given to the most 6 ignorant and degraded men—both natives and foreigners.

Having deprived her of this first right of a citizen, the elective 7 franchise, thereby leaving her without representation in the halls of legislation, he has oppressed her on all sides.

He has made her, if married, in the eye of the law, civilly dead. 8

He has taken from her all right in property, even to the wages 9 she earns.

He has made her, morally, an irresponsible being, as she can 10 commit many crimes with impunity, provided they be done in the presence of her husband. In the covenant of marriage, she is compelled to promise obedience to her husband, he becoming, to all intents and purposes, her master—the law giving him power to deprive her of her liberty, and to administer chastisement.

11   He has so framed the laws of divorce, as to what shall be the proper causes, and in case of separation, to whom the guardianship of the children shall be given, as to be wholly regardless of the happiness of women—the law, in all cases, going upon a false supposition of the supremacy of man, and giving all power into his hands.

12   After depriving her of all rights as a married woman, if single, and the owner of property, he has taxed her to support a government which recognizes her only when her property can be made profitable to it.

13   He has monopolized nearly all the profitable employments, and from those she is permitted to follow, she receives but a scanty remuneration. He closes against her all the avenues to wealth and distinction which he considers most honorable to himself. As a teacher of theology, medicine, or law, she is not known.

14   He has denied her the facilities for obtaining a thorough education, all colleges being closed against her.

15   He allows her in Church, as well as State, but a subordinate position, claiming Apostolic authority for her exclusion from the ministry, and, with some exceptions, from any public participation in the affairs of the Church.

16   He has created a false public sentiment by giving to the world a different code of morals for men and women, by which moral delinquencies which exclude women from society, are not only tolerated, but deemed of little account in man.

17   He has usurped the prerogative of Jehovah himself, claiming it as his right to assign for her a sphere of action, when that belongs to her conscience and to her God.

18   He has endeavored, in every way that he could, to destroy her confidence in her own powers, to lessen her self-respect, and to make her willing to lead a dependent and abject life.

19   Now in view of this entire disfranchisement of one-half the people of this country, their social and religious degradation—in view of the unjust laws above mentioned, and because women do feel themselves aggrieved, oppressed, and fraudulently deprived

of their most sacred rights, we insist that they have immediate admission to all the rights and privileges which belong to them as citizens of the United States.

In entering upon the great work before us, we anticipate no 20 small amount of misconception, misrepresentation, and ridicule; but we shall use every instrumentality within our power to effect our object. We shall employ agents, circulate tracts, petition the State and National legislatures, and endeavor to enlist the pulpit and the press in our behalf. We hope this Convention will be followed by a series of Conventions embracing every part of the country.

A Proposal I Never Thought I'd Consider

Sabaa Saleem

In spite of myself, I think I may agree to an arranged marriage.   1

Beginning next month, my parents will contact Muslim fam- 2 ily friends around the world with a list of criteria for a husband: a twentysomething, classically handsome, Urdu-speaking Muslim man who is 6 feet tall, with an MD and MBA, as well as a PhD in something respectable like molecular toxicology. He must have a good sense of family and a financial portfolio fat enough to take care of the next 15 generations. My parents will screen the candidates, and after I graduate from college next spring, they will introduce me to the few they deem best. Ultimately, the lucky man will have to pass my own stringent test: Does he own every Radiohead album and listen to them regularly?

Like so many other young South Asians in America, I am the 3 product of two cultures whose conflicting values pull at me with equal urgency. Never have I felt as torn between the two as I do about the question of marriage. I have been a Californian for all but the first year of my life, when my family lived in Britain, where I was born. I grew up in a small town in the Mojave Desert where conservative Republicans were as common as cacti. Inexplicably, I grew up liberal and a feminist.

4   My mother and father were born and raised in Pakistan, where religion is entrenched in the culture and the culture is explicitly unyielding. Though they left family and comfort decades ago for opportunity in the West, they brought strong religious faith and cultural expectations with them—and tried to instill sobriety and respect in my two older brothers and me. They have more or less succeeded, but they have also endured nearly 30 years of our stubborn refusal to conform. They have grudgingly accepted that; while respectful, their children are also independent, maybe even eccentric—qualities not admired by most traditional Pakistanis.

5   My parents would casually joke about my marriage while I was growing up. I was uneasy about it, but it seemed so far off that it was easy for me to laugh it off. "When pigs fly!" I'd say, and change the subject.

6   Now, almost everyone I know—friends, teachers, co-workers— expects me, as a child of the West, to reject the notion of arranged marriage, to proclaim my independence loudly. Sometimes, I still expect that, too. But as a young Muslim woman, I also expect myself to accept the obligations I have as my parents' daughter— regardless of the emotional cost to me.

7   Pakistani culture and Islam beckon me with security, familiarity and ease. By agreeing to an arranged marriage, I could more easily satisfy my religious obligation to abstain from intimacy with the opposite sex until marriage—not an easy feat, may I say. I would be participating in the ceremony of a culture 11,000 miles removed, a ceremony I've witnessed only twice. By doing so, I could spare my parents the stinging criticism they would face if their daughter chose her own path: barbs from three generations of extended family, all of whom accepted their own arranged marriages without argument—and some of whom complain about them to this day.

8   At the same time, Pakistani culture repels me with its expectation that I adhere to a tradition that essentially advocates handing me over to a man for safekeeping. From the endless gossip of aunts, uncles, cousins and friends, I know the courtship ritual well. I will briefly meet my parents' choices and pick those who interest me. With each man, after perhaps a month of chaperoned dating, phone calls, no physical contact and little understanding

of whether we would mesh, I am supposed to decide whether to marry him.

In the end, the decision will be mine. My parents would never 9 force me to marry a particular man. But they do expect me not to dawdle. Ideally, I should make a decision after no more than five or six meetings. I am supposed to pick a husband, accept my fate and hope the marriage is successful. Our engagement would likely last a year or two, during which we would get to know each other better—and maybe even grow fond of each other. (Breaking it off at that point would be possible, but that would reflect badly on me and on my family and would represent time wasted.) Still, I worry that my filial piety could lead me down an empty road— where independent minds and hearts are given up to the demands of a culture that I often find perplexing.

I am not alone in this struggle. My oldest brother and I have 10 mulled over the marriage question for hours and hours. My other brother, the middle child and black sheep of the family, long ago informed our parents that there would be no arranged marriage for him—in fact, there probably wouldn't be a marriage at all. My parents hope he'll come to his senses. And though their oldest child is 29—marrying age for men in Pakistan—my parents accept his excuse that he's just not ready. Maybe they focus less on him because my father was 31 when he married. Whatever the reason, until I get married, my parents' eyes are on me. Their priorities for me are that I get a bachelor's degree and marry—in that order. Thus, I decided to take an honors thesis class last year to postpone my graduation until next March, when UCLA will have to forcibly boot me out. I am searching for ways to extend my school days so that I can put off the marriage decision again. I have to admit, I'm beginning to feel a creeping sense of desperation because I was imbued with a sense of skepticism toward anything that is overly reliant on tradition rather than reason. But my skepticism is outweighed by an obligation to my mother and father, and to their happiness.

My parents are not evil people who have kept me in a box 11 my whole life, bent on handing me over to a man who will do the same. They've always treated me with love and respect and showed trust in my judgment. And the rules they applied to me when I was younger have remained a part of me, even when I have not wanted them to. For example, my parents never allowed me to date and generally frowned on any male friendships. Dating leads to intimacy, which would be out of the question. In high school, I was far quieter than I am now, and a tight curfew ensured my good behavior.

12   But the coed dorms, parties and freedom of college have presented a moral dilemma for me. I did not want to disappoint my parents. So I developed a complex method of discouraging in myself behavior that they, and Islam, would consider deviant. When I thought someone was about to ask me out, I used the idea that I wasn't sure about my sexuality as a ruse to get him to keep his distance. Or I ran off, claiming an appointment. But after four years of these tactics—which have not failed me yet—I find it harder to convince others, and myself, that I'm not interested.

13   Then I think of my parents and their leniency over the years and I stop having the conversation with myself in which I have doubts. Despite their strict upbringing, my parents do not ask me to wear the Islamic head cover. They did not insist that I attend a local college and continue to live at home, as many Muslim girls do. They do not admonish me when I stay out late, and they only occasionally flare up at my decision to forgo medicine for journalism. They remind me to eat and sleep and worry less about grades and career, and they encourage me to attend concerts and enjoy my youth.

14   My parents have given me every opportunity for happiness. And I know that their happiness depends on fulfilling their responsibilities as good Muslim parents. They must see their children married to other Muslims of whom they approve.

15   That took on a new urgency last January when my father, who has a bad heart, also had a stroke. A religious man, he now even more adamantly believes it is his duty to secure my spiritual well-being in whatever time he has left. If he succeeds in marrying me well, ideally to a Muslim from a good Pakistani family, then my soul will be at peace in the afterlife. Moreover, he will be enabling me to follow the rules set out by Islam—to respect my parents' wishes, to start a family and to hand down my religious morals to my children.

16   That holds nearly as much weight as performing his five daily prayers. For him, my marriage would be the crowning achievement

in a life nearly complete. I worry that, if his health deteriorates further and I am not married, I will be the cause of his having an incomplete life.

Similarly, my mother doesn't believe she can perform the pilgrimage to Mecca—of paramount importance to even moderately devout Muslims—with a clear conscience until I am married. If I refused to get married, my parents would be brokenhearted and confused. Like any child close to her parents, I could not watch them suffer. [17]

And so I find myself defending arranged marriage against those who see it as absurd or even barbaric. Yet I'm disturbed by the doubt these critics instill in me. My fifth year of college buys me more time to resolve my career insecurities. But if I can't even decide between writing or editing, philanthropy or graduate school, how can I commit myself to a man I'll know so little about? Beyond my parents' requirements, there are traits I need in the man I marry that cannot be discerned from a few meetings. Will he be able to hold his own in a discussion with me? Will he calmly accept that I will be at least a half-hour late to any important event? Will he make fun of Bollywood films with me? [18]

If we marry, it will no doubt be for life. Muslims accept divorce, but usually as a last resort, and many Pakistanis, including my extended family, see divorce as an escape for the weak-willed. [19]

And is it selfish and idealistic to want "true love"? My American instincts tell me that love comes before marriage, not a few years after—if I am lucky. Like a lot of South Asians raised in the United States, I hope for a "love-match"—where parents accept the Muslim their child has met on her own and has decided to marry. My parents have said that this route would please them most, because it would be a compromise between their ideals and mine. [20]

A month ago, I asked my mother about her determination to have me married soon, especially when her own marriage at 21 took her to London, away from the world she knew, preventing her from pursuing a career and establishing her independence. She said, "Do you think I want to you to leave us—to have a man at the center of your life? Maybe even to go away? I want my daughter close to me always, but this is my duty; I don't have a choice—I can't be selfish. I have to let you go." [21]

22   That day, I decided I would have an arranged marriage.

23   But now, I marvel at how quickly the summer has passed. I feel like hyperventilating when I think how quickly spring will come, and engagement and marriage will follow. I fantasize about ways to scare off suitors (bringing sock puppets to our first meeting, perhaps?). Briefly, I resolve to put off marriage, for a few years at least.

24   But then I think of my parents' anguish if I refuse to honor their wishes—I think of my father and the shadowy road ahead of him—and of how empty I will feel. And I wonder, if I have one foot in each world, is it possible to keep from being torn apart?

The Conservative Case for Gay Marriage

Andrew Sullivan

1   A long time ago, the *New Republic* ran a contest to discover the most boring headline ever written. Entrants had to beat the following snoozer, which had inspired the event: WORTHWHILE CANADIAN INITIATIVE. Little did the contest organizers realize that one day such a headline would be far from boring and, in its own small way, a social watershed.

2   Canada's federal government decided last week not to contest the rulings of three provincial courts that had all come to the conclusion that denying homosexuals the right to marry violated Canada's constitutional commitment to civic equality. What that means is that gay marriage has now arrived in the western hemisphere. And this isn't some euphemism. It isn't the quasi-marriage now celebrated in Vermont, whose "civil unions" approximate marriage but don't go by that name. It's just marriage—for all. Canada now follows the Netherlands and Belgium with full-fledged marital rights for gays and lesbians.

3   Could it happen in the U.S.? The next few weeks will give us many clues. The U.S. Supreme Court is due to rule any day now on whether it's legal for Texas and other states to prosecute

sodomy among gays but not straights. More critical, Massachusetts' highest court is due to rule very soon on whether the denial of marriage to gays is illicit discrimination against a minority. If Massachusetts rules that it is, then gay couples across America will be able to marry not only in Canada (where there are no residency or nationality requirements for marriage) but also in a bona fide American state. There will be a long process of litigation as various married couples try hard to keep their marriages legally intact from one state to another.

This move seems an eminently conservative one—in fact, almost an emblem of "compassionate conservatism." Conservatives have long rightly argued for the vital importance of the institution of marriage for fostering responsibility, commitment and the domestication of unruly men. Bringing gay men and women into this institution will surely change the gay subculture in subtle but profoundly conservative ways. When I grew up and realized I was gay, I had no concept of what my own future could be like. Like most other homosexuals, I grew up in a heterosexual family and tried to imagine how I too could one day be a full part of the family I loved. But I figured then that I had no such future. I could never have a marriage, never have a family, never be a full and equal part of the weddings and relationships and holidays that give families structure and meaning. When I looked forward, I saw nothing but emptiness and loneliness. No wonder it was hard to connect sex with love and commitment. No wonder it was hard to feel at home in what was, in fact, my home.

For today's generation of gay kids, all that changes. From the beginning, they will be able to see their future as part of family life—not in conflict with it. Their "coming out" will also allow them a "coming home." And as they date in adolescence and early adulthood, there will be some future anchor in their mind-set, some ultimate structure with which to give their relationships stability and social support. Many heterosexuals, I suspect, simply don't realize how big a deal this is. They have never doubted that one day they could marry the person they love. So they find it hard to conceive how deep a psychic and social wound the exclusion from marriage and family can be. But the polls suggest this is changing fast: the majority of people 30 and younger see gay marriage as inevitable and understandable. Many young straight couples simply don't see married gay peers next door as some sort of threat to their own lives. They can get along in peace.

6   As for religious objections, it's important to remember that the issue here is not religious. It's civil. Various religious groups can choose to endorse same-sex marriage or not as they see fit. Their freedom of conscience is as vital as gays' freedom to be treated equally under the civil law. And there's no real reason that the two cannot coexist. The Roman Catholic Church, for example, opposes remarriage after divorce. But it doesn't seek to make civil divorce and remarriage illegal for everyone. Similarly, churches can well decide this matter in their own time and on their own terms while allowing the government to be neutral between competing visions of the good life. We can live and let live.

7   And after all, isn't that what this really is about? We needn't all agree on the issue of homosexuality to believe that the government should treat every citizen alike. If that means living next door to someone of whom we disapprove, so be it. But disapproval needn't mean disrespect. And if the love of two people, committing themselves to each other exclusively for the rest of their lives, is not worthy of respect, then what is?

The Making of a Divorce Culture

Barbara Dafoe Whitehead

1   Divorce is now part of everyday American life. It is embedded in our laws and institutions, our manners and mores, our movies and television shows, our novels and children's storybooks, and our closest and most important relationships. Indeed, divorce has become so pervasive that many people naturally assume it has seeped into the social and cultural mainstream over a long period of time. Yet this is not the case. Divorce has become an American way of life only as the result of recent and revolutionary change.

2   The entire history of American divorce can be divided into two periods, one evolutionary and the other revolutionary. For most of the nation's history, divorce was a rare occurrence and an insignificant feature of family and social relationships. In the

first sixty years of the twentieth century, divorce became more common, but it was hardly commonplace. In 1960, the divorce rate stood at a still relatively modest level of nine per one thousand married couples. After 1960, however, the rate accelerated at a dazzling pace. It doubled in roughly a decade and continued its upward climb until the early 1980s, when it stabilized at the highest level among advanced Western societies. As a consequence of this sharp and sustained rise, divorce moved from the margins to the mainstream of American life in the space of three decades.

Ideas are important in revolutions, yet surprisingly little 3 attention has been devoted to the ideas that gave impetus to the divorce revolution. Of the scores of books on divorce published in recent decades, most focus on its legal, demographic, economic, or (especially) psychological dimensions. Few, if any, deal fully with its intellectual origins. Yet trying to comprehend the divorce revolution and its consequences without some sense of its ideological origins is like trying to understand the American Revolution without taking into account the thinking of John Locke, Thomas Jefferson, or Thomas Paine. This more recent revolution, like the revolution of our nation's founding, has its roots in a distinctive set of ideas and claims.

This book is about the ideas behind the divorce revolution 4 and how these ideas have shaped a culture of divorce. The making of a divorce culture has involved three overlapping changes: first, the emergence and widespread diffusion of a historically new and distinctive set of ideas about divorce in the last third of the twentieth century; second, the migration of divorce from a minor place within a system governed by marriage to a freestanding place as a major institution governing family relationships; and third, a widespread shift in thinking about the obligations of marriage and parenthood.

Beginning in the late 1950s, Americans began to change their 5 ideas about the individual's obligations to family and society. Broadly described, this change was away from an ethic of obligation to others and toward an obligation to self. I do not mean that people suddenly abandoned all responsibilities to others, but rather that they became more acutely conscious of their responsibility to attend to their own individual needs and interests. At least as important as the moral obligation to look after others, the new thinking suggested, was the moral obligation to look after oneself.

6   This ethical shift had a profound impact on ideas about the nature and purpose of the family. In the American tradition, the marketplace and the public square have represented the realms of life devoted to the pursuit of individual interest, choice, and freedom, while the family has been the realm defined by voluntary commitment, duty, and self-sacrifice. With the greater emphasis on individual satisfaction in family relationships, however, family well-being became subject to a new metric. More than in the past, satisfaction in this sphere came to be based on subjective judgments about the content and quality of individual happiness rather than on such objective measures as level of income, material nurture and support, or boosting children onto a higher rung on the socioeconomic ladder. People began to judge the strength and "health" of family bonds according to their capacity to promote individual fulfillment and personal growth. As a result, the conception of the family's role and place in the society began to change. The family began to lose its separate place and distinctive identity as the realm of duty, service, and sacrifice. Once the domain of the obligated self, the family was increasingly viewed as yet another domain for the expression of the unfettered self.

7   These broad changes figured centrally in creating a new conception of divorce which gained influential adherents and spread broadly and swiftly throughout the society—a conception that represented a radical departure from earlier notions. Once regarded mainly as a social, legal, and family event in which there were other stakeholders, divorce now became an event closely linked to the pursuit of individual satisfactions, opportunities, and growth.

8   The new conception of divorce drew upon some of the oldest, and most resonant, themes in the American political tradition. The nation, after all, was founded as the result of a political divorce, and revolutionary thinkers explicitly adduced a parallel between the dissolution of marital bonds and the dissolution of political bonds. In political as well as marital relationships, they argued, bonds of obligation were established voluntarily on the basis of mutual affection and regard. Once such bonds turned cold and oppressive, peoples, like individuals, had the right to dissolve them and to form more perfect unions.

In the new conception of divorce, this strain of eighteenth- 9
century political thought mingled with a strain of twentieth-
century psychotherapeutic thought. Divorce was not only an
individual right but also a psychological resource. The dissolution
of marriage offered the chance to make oneself over from the
inside out, to refurbish and express the inner self, and to acquire
certain valuable psychological assets and competencies, such as
initiative, assertiveness, and a stronger and better self-image.

The conception of divorce as both an individual right and an 10
inner experience merged with and reinforced the new ethic of obligation to the self. In family relationships, one had an obligation to
be attentive to one's own feelings and to work toward improving
the quality of one's inner life. This ethical imperative completed
the rationale for a sense of individual entitlement to divorce.
Increasingly, mainstream America saw the legal dissolution of marriage as a matter of individual choice, in which there were no other
stakeholders or larger social interests. This conception of divorce
strongly argued for removing the social, legal, and moral impedi-
ments to the free exercise of the individual right to divorce.

Traditionally, one major impediment to divorce was the pres- 11
ence of children in the family. According to well-established popular belief, dependent children had a stake in their parents'
marriage and suffered hardship as a result of the dissolution of
the marriage. Because children were vulnerable and dependent,
parents had a moral obligation to place their children's interests
in the marital partnership above their own individual satisfactions. This notion was swiftly abandoned after the 1960s. Influential voices in the society, including child-welfare professionals,
claimed that the happiness of individual parents, rather than an
intact marriage, was the key determinant of children's family
well-being. If divorce could make one or both parents happier,
then it was likely to improve the well-being of children as well.

In the following decades, the new conception of divorce spread 12
through the law, therapy, etiquette, the social sciences, popular
advice literature, and religion. Concerns that had dominated earlier
thinking on divorce were now dismissed as old-fashioned and
excessively moralistic. Divorce would not harm children but would
lead to greater happiness for children and their single parents. It
would not damage the institution of marriage but would make

possible better marriages and happier individuals. Divorce would not damage the social fabric by diminishing children's life chances but would strengthen the social fabric by improving the quality of affective bonds between parents and children, whatever form the structural arrangements of their families might happen to take.

13   As the sense of divorce as an individual freedom and entitlement grew, the sense of concern about divorce as a social problem diminished. Earlier in the century, each time the divorce rate increased sharply, it had inspired widespread public concern and debate about the harmful impact of divorce on families and the society. But in the last third of the century, as the divorce rate rose to once unthinkable levels, public anxiety about it all but vanished. At the very moment when divorce had its most profound impact on the society, weakening the institution of marriage, revolutionizing the structure of families and reorganizing parent-child relationships, it ceased to be a source of concern or debate.

14   The lack of attention to divorce became particularly striking after the 1980s, as a politically polarized debate over the state of the American family took shape. On one side, conservatives pointed to abortion, illegitimacy, and homosexuality as forces destroying the family. On the other, liberals cited domestic violence, economic insecurity, and inadequate public supports as the key problems afflicting the family. But politicians on both sides had almost nothing to say about divorce. Republicans did not want to alienate their upscale constituents or their libertarian wing, both of whom tended to favor easy divorce, nor did they want to call attention to the divorces among their own leadership. Democrats did not want to anger their large constituency among women who saw easy divorce as a hard-won freedom and prerogative, nor did they wish to seem unsympathetic to single mothers. Thus, except for bipartisan calls to get tougher with deadbeat dads, both Republicans and Democrats avoided the issue of divorce and its consequences as far too politically risky.

15   But the failure to address divorce carried a price. It allowed the middle class to view family breakdown as a "them" problem rather than an "us" problem. Divorce was not like illegitimacy or welfare dependency, many claimed. It was a matter of individual choice, imposing few, if any, costs or consequences on others. Thus, mainstream America could cling to the comfortable illusion

that the nation's family problems had to do with the behavior of unwed teenage mothers or poor women on welfare rather than with the instability of marriage and family life within its own ranks.

Nonetheless, after thirty years of persistently high levels 16 of divorce, this illusion, though still politically attractive, is increasingly difficult to sustain in the face of a growing body of experience and evidence. To begin with, divorce has indeed hurt children. It has created economic insecurity and disadvantage for many children who would not otherwise be economically vulnerable. It has led to more fragile and unstable family households. It has caused a mass exodus of fathers from children's households and, all too often, from their lives. It has reduced the levels of parental time and money invested in children. In sum, it has changed the very nature of American childhood. Just as no patient would have designed today's system of health care, so no child would have chosen today's culture of divorce.

Divorce figures prominently in the altered economic fortunes 17 of middle-class families. Although the economic crisis of the middle class is usually described as a problem caused by global economic changes, changing patterns in education and earnings, and ruthless corporate downsizing, it owes more to divorce than is commonly acknowledged. Indeed, recent data suggest that marriage may be a more important economic resource than a college degree. According to an analysis of 1994 income patterns, the median income of married-parent households whose heads have only a high school diploma is ten percent higher than the median income of college-educated single-parent households.[1]

---

[1]An analysis of income data provided by The Northeastern University Center for Labor Market Studies shows the following distribution by education and marital status:

MEDIAN INCOMES FOR U.S. FAMILIES WITH CHILDREN, 1994

Education of household head	Married Couple Families	Single Parent Families
College Graduate	$71,263	$36,006
High School Graduate	$40,098	$14,698

Based on 1994 Current Population Statistics. Families with one or more children under 18. Age of household head: 22–62.

Parents who are college graduates *and* married form the new economic elite among families with children. Consequently, those who are concerned about what the downsizing of corporations is doing to workers should also be concerned about what the downsizing of families through divorce is doing to parents and children.

18   Widespread divorce depletes social capital as well. Scholars tell us that strong and durable family and social bonds generate certain "goods" and services, including money, mutual assistance, information, caregiving, protection, and sponsorship. Because such bonds endure over time, they accumulate and form a pool of social capital which can be drawn down upon, when needed, over the entire course of a life. An elderly couple, married for fifty years, is likely to enjoy a substantial body of social and emotional capital, generated through their long-lasting marriage, which they can draw upon in caring for each other and for themselves as they age. Similarly, children who grow up in stable, two-parent married households are the beneficiaries of the social and emotional capital accumulated over time as a result of an enduring marriage bond. As many parents know, children continue to depend on these resources well into young adulthood. But as family bonds become increasingly fragile and vulnerable to disruption, they become less permanent and thus less capable of generating such forms of help, financial resources, and mutual support. In short, divorce consumes social capital and weakens the social fabric. At the very time that sweeping socioeconomic changes are mandating greater investment of social capital in children, widespread divorce is reducing the pool of social capital. As the new economic and social conditions raise the hurdles of child-rearing higher, divorce digs potholes in the tracks.

19   It should be stressed that this book is not intended as a brief against divorce as such. We must assume that divorce is necessary as a remedy for irretrievably broken marriages, especially those that are marred by severe abuse such as chronic infidelity, drug addiction, or physical violence. Nor is its argument directed against those who are divorced. It assumes that divorce is difficult, painful, and often unwanted by at least one spouse, and that divorcing couples require compassion and support from family, friends, and their religious communities. Nor should this book be taken as an appeal for a return to an earlier era of American

family life. The media routinely portray the debate over the family as one between nostalgists and realists, between those who want to turn back the clock to the fifties and those who want to march bravely and resolutely forward into the new century. But this is a lazy and misguided approach, driven more by the easy availability of archival photos and footage from 1950s television sitcoms than by careful consideration of the substance of competing arguments.

More fundamentally, this approach overlooks the key issue. 20 And that issue is not how today's families might stack up against those of an earlier era; indeed, no reliable empirical data for such a comparison exist. In an age of diverse family structures, the heart of the matter is what kinds of contemporary family arrangements have the greatest capacity to promote children's well-being, and how we can ensure that more children have the advantages of growing up in such families.

In the past year or so, there has been growing recognition of the 21 personal and social costs of three decades of widespread divorce. A public debate has finally emerged. Within this debate, there are two separate and overlapping discussions.

The first centers on a set of specific proposals that are 22 intended to lessen the harmful impact of divorce on children: a federal system of child-support collection, tougher child-support enforcement, mandatory counseling for divorcing parents, and reform of no-fault divorce laws in the states. What is striking about this discussion is its narrow focus on public policy, particularly on changes in the system of no-fault divorce. In this, as in so many other crucial discussions involving social and moral questions, the most vocal and visible participants come from the world of government policy, electoral politics, and issue advocacy. The media, which are tongue-tied unless they can speak in the language of left-right politics, reinforce this situation. And the public is offered needlessly polarized arguments that hang on a flat yes-or-no response to this or that individual policy measure. All too often, this discussion of divorce poses what *Washington Post* columnist E. J. Dionne aptly describes as false choices.

Notably missing is a serious consideration of the broader 23 moral assumptions and empirical claims that define our divorce culture. Divorce touches on classic questions in American public philosophy—on the nature of our most important human and social bonds, the duties and obligations imposed by bonds we voluntarily elect, the "just causes" for the dissolution of those bonds, and the differences between obligations volunteered and those that must be coerced. Without consideration of such questions, the effort to change behavior by changing a few public policies is likely to founder.

24   The second and complementary discussion does try to place divorce within a larger philosophical framework. Its proponents have looked at the decline in the well-being of the nation's children as the occasion to call for a collective sense of commitment by all Americans to all of America's children. They pose the challenging question: "What are Americans willing to do 'for the sake of *all* children'?" But while this is surely an important question, it addresses only half of the problem of declining commitment. The other half has to do with how we answer the question: "What are individual parents obliged to do 'for the sake of their own children'?"

25   Renewing a *social* ethic of commitment to children is an urgent goal, but it cannot be detached from the goal of strengthening the *individual* ethic of commitment to children. The state of one affects the standing of the other. A society that protects the rights of parents to easy, unilateral divorce, and flatly rejects the idea that parents should strive to preserve a marriage "for the sake of the children," faces a problem when it comes to the question of public sacrifice "for the sake of the children." To put it plainly, many of the ideas we have come to believe and vigorously defend about adult prerogatives and freedoms in family life are undermining the foundations of altruism and support for children.

26   With each passing year, the culture of divorce becomes more deeply entrenched. American children are routinely schooled in divorce. Mr. Rogers teaches toddlers about divorce. An entire children's literature is devoted to divorce. Family movies and videos for children feature divorced families. *Mrs. Doubtfire*, originally a children's book about divorce and then a hit movie, is aggressively marketed as a holiday video for kids. Of course, these books and movies are designed to help children deal with the social reality and psychological trauma of divorce. But they

also carry an unmistakable message about the impermanence and unreliability of family bonds. Like romantic love, the children's storybooks say, family love comes and goes. Daddies disappear. Mommies find new boyfriends. Mommies' boyfriends leave. Grandparents go away. Even pets must be left behind.

More significantly, in a society where nearly half of all children are likely to experience parental divorce, family breakup becomes a defining event of American childhood itself. Many children today know nothing but divorce in their family lives. And although children from divorced families often say they want to avoid divorce if they marry, young adults whose parents divorced are more likely to get divorced themselves and to bear children outside of marriage than young adults from stable married-parent familes. 27

Precisely because the culture of divorce has generational momentum, this book offers no easy optimism about the prospects for change. But neither does it counsel passive resignation or acceptance of the culture's relentless advance. What it does offer is a critique of the ideas behind current divorce trends. Its argument is directed against the ideas about divorce that have gained ascendancy, won our support, and lodged in our consciousness as "proven" and incontrovertible. It challenges the popular idea of divorce as an individual right and freedom to be exercised in the pursuit of individual goods and satisfactions, without due regard for other stakeholders in the marital partnership, especially children. This may be a fragile and inadequate response to a profoundly consequential set of changes, but it seeks the abandonment of ideas that have misled us and failed our children. 28

In a larger sense, this book is both an appreciation and a criticism of what is peculiarly American about divorce. Divorce has spread throughout advanced Western societies at roughly the same pace and over roughly the same period of time. Yet nowhere else has divorce been so deeply imbued with the larger themes of a nation's political traditions. Nowhere has divorce so fully reflected the spirit and susceptibilities of a people who share an extravagant faith in the power of the individual and in the power of positive thinking. Divorce in America is not unique, but what we have made of divorce is uniquely American. In exploring the 29 cultural roots of divorce, therefore, we look at ourselves, at what is best and worst in our traditions, what is visionary and what is blind, and how the two are sometimes tragically commingled and confused.

Making the Case for Teaching Our Boys to . . . 'Bring Me Home a Black Girl'

Audrey Edwards

1   The first time I saw my stepson, Ugo, make a move on a girl, he was about 7, and so was she—a dark-skinned little cutie standing at the juke-box in a Brooklyn family diner looking for a song to play. In a flash, Ugo was at her side, shy but bold at the same time. He pretended to be looking for a song, too, but he was mainly just looking at her, instantly in puppy love. "That's right," I said to him, fairly loudly and pointedly. "When it's time to get married, I want you to bring me home a girl just like that—a Black girl." The girl's parents, sitting at a table nearby, looked at me in surprise and then suddenly beamed. Ugo's father, sitting with me, just nodded and grinned.

2   "Bring me home a Black girl." It's one of those commandments Ugo has heard from me most of his life, right up there with "Don't do drugs," "Finish school" and "Use a condom." Over the years he has rolled his eyes, sighed in exasperation, muttered that I was racist or been mortified whenever I'd blurt out things like "Dark, light, shades in between—it don't matter to me as long as she's Black." But Ugo has also grown up to be very clear about what that edict really means: Don't even think about marrying a White girl.

3   I myself became clear about this—or clear about a mother's role in imparting to male children what's expected when it comes to marriage—when I interviewed the son of a Black magazine publisher ten years ago. The publisher had three sons and a Black

wife who had made it clear to her boys that they were not to bring home any White girls. "We could have them as friends," the eldest son recalled, "but we were definitely not to marry them."

In all the grousing and hand wringing we do over brothers' 4 marrying outside the race, it had never occurred to me that the issue might be addressed by something as simple and basic as child rearing. We tell our sons almost every day what we expect when it comes to their behavior, but we seldom, if ever, tell them what we expect when it comes to that most serious of decisions: choosing a partner. Oh, we may ask vague, cursory questions about the women they bring home: Can she cook? What work does she do? Who are her people? But rarely do we come right out and make the case for marrying Black. Truth be told, we're much more likely to make the case for marrying "light" or marrying someone with "good hair" so we can have "pretty grandbabies." Or we might argue, shouldn't people be allowed to marry whomever they want? Wasn't that one of the goals of integration?

If we were playing on an equal field, yes, we'd all be free 5 to marry anyone. But the fact is, we're not. For Black women, one of the inequities on the current playing field has been the rate at which Black men are marrying outside the race. While most Black men still marry Black women, according to a joint survey by the U.S. Census Bureau and the Bureau of Labor Statistics, the number of Black men marrying White women has increased tenfold in the last 40 years, up from 25,000 in 1960 to 268,000 today. That's more than double the number of Black women who marry White men.

Where Black people are concerned, the increasing numbers of 6 interracial unions could eventually lead to what sex therapist Gwendolyn Goldsby Grant, Ed.D., calls annihilation through integration, a weakening of the culture and economic resources of the Black community. So the question becomes, How do we ensure our cultural and economic survival as a people? One way is to start early and plainly telling our boys to marry Black girls. We need to put the emphasis on our boys because they are more likely than our girls to choose a White partner. Add to that the fact that men still take the lead when it comes to choosing a marriage partner, and it becomes obvious that molding our boys' attitudes is critical.

7   Of course, we may first have to get past what we think telling Black boys to marry Black means. "Somehow Black people are taught that to be ethnocentric is to be racist," says Grant. "But to want to be with people who share your values, religion and culture is very normal. It is not anti–anybody else."

8   Indeed, it seems almost anti-self to want to mate with someone from a culture that has historically denigrated, despised and oppressed you—and continues to do so. "People don't consciously say, 'I don't value myself, so I'm going to seek an image outside my culture,' but the choices you make reflect what you believe," Grant explains. "This is why images are so important. Our children must see themselves positively reflected in the world, and if they don't, they start valuing the dominant culture. And when you worship the dominant culture and pay no attention to your own, you're not making choices for your highest good. You're confused."

9   As Maxwell C. Manning, an assistant professor of social work at Howard University, points out, "If you look at strong cultures, like the Jews, you'll find they have a high rate of marrying within their group. That's how they remain strong." Manning, who says he would be surprised if his own 21-year-old son "walked in the door with a White woman," notes that when as a young man he dated several White women, his parents were very upset. "That told me I should never think about marrying White," he recalls.

10   "I really wanted to be connected to my community," he continues. "Carrying the name and the culture is so important, and I think that would have been more difficult had I married a White woman." The expectations of Manning's parents no doubt influenced his choosing a Black woman when it came time to marry, just as his expectations for his son may well lead him to choose a Black woman as his wife.

11   How parents communicate to their children the importance of marrying within the group will vary, whether it's an in-your-face admonishment like the kind I've always given my stepson, or simply letting your child know, as Manning's parents did, that you're not pleased when he dates White girls. What's most important, says Manning, "is that we communicate to children what our values are. And one of the values should be to marry within the race to further our heritage and our culture."

But culture and heritage are only two factors in a complicated 12
race equation. For me it's just as important that Ugo affirm the
beauty and desirability of Black women by choosing to marry one.
When he zeroed in on that little Black girl at the jukebox many
years ago, he was displaying what I thought was natural—
an instinctive attraction to someone who looked like him. But
according to experts, by age 7, Black children have already been
bombarded by media images that can negatively shape how
they view themselves and the partners you'd think they would
naturally be drawn to.

That's why it's so important that we constantly affirm our 13
children, helping them to appreciate their own intelligence,
beauty and strength. Whether it's in the artwork on your walls,
the posters in your child's room or the books and magazines lying
around the house, positive Black media images should be as inte-
gral a part of a Black child's life as the images coming in through
television, videos and other media.

Fortunately for Ugo, his African grandmother and mother 14
and his Afrocentric Black American father have all contributed to
his being grounded in a strong Black identity. But that doesn't mean
he hasn't also been shaped by seeing his two handsome Black male
cousins have relationships and children with White women. So I
try to be as relentless in countering the White-is-right images he's
assaulted with as our society has been in perpetuating them.

Clearly, one of the most insistent images going is that White 15
women are the most beautiful and therefore should be the most
desired. If you buy into this notion, then Black women can never
be fully prized—and this is the message we get every time a
brother dates or marries a woman who is not Black. Maybe we
shouldn't take such behavior personally, but it's damn hard not
to. Black women are more likely than women of any other race to
remain without a partner. So when Black men marry out of the
race, it not only further diminishes the number of brothers available to Black women, but it also undermines our very confidence
as desirable women. I don't want this to be a message Ugo ever
sends out. He knows that if he wants to keep Mommy Audrey
happy, he will bring me home a Black girl.

This is the message senior marketing executive Valerie 16
Williams has also given her 15-year-old son. "I tell him I want to

have grandchildren who look like me," says Williams, who is frank on racial matters. "I don't want to be sitting around the dinner table at Thanksgiving feeling I have to bite my tongue." Nor does Williams think it's possible to escape issues of race and White supremacy in interracial unions, no matter how great the love may be. "I don't care what anybody says," she argues, "there's not a White person in America who doesn't feel superior to a former slave. Why would I want my son to marry someone who will probably always subconsciously feel she's better than him just because she's White?"

17   We often forget that relationships are also built on economic foundations and that Black-earned money leaves the community whenever a Black man marries out of the race. This is what rankles whenever we see wealthy Black athletes, entertainers or CEOs of Fortune 500 companies choose to lay their riches at the feet of White women by marrying them. So I have no doubt what motivated the Black publisher's wife to insist all those years ago that her three sons never think about marrying out of the race. Her husband had spent half his life building a multimillion-dollar business, and she did not want the wealth he would leave to his sons to pass out of Black hands. The publisher's wife was very clear about that. And her sons all married beautiful Black women and gave her beautiful Black grandchildren who look like her and will keep the money where it should be—in the Black family. In the Black community.

18   Last spring, while touring with Ugo the predominantly White college he would attend in the fall, I felt a moment of panic. Too many of the White girls, it seemed, were grinning in his direction. He is 19 now, strapping, handsome and a magnet for women of other races who find Black men as irresistible as we do. "Ugo," I instinctively blurted out, clutching his arm. "Please. Bring me home—" "Don't worry," he interrupted, putting his arm around me with calm reassurance. "I will."

Chapter 8

Responsibility and the Economy: Should Money Have a Mind of Its Own?

A Modest Proposal

Jonathan Swift

It is a melancholy object to those who walk through this great 1 town or travel in the country, when they see the streets, the roads, and cabin doors, crowded with beggars of the female sex, followed by three, four, or six children, all in rags and importuning every passenger for an alms. These mothers, instead of being able to work for their honest livelihood, are forced to employ all their time in strolling to beg sustenance for their helpless infants, who, as they grow up, either turn thieves for want of work, or leave their dear native country to fight for the Pretender in Spain, or sell themselves to the Barbadoes.

I think it is agreed by all parties that this prodigious num- 2 ber of children in the arms, or on the backs, or at the heels of their mothers, and frequently of their fathers, is in the present deplorable state of the kingdom a very great additional grievance; and therefore whoever could find out a fair, cheap, and easy method of making these children sound, useful members of the commonwealth would deserve so well of the public as to have his statue set up for a preserver of the nation.

But my intention is very far from being confined to provide 3 only for the children of professed beggars; it is of a much greater extent, and shall take in the whole number of infants at a certain age who are born of parents in effect as little able to support them as those who demand our charity in the streets.

4   As to my own part, having turned my thoughts for many years upon this important subject, and maturely weighed the several schemes of other projectors, I have always found them grossly mistaken in their computation. It is true, a child just dropped from its dam may be supported by her milk for a solar year, with little other nourishment; at most not above the value of two shillings, which the mother may certainly get, or the value in scraps, by her lawful occupation of begging; and it is exactly at one year old that I propose to provide for them in such a manner as instead of being a charge upon their parents or the parish, or wanting food and raiment for the rest of their lives, they shall on the contrary contribute to the feeding, and partly to the clothing, of many thousands.

5   There is likewise another great advantage in my scheme, that it will prevent those involuntary abortions, and that horrid practice of women murdering their bastard children, alas, too frequent among us, sacrificing the poor innocent babes, I doubt, more to avoid the expense than the shame, which would move tears and pity in the most savage and inhuman breast.

6   The number of souls in this kingdom being usually reckoned one million and a half, of these I calculate there may be about two hundred thousand couples whose wives are breeders, from which number I subtract thirty thousand couples who are able to maintain their own children, although I apprehend there cannot be so many under the present distress of the kingdom; but this being granted, there will remain an hundred and seventy thousand breeders. I again subtract fifty thousand for those women who miscarry, or whose children die by accident or disease within the year. There only remain an hundred and twenty thousand children of poor parents annually born. The question therefore is, how this number shall be reared and provided for, which, as I have already said, under the present situation of affairs, is utterly impossible by all the methods hitherto proposed. For we can neither employ them in handicraft nor agriculture; we neither build houses (I mean in the country) nor cultivate land. They can very seldom pick up livelihood by stealing till they arrive at six years old, except where they are of towardly parts; although I confess they learn the rudiments much earlier,

during which time they can however be looked upon only as pro-bationers, as I have been informed by a principal gentleman in the county of Cavan, who protested to me that he never knew above one or two instances under the age of six, even in a part of the king-dom so renowned for the quickest proficiency in that art.

I am assured by our merchants that a boy or a girl before 7 twelve years old is no salable commodity; and even when they come to this age, they will not yield above three pounds, or three pounds and half a crown at most on the Exchange; which cannot turn to account either to the parents or the kingdom, the charge of nutriment and rags having been at least four times that value.

I shall now therefore humbly propose my own thoughts, 8 which I hope will not be liable to the least objection.

I have been assured by a very knowing American of my 9 acquaintance in London, that a young healthy child well nursed is at a year old a most delicious, nourishing, and wholesome food, whether stewed, roasted, baked, or boiled; and I make no doubt that it will equally serve in fricasee or a ragout.

I do therefore humbly offer it to public consideration that of 10 the hundred and twenty thousand children, already computed, twenty thousand may be reserved for breed, whereof only one fourth part to be males, which is more than we allow to sheep, black cattle, or swine; and my reason is that these children are sel-dom the fruits of marriage, a circumstance not much regarded by our savages, therefore one male will be sufficient to serve four females. That the remaining hundred thousand may at a year old be offered in sale to the persons of quality and fortune through the kingdom, always advising the mother to let them suck plentifully in the last month, so as to render them plump and fat for a good table. A child will make two dishes at an entertainment for friends; and when the family dines alone, the fore or hind quarter will make a reasonable dish, and seasoned with a little pepper or salt will be very good boiled on the fourth day, especially in winter.

I have reckoned upon a medium that a child just born will 11 weigh twelve pounds, and in a solar year if tolerably nursed increaseth to twenty-eight pounds.

I grant this food will be somewhat dear, and therefore very 12 proper for landlords, who, as they have already devoured most of the parents, seem to have the best title to the children.

13   Infant's flesh will be in season throughout the year, but more plentiful in March, and a little before and after. For we are told by a grave author, an eminent French physician, that fish being a prolific diet, there are more children born in Roman Catholic countries about nine months after Lent, than at any other season; therefore, reckoning a year after Lent, the markets will be more glutted than usual, because the number of popish infants is at least three to one in this kingdom; and therefore it will have one other collateral advantage, by lessening the number of Papists among us.

14   I have already computed the charge of nursing a beggar's child (in which list I reckon all cottagers, laborers, and four fifths of the farmers) to be about two shillings per annum, rags included; and I believe no gentleman would repine to give ten shillings for the carcass of a good fat child, which, as I have said, will make four dishes of excellent nutritive meat, when he hath only some particular friend or his own family to dine with him. Thus the squire will learn to be a good landlord, and grow popular among the tenants; the mother will have eight shillings net profit, and be fit for work till she produces another child.

15   Those who are more thrifty (as I must confess the times require) may flay the carcass; the skin of which artificially dressed will make admirable gloves for ladies, and summer boots for fine gentlemen.

16   As to our city of Dublin, shambles may be appointed for this purpose in the most convenient parts of it, and butchers we may be assured will not be wanting; although I rather recommend buying the children alive, and dressing them hot from the knife as we do roasting pigs.

17   A very worthy person, a true lover of his country, and whose virtues I highly esteem, was lately pleased in discoursing on this matter to offer a refinement upon my scheme. He said that many gentlemen of his kingdom, having of late destroyed their deer, he conceived that the want of venison might be well supplied by the bodies of young lads and maidens, not exceeding fourteen years of age nor under twelve, so great a number of both sexes in every county being now ready to starve for want of work and service; and these to be disposed of by their parents, if alive, or otherwise by their nearest relations. But with due deference to so excellent a friend and so deserving a patriot, I cannot be altogether in his

sentiments; for as to the males, my American acquaintance assured me from frequent experience that their flesh was generally tough and lean, like that of our schoolboys, by continual exercise, and their taste disagreeable; and to fatten them would not answer the charge. Then as to the females, it would, I think with humble submission, be a loss to the public, because they soon would become breeders themselves; and besides, it is not improbable that some scrupulous people might be apt to censure such a practice (although indeed very unjustly) as a little bordering upon cruelty; which, I confess, hath always been with me the strongest objection against any project, how well soever intended.

But in order to justify my friend, he confessed that this expedient was put into his head by the famous Psalmanazar, a native of the island Formosa, who came from thence to London above twenty years ago, and in conversation told my friend that in his country when any young person happened to be put to death, the executioner sold the carcass to the persons of quality as a prime dainty; and that in his time the body of a plump girl of fifteen, who was crucified for an attempt to poison the emperor, was sold to his Imperial Majesty's prime minister of state, and other great mandarins of the court, in joints from the gibbet, at four hundred crowns. Neither indeed can I deny that if the same use were made of several plump young girls in this town, who without one single groat to their fortunes cannot stir abroad without a chair, and appear at the playhouse and assemblies in foreign fineries which they never will pay for, the kingdom would not be the worse. 18

Some persons of a desponding spirit are in great concern about that vast number of poor people who are aged, diseased, or maimed, and I have been desired to employ my thoughts what course may be taken to ease the nation of so grievous an encumbrance. But I am not in the least pain upon that matter, because it is very well known that they are every day dying and rotting by cold and famine, and filth and vermin, as fast as can be reasonably expected. And as to the younger laborers, they are now in almost as hopeful a condition. They cannot get work, and consequently pine away for want of nourishment to a degree that if any time they are accidentally hired to common labor, they have not strength to perform it; and thus the country and themselves are happily delivered from the evils to come. 19

20   I have too long digressed, and therefore shall return to my subject. I think the advantages by the proposal which I have made are obvious and many, as well as of the highest importance.

21   For first, as I have already observed, it would greatly lessen the number of Papists, with whom we are yearly overrun, being the principal breeders of the nation as well as our most dangerous enemies; and who stay at home on purpose to deliver the kingdom to the Pretender, hoping to take their advantage by the absence of so many good Protestants, who have chosen rather to leave their country than to stay at home and pay tithes against their conscience to an Episcopal curate.

22   Secondly, the poorer tenants will have something valuable of their own, which by law may be made liable to distress, and help to pay their landlord's rent, their corn and cattle being already seized and money a thing unknown.

23   Thirdly, whereas the maintenance of an hundred thousand children, from two years old and upwards, cannot be computed at less than ten shillings a piece per annum, the nation's stock will be thereby increased fifty thousand pounds per annum, besides the profit of a new dish introduced to the tables of all gentlemen of fortune in the kingdom who have any refinement in taste. And the money will circulate among ourselves, the goods being entirely of our own growth and manufacture.

24   Fourthly, the constant breeders, besides the gain of eight shillings sterling per annum by the sale of their children, will be rid of the charge for maintaining them after the first year.

25   Fifthly, this food would likewise bring great custom to taverns, where the vintners will certainly be so prudent as to procure the best receipts for dressing it to perfection, and consequently have their houses frequented by all the fine gentlemen, who justly value themselves upon their knowledge in good eating; and a skillful cook, who understands how to oblige his guests, will contrive to make it as expensive as they please.

26   Sixthly, this would be a great inducement to marriage, which all wise nations have either encouraged by rewards or enforced by laws and penalties. It would increase the care and tenderness of mothers toward their children, when they were sure of a settlement for life to the poor babes, provided in some sort by the public, to their annual profit instead of expense. We should see an

honest emulation among the married women, which of them could bring the fattest child to the market. Men would become as fond of their wives during the time of pregnancy as they are now of their mares in foal, their cows in calf, or sows when they are ready to farrow; nor offer to beat or kick them (as is too frequent a practice) for fear of a miscarriage.

Many other advantages might be enumerated. For instance, 27 the addition of some thousand carcasses in our exportation of barreled beef, the propagation of swine's flesh, and improvements in the art of making good bacon, so much wanted among us by the great destruction of pigs, too frequent at our tables, which are no way comparable in taste or magnificence to a well-grown, fat, yearling child, which roasted whole will make a considerable figure at a lord mayor's feast or any other public entertainment. But this and many others I omit, being studious of brevity.

Supposing that one thousand families in this city would be 28 constant customers for infants' flesh, besides others who might have it at merry meetings, particularly weddings and christenings, I compute that Dublin would take off annually about twenty thousand carcasses, and the rest of the kingdom (where probably they will be sold somewhat cheaper) the remaining eighty thousand.

I can think of no one objection that will possibly be raised 29 against this proposal, unless it should be urged that the number of people will be thereby much lessened in the kingdom. This I freely own, and it was indeed one principal design in offering it to the world. I desire the reader will observe; that I calculate my remedy for this one individual kingdom of Ireland and for no other that ever was, is, or I think ever can be upon earth. Therefore, let no man talk to me of other expedients: of taxing our absentees at five shillings a pound: of using neither clothes nor household furniture except what is of our own growth and manufacture: of utterly rejecting the materials and instruments that promote foreign luxury: of curing the expensiveness of pride, vanity, idleness, and gaming in our women: of introducing a vein of parsimony, prudence, and temperance: of learning to love our country, in the want of which we differ even from Lowlanders and the inhabitants of Topinamboo: of quitting our animosities and factions, nor acting any longer like the Jews, who were murdering one another at the very moment their city was taken: of being a little cautious not to sell our country and conscience for nothing: of teaching landlords to have at least one degree of mercy toward their tenants: lastly, of putting a spirit of honesty, industry, and skill into our shopkeepers; who, if a resolution could now be taken to buy only our native goods, would immediately unite to cheat and exact upon us in the price, the measure, and the goodness, nor could ever yet be brought to make one fair proposal of just dealing, though often and earnestly invited to it.

30   Therefore, I repeat, let no man talk to me of these and the like expedients, till he hath at least some glimpse of hope that there will ever be some hearty and sincere attempt to put them in practice.

31   But as to myself, having been wearied out for many years with offering vain, idle, visionary thoughts, and at length utterly despairing of success, I fortunately fell upon this proposal, which, as it is wholly new, so it hath something solid and real, of no expense and little trouble, full in our own power, and whereby we can incur no danger in disobliging England. For this kind of commodity will not bear exportation, the flesh being of too tender a consistence to admit a long continuance in salt, although perhaps I could name a country which would be glad to eat up our whole nation without it.

32   After all, I am not so violently bent upon my own opinion as to reject any offer proposed by wise men, which shall be found equally innocent, cheap, easy, and effectual. But before something of that kind shall be advanced in contradiction to my scheme, and offering a better, I desire the author or authors will be pleased maturely to consider two points. First, as things now stand, how they will be able to find food and raiment for an hundred thousand useless mouths and backs. And secondly, there being a round million of creatures in human figure throughout this kingdom, whose sole subsistence put into a common stock would leave them in debt two millions of pounds sterling, adding those who are beggars by profession to the bulk of farmers, cottagers, and laborers, with their wives and children who are beggars in effect; I desire those politicians who dislike my overture, and may perhaps be so bold to attempt an answer, that they will first ask the parents of these mortals whether they would not at this day think it a great happiness to have been sold for food at a year old

in this manner I prescribe, and thereby have avoided such a perpetual scene of misfortunes as they have since gone through by the oppression of landlords, the impossibility of paying rent without money or trade, the want of common sustenance, with neither house nor clothes to cover them from the inclemencies of the weather, and the most inevitable prospect of entailing the like or greater miseries upon their breed forever.

I profess, in the sincerity of my heart, that I have not the least 33 personal interest in endeavoring to promote this necessary work, having no other motive than the public good of my country, by advancing our trade, providing for infants, relieving the poor, and giving some pleasure to the rich. I have no children by which I can propose to get a single penny; the youngest being nine years old, and my wife past childbearing.

In Praise of Idleness

Bertrand Russell

Like most of my generation, I was brought up on the saying: 1 "Satan finds some mischief for idle hands to do." Being a highly virtuous child, I believed all that I was told, and acquired a conscience which has kept me working hard down to the present moment. But although my conscience has controlled my actions, my opinions have undergone a revolution. I think that there is far too much work done in the world, that immense harm is caused by the belief that work is virtuous, and that what needs to be preached in modern industrial countries is quite different from what always has been preached. Everyone knows the story of the traveller in Naples who saw twelve beggars lying in the sun (it was before the days of Mussolini), and offered a lira to the laziest of them. Eleven of them jumped up to claim it, so he gave it to the twelfth. This traveller was on the right lines. But in countries which do not enjoy Mediterranean sunshine, idleness is more difficult, and a great public propaganda will be required to inaugurate it. I hope that, after reading the following pages, the leaders of the YMCA will start a campaign to induce good young men to do nothing. If so, I shall not have lived in vain.

2   Before advancing my own arguments for laziness, I must dispose of one which I cannot accept. Whenever a person who already has enough to live on proposes to engage in some everyday kind of job, such as school-teaching or typing, he or she is told that such conduct takes the bread out of other people's mouths, and is therefore wicked. If this argument were valid, it would only be necessary for us all to be idle in order that we should all have our mouths full of bread. What people who say such things forget is that what a man earns he usually spends, and in spending he gives employment. As long as a man spends his income, he puts just as much bread into people's mouths in spending as he takes out of other people's mouths in earning. The real villain, from this point of view, is the man who saves. If he merely puts his savings in a stocking, like the proverbial French peasant, it is obvious that they do not give employment. If he invests his savings, the matter is less obvious, and different cases arise.

3   One of the commonest things to do with savings is to lend them to some Government. In view of the fact that the bulk of the public expenditure of most civilised Governments consists in payment for past wars or preparation for future wars, the man who lends his money to a Government is in the same position as the bad men in Shakespeare who hire murderers. The net result of the man's economical habits is to increase the armed forces of the State to which he lends his savings. Obviously it would be better if he spent the money, even if he spent it in drink or gambling.

4   But, I shall be told, the case is quite different when savings are invested in industrial enterprises. When such enterprises succeed, and produce something useful, this may be conceded. In these days, however, no one will deny that most enterprises fail. That means that a large amount of human labour, which might have been devoted to producing something that could be enjoyed, was expended on producing machines which, when produced, lay idle and did no good to anyone. The man who invests his savings in a concern that goes bankrupt is therefore injuring others as well as himself. If he spent his money, say, in giving parties for his friends, they (we may hope) would get pleasure, and so would all those upon whom he spent money, such as the butcher, the baker, and the bootlegger. But if he spends it (let us say) upon

laying down rails for surface cars in some place where surface cars turn out not to be wanted, he has diverted a mass of labour into channels where it gives pleasure to no one. Nevertheless, when he becomes poor through failure of his investment he will be regarded as a victim of undeserved misfortune, whereas the gay spendthrift, who has spent his money philanthropically, will be despised as a fool and a frivolous person.

All this is only preliminary. I want to say, in all seriousness, 5 that a great deal of harm is being done in the modern world by belief in the virtuousness of work, and that the road to happiness and prosperity lies in an organised diminution of work.

First of all: what is work? Work is of two kinds: first, altering 6 the position of matter at or near the earth's surface relatively to other such matter; second, telling other people to do so. The first kind is unpleasant and ill paid; the second is pleasant and highly paid. The second kind is capable of indefinite extension: there are not only those who give orders, but those who give advice as to what orders should be given. Usually two opposite kinds of advice are given simultaneously by two organised bodies of men; this is called politics. The skill required for this kind of work is not knowledge of the subjects as to which advice is given, but knowledge of the art of persuasive speaking and writing, i.e. of advertising.

Throughout Europe, though not in America, there is a third 7 class of men, more respected than either of the classes of workers. There are men who, through ownership of land, are able to make others pay for the privilege of being allowed to exist and to work. These landowners are idle, and I might therefore be expected to praise them. Unfortunately, their idleness is only rendered possible by the industry of others; indeed their desire for comfortable idleness is historically the source of the whole gospel of work. The last thing they have ever wished is that others should follow their example.

From the beginning of civilisation until the Industrial Revo- 8 lution, a man could, as a rule, produce by hard work little more than was required for the subsistence of himself and his family, although his wife worked at least as hard as he did, and his children added their labour as soon as they were old enough to do so. The small surplus above bare necessaries was not left to those who produced it, but was appropriated by warriors and priests. In times of famine there was no surplus; the warriors and priests, however, still secured as much as at other times, with the result that many of the workers died of hunger. This system persisted in Russia until 1917, and still persists in the East; in England, in spite of the Industrial Revolution, it remained in full force throughout the Napoleonic wars, and until a hundred years ago, when the new class of manufacturers acquired power. In America, the system came to an end with the Revolution, except in the South, where it persisted until the Civil War. A system which lasted so long and ended so recently has naturally left a profound impress upon men's thoughts and opinions. Much that we take for granted about the desirability of work is derived from this system, and, being pre-industrial, is not adapted to the modern world.

9   Modern technique has made it possible for leisure, within limits, to be not the prerogative of small privileged classes, but a right evenly distributed throughout the community. The morality of work is the morality of slaves, and the modern world has no need of slavery.

10   It is obvious that, in primitive communities, peasants, left to themselves, would not have parted with the slender surplus upon which the warriors and priests subsisted, but would have either produced less or consumed more. At first, sheer force compelled them to produce and part with the surplus. Gradually, however, it was found possible to induce many of them to accept an ethic according to which it was their duty to work hard, although part of their work went to support others in idleness. By this means the amount of compulsion required was lessened, and the expenses of government were diminished. To this day, 99 per cent of British wage-earners would be genuinely shocked if it were proposed that the King should not have a larger income than a working man. The conception of duty, speaking historically, has been a means used by the holders of power to induce others to live for the interests of their masters rather than for their own. Of course the holders of power conceal this fact from themselves by managing to believe that their interests are identical with the larger interests of humanity. Sometimes this is true; Athenian slave-owners, for instance, employed part of their leisure in

making a permanent contribution to civilisation which would have been impossible under a just economic system. Leisure is essential to civilisation, and in former times leisure for the few was only rendered possible by the labours of the many. But their labours were valuable, not because work is good, but because leisure is good. And with modern technique it would be possible to distribute leisure justly without injury to civilisation.

Modern technique has made it possible to diminish enormously the amount of labour required to secure the necessaries of life for everyone. This was made obvious during the war. At that time all the men in the armed forces, and all the men and women engaged in the production of munitions, all the men and women engaged in spying, war propaganda, or Government offices connected with the war, were withdrawn from productive occupations. In spite of this, the general level of well-being among unskilled wage-earners on the side of the Allies was higher than before or since. The significance of this fact was concealed by finance: borrowing made it appear as if the future was nourishing the present. But that, of course, would have been impossible; a man cannot eat a loaf of bread that does not yet exist. The war showed conclusively that, by the scientific organisation of production, it is possible to keep modern populations in fair comfort on a small part of the working capacity of the modern world. If, at the end of the war, the scientific organisation, which had been created in order to liberate men for fighting and munition work, had been preserved, and the hours of the week had been cut down to four, all would have been well. Instead of that the old chaos was restored, those whose work was demanded were made to work long hours, and the rest were left to starve as unemployed. Why? Because work is a duty, and a man should not receive wages in proportion to what he has produced, but in proportion to his virtue as exemplified by his industry.

This is the morality of the Slave State, applied in circumstances totally unlike those in which it arose. No wonder the result has been disastrous. Let us take an illustration. Suppose that, at a given moment, a certain number of people are engaged in the manufacture of pins. They make as many pins as the world needs, working (say) eight hours a day. Someone makes an invention by which the same number of men can make twice as many pins: pins are already so cheap that hardly any more will be bought at a lower price. In a sensible world, everybody concerned in the manufacturing of pins would take to working four hours instead of eight, and everything else would go on as before. But in the actual world this would be thought demoralising. The men still work eight hours, there are too many pins, some employers go bankrupt, and half the men previously concerned in making pins are thrown out of work. There is, in the end, just as much leisure as on the other plan, but half the men are totally idle while half are still overworked. In this way, it is insured that the unavoidable leisure shall cause misery all round instead of being a universal source of happiness. Can anything more insane be imagined?

13   The idea that the poor should have leisure has always been shocking to the rich. In England, in the early nineteenth century, fifteen hours was the ordinary day's work for a man; children sometimes did as much, and very commonly did twelve hours a day. When meddlesome busybodies suggested that perhaps these hours were rather long, they were told that work kept adults from drink and children from mischief. When I was a child, shortly after urban working men had acquired the vote, certain public holidays were established by law, to the great indignation of the upper classes. I remember hearing an old Duchess say: "What do the poor want with holidays? They ought to work." People nowadays are less frank, but the sentiment persists, and is the source of much of our economic confusion.

14   Let us, for a moment, consider the ethics of work frankly, without superstition. Every human being, of necessity, consumes, in the course of his life, a certain amount of the produce of human labour. Assuming, as we may, that labour is on the whole disagreeable, it is unjust that a man should consume more than he produces. Of course he may provide services rather than commodities, like a medical man, for example; but he should provide something in return for his board and lodging. To this extent, the duty of work must be admitted, but to this extent only.

15   I shall not dwell upon the fact that, in all modern societies outside the USSR, many people escape even this minimum amount of work, namely all those who inherit money and all those who marry money. I do not think the fact that these people

are allowed to be idle is nearly so harmful as the fact that wage-earners are expected to overwork or starve.

If the ordinary wage-earner worked four hours a day, there 16 would be enough for everybody and no unemployment—assuming a certain very moderate amount of sensible organisation. This idea shocks the well-to-do, because they are convinced that the poor would not know how to use so much leisure. In America men often work long hours even when they are well off; such men, naturally, are indignant at the idea of leisure for wage-earners, except as the grim punishment of unemployment; in fact, they dislike leisure even for their sons. Oddly enough, while they wish their sons to work so hard as to have no time to be civilised, they do not mind their wives and daughters having no work at all. The snobbish admiration of uselessness, which, in an aristocratic society, extends to both sexes, is, under a plutocracy, confined to women; this, however, does not make it any more in agreement with common sense.

The wise use of leisure, it must be conceded, is a product of 17 civilisation and education. A man who has worked long hours all his life will become bored if he becomes suddenly idle. But without a considerable amount of leisure a man is cut off from many of the best things. There is no longer any reason why the bulk of the population should suffer this deprivation; only a foolish asceticism, usually vicarious, makes us continue to insist on work in excessive quantities now that the need no longer exists.

In the new creed which controls the government of Russia, 18 while there is much that is very different from the traditional teaching of the West, there are some things that are quite unchanged. The attitude of the governing classes, and especially of those who conduct educational propaganda, on the subject of the dignity of labour, is almost exactly that which the governing classes of the world have always preached to what were called the "honest poor". Industry, sobriety, willingness to work long hours for distant advantages, even submissiveness to authority, all these reappear; moreover authority still represents the will of the Ruler of the Universe, Who, however, is now called by a new name, Dialectical Materialism.

The victory of the proletariat in Russia has some points in 19 common with the victory of the feminists in some other countries.

For ages, men had conceded the superior saintliness of women, and had consoled women for their inferiority by maintaining that saintliness is more desirable than power. At last the feminists decided that they would have both, since the pioneers among them believed all that the men had told them about the desirability of virtue, but not what they had told them about the worthlessness of political power. A similar thing has happened in Russia as regards manual work. For ages, the rich and their sycophants have written in praise of "honest toil", have praised the simple life, have professed a religion which teaches that the poor are much more likely to go to heaven than the rich, and in general have tried to make manual workers believe that there is some special nobility about altering the position of matter in space, just as men tried to make women believe that they derived some special nobility from their sexual enslavement. In Russia, all this teaching about the excellence of manual work has been taken seriously, with the result that the manual worker is more honoured than anyone else. What are, in essence, revivalist appeals are made, but not for the old purposes: they are made to secure shock workers for special tasks. Manual work is the ideal which is held before the young, and is the basis of all ethical teaching.

20   For the present, possibly, this is all to the good. A large country, full of natural resources, awaits development, and has to be developed with very little use of credit. In these circumstances, hard work is necessary, and is likely to bring a great reward. But what will happen when the point has been reached where everybody could be comfortable without working long hours?

21   In the West, we have various ways of dealing with this problem. We have no attempt at economic justice, so that a large proportion of the total produce goes to a small minority of the population, many of whom do no work at all. Owing to the absence of any central control over production, we produce hosts of things that are not wanted. We keep a large percentage of the working population idle, because we can dispense with their labour by making the others overwork. When all these methods prove inadequate, we have a war: we cause a number of people to manufacture high explosives, and a number of others to explode them, as if we were children who had just discovered fireworks. By a combination of all these devices we manage, though

with difficulty, to keep alive the notion that a great deal of severe manual work must be the lot of the average man.

In Russia, owing to more economic justice and central control 22 over production, the problem will have to be differently solved. The rational solution would be, as soon as the necessaries and elementary comforts can be provided for all, to reduce the hours of labour gradually, allowing a popular vote to decide, at each stage, whether more leisure or more goods were to be preferred. But, having taught the supreme virtue of hard work, it is difficult to see how the authorities can aim at a paradise in which there will be much leisure and little work. It seems more likely that they will find continually fresh schemes, by which present leisure is to be sacrificed to future productivity. I read recently of an ingenious plan put forward by Russian engineers, for making the White Sea and the northern coasts of Siberia warm, by putting a dam across the Kara Sea. An admirable project, but liable to postpone proletarian comfort for a generation, while the nobility of toil is being displayed amid the ice-fields and snowstorms of the Arctic Ocean. This sort of thing, if it happens, will be the result of regarding the virtue of hard work as an end in itself, rather than as a means to a state of affairs in which it is no longer needed.

The fact is that moving matter about, while a certain amount 23 of it is necessary to our existence, is emphatically not one of the ends of human life. If it were, we should have to consider every navvy superior to Shakespeare. We have been misled in this matter by two causes. One is the necessity of keeping the poor contented, which has led the rich, for thousands of years, to preach the dignity of labour, while taking care themselves to remain undignified in this respect. The other is the new pleasure in mechanism, which makes us delight in the astonishingly clever changes that we can produce on the earth's surface. Neither of these motives makes any great appeal to the actual worker. If you ask him what he thinks the best part of his life, he is not likely to say: "I enjoy manual work because it makes me feel that I am fulfilling man's noblest task, and because I like to think how much man can transform his planet. It is true that my body demands periods of rest, which I have to fill in as best I may, but I am never so happy as when the morning comes and I can return to the toil from which my contentment springs." I have never heard working men say this sort of thing. They consider work, as it should be considered, a necessary means to a livelihood, and it is from their leisure that they derive whatever happiness they may enjoy.

24   It will be said that, while a little leisure is pleasant, men would not know how to fill their days if they had only four hours of work out of the twenty-four. In so far as this is true in the modern world, it is a condemnation of our civilisation; it would not have been true at any earlier period. There was formerly a capacity for light-heartedness and play which has been to some extent inhibited by the cult of efficiency. The modern man thinks that everything ought to be done for the sake of something else, and never for its own sake. Serious-minded persons, for example, are continually condemning the habit of going to the cinema, and telling us that it leads the young into crime. But all the work that goes to producing a cinema is respectable, because it is work, and because it brings a money profit. The notion that the desirable activities are those that bring a profit has made everything topsy-turvy. The butcher who provides you with meat and the baker who provides you with bread are praiseworthy, because they are making money; but when you enjoy the food they have provided, you are merely frivolous, unless you eat only to get strength for your work. Broadly speaking, it is held that getting money is good and spending money is bad. Seeing that they are two sides of one transaction, this is absurd; one might as well maintain that keys are good, but keyholes are bad. Whatever merit there may be in the production of goods must be entirely derivative from the advantage to be obtained by consuming them. The individual, in our society, works for profit; but the social purpose of his work lies in the consumption of what he produces. It is this divorce between the individual and the social purpose of production that makes it so difficult for men to think clearly in a world in which profit-making is the incentive to industry. We think too much of production, and too little of consumption. One result is that we attach too little importance to enjoyment and simple happiness, and that we do not judge production by the pleasure that it gives to the consumer.

25   When I suggest that working hours should be reduced to four, I am not meaning to imply that all the remaining time should necessarily be spent in pure frivolity. I mean that four hours' work a

day should entitle a man to the necessities and elementary comforts of life, and that the rest of his time should be his to use as he might see fit. It is an essential part of any such social system that education should be carried further than it usually is at present, and should aim, in part, at providing tastes which would enable a man to use leisure intelligently. I am not thinking mainly of the sort of things that would be considered "highbrow". Peasant dances have died out except in remote rural areas, but the impulses which caused them to be cultivated must still exist in human nature. The pleasures of urban populations have become mainly passive: seeing cinemas, watching football matches, listening to the radio, and so on. This results from the fact that their active energies are fully taken up with work; if they had more leisure, they would again enjoy pleasures in which they took an active part.

In the past, there was a small leisure class and a larger working class. The leisure class enjoyed advantages for which there was no basis in social justice; this necessarily made it oppressive, limited its sympathies, and caused it to invent theories by which to justify its privileges. These facts greatly diminished its excellence, but in spite of this drawback it contributed nearly the whole of what we call civilisation. It cultivated the arts and discovered the sciences; it wrote the books, invented the philosophies, and refined social relations. Even the liberation of the oppressed has usually been inaugurated from above. Without the leisure class, mankind would never have emerged from barbarism. 26

The method of a leisure class without duties was, however, extraordinarily wasteful. None of the members of the class had to be taught to be industrious, and the class as a whole was not exceptionally intelligent. The class might produce one Darwin, but against him had to be set tens of thousands of country gentlemen who never thought of anything more intelligent than fox-hunting and punishing poachers. At present, the universities are supposed to provide, in a more systematic way, what the leisure class provided accidentally and as a by-product. This is a great improvement, but it has certain drawbacks. University life is so different from life in the world at large that men who live in academic milieu tend to be unaware of the preoccupations and problems of ordinary men and women; moreover their ways of expressing 27 themselves are usually such as to rob their opinions of the influence that they ought to have upon the general public. Another disadvantage is that in universities studies are organised, and the man who thinks of some original line of research is likely to be discouraged. Academic institutions, therefore, useful as they are, are not adequate guardians of the interests of civilisation in a world where everyone outside their walls is too busy for unutilitarian pursuits.

28   In a world where no one is compelled to work more than four hours a day, every person possessed of scientific curiosity will be able to indulge it, and every painter will be able to paint without starving, however excellent his pictures may be. Young writers will not be obliged to draw attention to themselves by sensational pot-boilers, with a view to acquiring the economic independence needed for monumental works, for which, when the time at last comes, they will have lost the taste and capacity. Men who, in their professional work, have become interested in some phase of economics or government, will be able to develop their ideas without the academic detachment that makes the work of university economists often seem lacking in reality. Medical men will have the time to learn about the progress of medicine, teachers will not be exasperatedly struggling to teach by routine methods things which they learnt in their youth, which may, in the interval, have been proved to be untrue.

29   Above all, there will be happiness and joy of life, instead of frayed nerves, weariness, and dyspepsia. The work exacted will be enough to make leisure delightful, but not enough to produce exhaustion. Since men will not be tired in their spare time, they will not demand only such amusements as are passive and vapid. At least one per cent will probably devote the time not spent in professional work to pursuits of some public importance, and, since they will not depend upon these pursuits for their livelihood, their originality will be unhampered, and there will be no need to conform to the standards set by elderly pundits. But it is not only in these exceptional cases that the advantages of leisure will appear. Ordinary men and women, having the opportunity of a happy life, will become more kindly and less persecuting and less inclined to view others with suspicion. The taste for war will die out, partly for this reason, and partly because it will involve long and severe

work for all. Good nature is, of all moral qualities, the one that the world needs most, and good nature is the result of ease and security, not of a life of arduous struggle. Modern methods of production have given us the possibility of ease and security for all; we have chosen, instead, to have overwork for some and starvation for others. Hitherto we have continued to be as energetic as we were before there were machines; in this we have been foolish, but there is no reason to go on being foolish forever.

Famine, Affluence, and Morality

Peter Singer

As I write this, in November 1971, people are dying in East Bengal from lack of food, shelter, and medical care. The suffering and death that are occurring there now are not inevitable, not unavoidable in any fatalistic sense of the term. Constant poverty, a cyclone, and a civil war have turned at least nine million people into destitute refugees; nevertheless, it is not beyond the capacity of the richer nations to give enough assistance to reduce any further suffering to very small proportions. The decisions and actions of human beings can prevent this kind of suffering. Unfortunately, human beings have not made the necessary decisions. At the individual level, people have, with very few exceptions, not responded to the situation in any significant way. Generally speaking, people have not given large sums to relief funds; they have not written to their parliamentary representatives demanding increased government assistance; they have not demonstrated in the streets, held symbolic fasts, or done anything else directed toward providing the refugees with the means to satisfy their essential needs. At the government level, no government has given the sort of massive aid that would enable the refugees to survive for more than a few days. Britain, for instance, has given rather more than most countries. It has, to date, given £14,750,000. For comparative purposes, Britain's share of the nonrecoverable development costs of the Anglo-French Concorde project is already in excess of £275,000,000, and on present estimates will reach £440,000,000. The implication is that the British government values a supersonic transport more than thirty times as highly as it values the lives of the nine million refugees. Australia is another country which, on a per capita basis, is well up in the "aid to Bengal" table. Australia's aid, however, amounts to less than one-twelfth of the cost of Sydney's new opera house. The total amount given, from all sources, now stands at about £65,000,000. The estimated cost of keeping the refugees alive for one year is £464,000,000. Most of the refugees have now been in the camps for more than six months. The World Bank has said that India needs a minimum of £300,000,000 in assistance from other countries before the end of the year. It seems obvious that assistance on this scale will not be forthcoming. India will be forced to choose between letting the refugees starve or diverting funds from her own development program, which will mean that more of her own people will starve in the future.[1]

2   These are the essential facts about the present situation in Bengal. So far as it concerns us here, there is nothing unique about this situation except its magnitude. The Bengal emergency is just the latest and most acute of a series of major emergencies in various parts of the world, arising both from natural and from manmade causes. There are also many parts of the world in which people die from malnutrition and lack of food independent of any special emergency. I take Bengal as my example only because it is the present concern, and because the size of the problem has ensured that it has been given adequate publicity. Neither individuals nor governments can claim to be unaware of what is happening there.

What are the moral implications of a situation like this? In what follows, I shall argue that the way people in relatively affluent countries react to a situation like that in Bengal cannot be justified; indeed, the whole way we look at moral issues—our moral conceptual scheme—needs to be altered, and with it, the way of life that has come to be taken for granted in our society.

3   In arguing for this conclusion I will not, of course, claim to be morally neutral. I shall, however, try to argue for the moral position that I take, so that anyone who accepts certain assumptions, to be made explicit, will, I hope, accept my conclusion.

I begin with the assumption that suffering and death from 4 lack of food, shelter, and medical care are bad. I think most people will agree about this, although one may reach the same view by different routes. I shall not argue for this view. People can hold all sorts of eccentric positions, and perhaps from some of them it would not follow that death by starvation is in itself bad. It is difficult, perhaps impossible, to refute such positions, and so for brevity I will henceforth take this assumption as accepted. Those who disagree need read no further.

My next point is this: if it is in our power to prevent something 5 bad from happening, without thereby sacrificing anything of comparable moral importance, we ought, morally, to do it. By "without sacrificing anything of comparable moral importance" I mean without causing anything else comparably bad to happen, or doing something that is wrong in itself, or failing to promote some moral good, comparable in significance to the bad thing that we can prevent. This principle seems almost as uncontroversial as the last one. It requires us only to prevent what is bad, and to promote what is good, and it requires this of us only when we can do it without sacrificing anything that is, from the moral point of view, comparably important. I could even, as far as the application of my argument to the Bengal emergency is concerned, qualify the point so as to make it: if it is in our power to prevent something very bad from happening, without thereby sacrificing anything morally significant, we ought, morally, to do it. An application of this principle would be as follows: if I am walking past a shallow pond and see a child drowning in it, I ought to wade in and pull the child out. This will mean getting my clothes muddy, but this is insignificant, while the death of the child would presumably be a very bad thing.

The uncontroversial appearance of the principle just stated is 6 deceptive. If it were acted upon, even in its qualified form, our lives, our society, and our world would be fundamentally changed. For the principle takes, firstly, no account of proximity or distance. It makes no moral difference whether the person I can help is a neighbor's child ten yards from me or a Bengali whose name I shall never know, ten thousand miles away. Secondly, the principle makes no distinction between cases in which I am the only person who could possibly do anything and cases in which I am just one among millions in the same position.

7   I do not think I need to say much in defense of the refusal to take proximity and distance into account. The fact that a person is physically near to us, so that we have personal contact with him, may make it more likely that we *shall* assist him, but this does not show that we *ought* to help him rather than another who happens to be further away. If we accept any principle of impartiality, universalizability, equality, or whatever, we cannot discriminate against someone merely because he is far away from us (or we are far away from him). Admittedly, it is possible that we are in a better position to judge what needs to be done to help a person near to us than one far away, and perhaps also to provide the assistance we judge to be necessary. If this were the case, it would be a reason for helping those near to us first. This may once have been a justification for being more concerned with the poor in one's town than with famine victims in India. Unfortunately for those who like to keep their moral responsibilities limited, instant communication and swift transportation have changed the situation. From the moral point of view, the development of the world into a "global village" has made an important, though still unrecognized, difference to our moral situation. Expert observers and supervisors, sent out by famine relief organizations or permanently stationed in famine-prone areas, can direct our aid to a refugee in Bengal almost as effectively as we could get it to someone in our own block. There would seem, therefore, to be no possible justification for discriminating on geographical grounds.

8   There may be a greater need to defend the second implication of my principle—that the fact that there are millions of other people in the same position, in respect to the Bengali refugees, as I am, does not make the situation significantly different from a situation in which I am the only person who can prevent something very bad from occurring. Again, of course, I admit that there is a psychological difference between the cases; one feels less guilty about doing nothing if one can point to others, similarly placed, who have also done nothing. Yet this can make no real difference to our moral obligations.[2] Should I consider that I am less obliged to pull the drowning child out of the pond if on looking around I see other people, no further away than I am, who have also noticed the child but are doing nothing? One has only to ask this question to see the absurdity of the view that numbers lessen obligation. It is a

view that is an ideal excuse for inactivity; unfortunately most of the major evils—poverty, overpopulation, pollution—are problems in which everyone is almost equally involved.

The view that numbers do make a difference can be made   9 plausible if stated in this way: if everyone in circumstances like mine gave £5 to the Bengal Relief Fund, there would be enough to provide food, shelter, and medical care for the refugees; there is no reason why I should give more than anyone else in the same circumstances as I am; therefore I have no obligation to give more than £5. Each premise in this argument is true, and the argument looks sound. It may convince us, unless we notice that it is based on a hypothetical premise, although the conclusion is not stated hypothetically. The argument would be sound if the conclusion were: if everyone in circumstances like mine were to give £5, I would have no obligation to give more than £5. If the conclusion were so stated, however, it would be obvious that the argument has no bearing on a situation in which it is not the case that everyone else gives £5. This, of course, is the actual situation. It is more or less certain that not everyone in circumstances like mine will give £5. So there will not be enough to provide the needed food, shelter, and medical care. Therefore by giving more than £5 I will prevent more suffering than I would if I gave just £5.

It might be thought that this argument has an absurd conse-   10 quence. Since the situation appears to be that very few people are likely to give substantial amounts, it follows that I and everyone else in similar circumstances ought to give as much as possible, that is, at least up to the point at which by giving more one would begin to cause serious suffering for oneself and one's dependents—perhaps even beyond this point to the point of marginal utility, at which by giving more one would cause oneself and one's dependents as much suffering as one would prevent in Bengal. If everyone does this, however, there will be more than can be used for the benefit of the refugees, and some of the sacrifice will have been unnecessary. Thus, if everyone does what he ought to do, the result will not be as good as it would be if everyone did a little less than he ought to do, or if only some do all that they ought to do.

The paradox here arises only if we assume that the actions in   11 question—sending money to the relief funds—are performed more or less simultaneously, and are also unexpected. For if it is to be expected that everyone is going to contribute something, then clearly each is not obliged to give as much as he would have been obliged to had others not been giving too. And if everyone is not acting more or less simultaneously, then those giving later will know how much more is needed, and will have no obligation to give more than is necessary to reach this amount. To say this is not to deny the principle that people in the same circumstances have the same obligations, but to point out that the fact that others have given, or may be expected to give, is a relevant circumstance: those giving after it has become known that many others are giving and those giving before are not in the same circumstances. So the seemingly absurd consequence of the principle I have put forward can occur only if people are in error about the actual circumstances—that is, if they think they are giving when others are not, but in fact they are giving when others are. The result of everyone doing what he really ought to do cannot be worse than the result of everyone doing less than he ought to do, although the result of everyone doing what he reasonably believes he ought to do could be.

12   If my argument so far has been sound, neither our distance from a preventable evil nor the number of other people who, in respect to that evil, are in the same situation as we are, lessens our obligation to mitigate or prevent that evil. I shall therefore take as established the principle I asserted earlier. As I have already said, I need to assert it only in its qualified form: if it is in our power to prevent something very bad from happening, without thereby sacrificing anything else morally significant, we ought, morally, to do it.

13   The outcome of this argument is that our traditional moral categories are upset. The traditional distinction between duty and charity cannot be drawn, or at least, not in the place we normally draw it. Giving money to the Bengal Relief Fund is regarded as an act of charity in our society. The bodies which collect money are known as "charities." These organizations see themselves in this way—if you send them a check, you will be thanked for your "generosity." Because giving money is regarded as an act of charity, it is not thought that there is anything wrong with not giving. The charitable man may be praised, but the man who is

not charitable is not condemned. People do not feel in any way ashamed or guilty about spending money on new clothes or a new car instead of giving it to famine relief. (Indeed, the alternative does not occur to them.) This way of looking at the matter cannot be justified. When we buy new clothes not to keep ourselves warm but to look "well-dressed" we are not providing for any important need. We would not be sacrificing anything significant if we were to continue to wear our old clothes, and give the money to famine relief. By doing so, we would be preventing another person from starving. It follows from what I have said earlier that we ought to give money away, rather than spend it on clothes which we do not need to keep us warm. To do so is not charitable, or generous. Nor is it the kind of act which philosophers and theologians have called "supererogatory"—an act which it would be good to do, but not wrong not to do. On the contrary, we ought to give the money away, and it is wrong not to do so.

I am not maintaining that there are no acts which are charitable, or that there are no acts which it would be good to do but not wrong not to do. It may be possible to redraw the distinction between duty and charity in some other place. All I am arguing here is that the present way of drawing the distinction, which makes it an act of charity for a man living at the level of affluence which most people in the "developed nations" enjoy to give money to save someone else from starvation, cannot be supported. It is beyond the scope of my argument to consider whether the distinction should be redrawn or abolished altogether. There would be many other possible ways of drawing the distinction—for instance, one might decide that it is good to make other people as happy as possible, but not wrong not to do so. 14

Despite the limited nature of the revision in our moral conceptual scheme which I am proposing, the revision would, given the extent of both affluence and famine in the world today, have radical implications. These implications may lead to further objections, distinct from those I have already considered. I shall discuss two of these. 15

One objection to the position I have taken might be simply that it is too drastic a revision of our moral scheme. People do not ordinarily judge in the way I have suggested they should. Most people 16 reserve their moral condemnation for those who violate some moral norm, such as the norm against taking another person's property. They do not condemn those who indulge in luxury instead of giving to famine relief. But given that I did not set out to present a morally neutral description of the way people make moral judgments, the way people do in fact judge has nothing to do with the validity of my conclusion. My conclusion follows from the principle which I advanced earlier, and unless that principle is rejected, or the arguments are shown to be unsound, I think the conclusion must stand, however strange it appears. It might, nevertheless, be interesting to consider why our society, and most other societies, do judge differently from the way I have suggested they should. In a well-known article, J. O. Urmson suggests that the imperatives of duty, which tell us what we must do, as distinct from what it would be good to do but not wrong not to do, function so as to prohibit behavior that is intolerable if men are to live together in society. This may explain the origin and continued existence of the present division between acts of duty and acts of charity. Moral attitudes are shaped by the needs of society, and no doubt society needs people who will observe the rules that make social existence tolerable. From the point of view of a particular society, it is essential to prevent violations of norms against killing, stealing, and so on. It is quite inessential, however, to help people outside one's own society.

17   If this is an explanation of our common distinction between duty and supererogation, however, it is not a justification of it. The moral point of view requires us to look beyond the interests of our own society. Previously, as I have already mentioned, this may hardly have been feasible, but it is quite feasible now. From the moral point of view, the prevention of the starvation of millions of people outside our society must be considered at least as pressing as the upholding of property norms within our society.

18   It has been argued by some writers, among them Sidgwick and Urmson, that we need to have a basic moral code which is not too far beyond the capacities of the ordinary man, for otherwise there will be a general breakdown of compliance with the moral code. Crudely stated, this argument suggests that if we tell people that they ought to refrain from murder and give everything they do not really need to famine relief, they will do neither, whereas if we

tell them that they ought to refrain from murder and that it is good to give to famine relief but not wrong not to do so, they will at least refrain from murder. The issue here is: Where should we draw the line between conduct that is required and conduct that is good although not required, so as to get the best possible result? This would seem to be an empirical question, although a very difficult one. One objection to the Sidgwick–Urmson line of argument is that it takes insufficient account of the effect that moral standards can have on the decisions we make. Given a society in which a wealthy man who gives 5 percent of his income to famine relief is regarded as most generous, it is not surprising that a proposal that we all ought to give away half our incomes will be thought to be absurdly unrealistic. In a society which held that no man should have more than enough while others have less than they need, such a proposal might seem narrow-minded. What it is possible for a man to do and what he is likely to do are both, I think, very greatly influenced by what people around him are doing and expecting him to do. In any case, the possibility that by spreading the idea that we ought to be doing very much more than we are to relieve famine we shall bring about a general breakdown of moral behavior seems remote. If the stakes are an end to widespread starvation, it is worth the risk. Finally, it should be emphasized that these considerations are relevant only to the issue of what we should require from others, and not to what we ourselves ought to do.

The second objection to my attack on the present distinction between duty and charity is one which has from time to time been made against utilitarianism. It follows from some forms of utilitarian theory that we all ought, morally, to be working full time to increase the balance of happiness over misery. The position I have taken here would not lead to this conclusion in all circumstances, for if there were no bad occurrences that we could prevent without sacrificing something of comparable moral importance, my argument would have no application. Given the present conditions in many parts of the world, however, it does follow from my argument that we ought, morally, to be working full time to relieve great suffering of the sort that occurs as a result of famine or other disasters. Of course, mitigating circumstances can be adduced—for instance, that if we wear ourselves out through overwork, we shall be less effective than we would otherwise have been. Nevertheless, when all considerations of this sort have been taken into account, the conclusion remains: we ought to be preventing as much suffering as we can without sacrificing something else of comparable moral importance. This conclusion is one which we may be reluctant to face. I cannot see, though, why it should be regarded as a criticism of the position for which I have argued, rather than a criticism of our ordinary standards of behavior. Since most people are self-interested to some degree, very few of us are likely to do everything that we ought to do. It would, however, hardly be honest to take this as evidence that it is not the case that we ought to do it.

20   It may still be thought that my conclusions are so wildly out of line with what everyone else thinks and has always thought that there must be something wrong with the argument somewhere. In order to show that my conclusions, while certainly contrary to contemporary Western moral standards, would not have seemed so extraordinary at other times and in other places, I would like to quote a passage from a writer not normally thought of as a way-out radical, Thomas Aquinas.

21   Now, according to the natural order instituted by divine providence, material goods are provided for the satisfaction of human needs. Therefore the division and appropriation of property, which proceeds from human law, must not hinder the satisfaction of man's necessity from such goods. Equally, whatever a man has in superabundance is owed, of natural right, to the poor for their sustenance. So Ambrosius says, and it is also to be found in the *Decretum Gratiani:* "The bread which you withhold belongs to the hungry; the clothing you shut away, to the naked; and the money you bury in the earth is the redemption and freedom of the penniless."

22   I now want to consider a number of points, more practical than philosophical, which are relevant to the application of the moral conclusion we have reached. These points challenge not the idea that we ought to be doing all we can to prevent starvation, but the idea that giving away a great deal of money is the best means to this end.

23   It is sometimes said that overseas aid should be a government responsibility, and that therefore one ought not to give to privately

run charities. Giving privately, it is said, allows the government and the noncontributing members of society to escape their responsibilities.

This argument seems to assume that the more people there 24 are who give to privately organized famine relief funds, the less likely it is that the government will take over full responsibility for such aid. This assumption is unsupported, and does not strike me as at all plausible. The opposite view—that if no one gives voluntarily, a government will assume that its citizens are uninterested in famine relief and would not wish to be forced into giving aid—seems more plausible. In any case, unless there were a definite probability that by refusing to give one would be helping to bring about massive government assistance, people who do refuse to make voluntary contributions are refusing to prevent a certain amount of suffering without being able to point to any tangible beneficial consequence of their refusal. So the onus of showing how their refusal will bring about government action is on those who refuse to give.

I do not, of course, want to dispute the contention that gov- 25 ernments of affluent nations should be giving many times the amount of genuine, no-strings-attached aid that they are giving now. I agree, too, that giving privately is not enough, and that we ought to be campaigning actively for entirely new standards for both public and private contributions to famine relief. Indeed, I would sympathize with someone who thought that campaigning was more important than giving oneself, although I doubt whether preaching what one does not practice would be very effective. Unfortunately, for many people the idea that "it's the government's responsibility" is a reason for not giving which does not appear to entail any political action either.

Another, more serious reason for not giving to famine relief 26 funds is that until there is effective population control, relieving famine merely postpones starvation. If we save the Bengal refugees now, others, perhaps the children of these refugees, will face starvation in a few years' time. In support of this, one may cite the now well-known facts about the population explosion and the relatively limited scope for expanded production.

This point, like the previous one, is an argument against 27 relieving suffering that is happening now, because of a belief about what might happen in the future; it is unlike the previous point in that very good evidence can be adduced in support of this belief about the future. I will not go into the evidence here. I accept that the earth cannot support indefinitely a population rising at the present rate. This certainly poses a problem for anyone who thinks it important to prevent famine. Again, however, one could accept the argument without drawing the conclusion that it absolves one from any obligation to do anything to prevent famine. The conclusion that should be drawn is that the best means of preventing famine, in the long run, is population control. It would then follow from the position reached earlier that one ought to be doing all one can to promote population control (unless one held that all forms of population control were wrong in themselves, or would have significantly bad consequences). Since there are organizations working specifically for population control, one would then support them rather than more orthodox methods of preventing famine.

28   A third point raised by the conclusion reached earlier relates to the question of just how much we all ought to be giving away. One possibility, which has already been mentioned, is that we ought to give until we reach the level of marginal utility—that is, the level at which, by giving more, I would cause as much suffering to myself or my dependents as I would relieve by my gift. This would mean, of course, that one would reduce oneself to very near the material circumstances of a Bengali refugee. It will be recalled that earlier I put forward both a strong and a moderate version of the principle of preventing bad occurrences. The strong version, which required us to prevent bad things from happening unless in doing so we would be sacrificing something of comparable moral significance, does seem to require reducing ourselves to the level of marginal utility. I should also say that the strong version seems to me to be the correct one. I proposed the more moderate version— that we should prevent bad occurrences unless, to do so, we had to sacrifice something morally significant—only in order to show that, even on this surely undeniable principle, a great change in our way of life is required. On the more moderate principle, it may not follow that we ought to reduce ourselves to the level of marginal utility, for one might hold that to reduce oneself and one's family to this level is to cause something significantly bad to

happen. Whether this is so I shall not discuss, since, as I have said, I can see no good reason for holding the moderate version of the principle rather than the strong version. Even if we accepted the principle only in its moderate form, however, it should be clear that we would have to give away enough to ensure that the consumer society, dependent as it is on people spending on trivia rather than giving to famine relief, would slow down and perhaps disappear entirely. There are several reasons why this would be desirable in itself. The value and necessity of economic growth are now being questioned not only by conservationists, but by economists as well. There is no doubt, too, that the consumer society has had a distorting effect on the goals and purposes of its members. Yet looking at the matter purely from the point of view of overseas aid, there must be a limit to the extent to which we should deliberately slow down our economy; for it might be the case that if we gave away, say, 40 percent of our Gross National Product, we would slow down the economy so much that in absolute terms we would be giving less than if we gave 25 percent of the much larger GNP that we would have if we limited our contribution to this smaller percentage.

I mention this only as an indication of the sort of factor that 29 one would have to take into account in working out an ideal. Since Western societies generally consider 1 percent of the GNP an acceptable level for overseas aid, the matter is entirely academic. Nor does it affect the question of how much an individual should give in a society in which very few are giving substantial amounts.

It is sometimes said, though less often now than it used to be, 30 that philosophers have no special role to play in public affairs, since most public issues depend primarily on an assessment of facts. On questions of fact, it is said, philosophers as such have no special expertise, and so it has been possible to engage in philosophy without committing oneself to any position on major public issues. No doubt there are some issues of social policy and foreign policy about which it can truly be said that a really expert assessment of the facts is required before taking sides or acting, but the issue of famine is surely not one of these. The facts about the existence of suffering are beyond dispute. Nor, I think, is it disputed that we can do something about it, either through orthodox methods of famine relief or through population control or both. This is therefore an issue on which philosophers are competent to take a position. The issue is one which faces everyone who has more money than he needs to support himself and his dependents, or who is in a position to take some sort of political action. These categories must include practically every teacher and student of philosophy in the universities of the Western world. If philosophy is to deal with matters that are relevant to both teachers and students, this is an issue that philosophers should discuss.

31   Discussion, though, is not enough. What is the point of relating philosophy to public (and personal) affairs if we do not take our conclusions seriously? In this instance, taking our conclusion seriously means acting upon it. The philosopher will not find it any easier than anyone else to alter his attitudes and way of life to the extent that, if I am right, is involved in doing everything that we ought to be doing. At the very least, though, one can make a start. The philosopher who does so will have to sacrifice some of the benefits of the consumer society, but he can find compensation in the satisfaction of a way of life in which theory and practice, if not yet in harmony, are at least coming together.

POSTSCRIPT

32   The crisis in Bangladesh that spurred me to write the above article is now of historical interest only, but the world food crisis is, if anything, still more serious. The huge grain reserves that were then held by the United States have vanished. Increased oil prices have made both fertilizer and energy more expensive in developing countries, and have made it difficult for them to produce more food. At the same time, their population has continued to grow. Fortunately, as I write now, there is no major famine anywhere in the world; but poor people are still starving in several countries, and malnutrition remains very widespread. The need for assistance is, therefore, just as great as when I first wrote, and we can be sure that without it there will, again, be major famines.

33   The contrast between poverty and affluence that I wrote about is also as great as it was then. True, the affluent nations have experienced a recession, and are perhaps not as prosperous as

they were in 1971. But the poorer nations have suffered as least as much from the recession, in reduced government aid (because if governments decide to reduce expenditure, they regard foreign aid as one of the expendable items, ahead of, for instance, defense or public construction projects) and in increased prices for goods and materials they need to buy. In any case, compared with the difference between the affluent nations and the poor nations, the whole recession was trifling; the poorest in the affluent nations remained incomparably better off than the poorest in the poor nations.

So the case for aid, on both a personal and a governmental level, remains as great now as it was in 1971, and I would not wish to change the basic argument that I put forward then. 34

There are, however, some matters of emphasis that I might put differently if I were to rewrite the article, and the most important of these concerns the population problem. I still think that, as I wrote then, the view that famine relief merely postpones starvation unless something is done to check population growth is not an argument against aid, it is only an argument against the type of aid that should be given. Those who hold this view have the same obligation to give to prevent starvation as those who do not; the difference is that they regard assisting population control schemes as a more effective way of preventing starvation in the long run. I would now, however, have given greater space to the discussion of the population problem; for I now think that there is a serious case for saying that if a country refuses to take any steps to slow the rate of its population growth, we should not give it aid. This is, of course, a very drastic step to take, and the choice it represents is a horrible choice to have to make; but if, after a dispassionate analysis of all the available information, we come to the conclusion that without population control we will not, in the long run, be able to prevent famine or other catastrophes, then it may be more humane in the long run to aid those countries that are prepared to take strong measures to reduce population growth, and to use our aid policy as a means of pressuring other countries to take similar steps. 35

It may be objected that such a policy involves an attempt to coerce a sovereign nation. But since we are not under an obligation to give aid unless that aid is likely to be effective in reducing 36 starvation or malnutrition, we are not under an obligation to give aid to countries that make no effort to reduce a rate of population growth that will lead to catastrophe. Since we do not force any nation to accept our aid, simply making it clear that we will not give aid where it is not going to be effective cannot properly be regarded as a form of coercion.

37   I should also make it clear that the kind of aid that will slow population growth is not just assistance with the setting up of facilities for dispensing contraceptives and performing sterilizations. It is also necessary to create the conditions under which people do not wish to have so many children. This will involve, among other things, providing greater economic security for people, particularly in their old age, so that they do not need the security of a large family to provide for them. Thus, the requirements of aid designed to reduce population growth and aid designed to eliminate starvation are by no means separate; they overlap, and the latter will often be a means to the former. The obligation of the affluent is, I believe, to do both. Fortunately, there are now many people in the foreign aid field, including those in the private agencies, who are aware of this.

38   One other matter that I should now put forward slightly differently is that my argument does, of course, apply to assistance with development, particularly agricultural development, as well as to direct famine relief. Indeed, I think the former is usually the better long-term investment. Although this was my view when I wrote the article, the fact that I started from a famine situation, where the need was for immediate food, has led some readers to suppose that the argument is only about giving food and not about other types of aid. This is quite mistaken, and my view is that the aid should be of whatever type is most effective.

39   On a more philosophical level, there has been some discussion of the original article which has been helpful in clarifying the issues and pointing to the areas in which more work on the argument is needed. In particular, as John Arthur has shown in "Rights and the Duty to Bring Aid" something more needs to be said about the notion of "moral significance." The problem is that to give an account of this notion involves nothing less than a full-fledged ethical theory; and while I am myself

inclined toward a utilitarian view, it was my aim in writing "Famine, Affluence, and Morality" to produce an argument which would appeal not only to utilitarians, but also to anyone who accepted the initial premises of the argument, which seemed to me likely to have a very wide acceptance. So I tried to get around the need to produce a complete ethical theory by allowing my readers to fill in their own version—within limits—of what is morally significant, and then see what the moral consequences are. This tactic works reasonably well with those who are prepared to agree that such matters as being fashionably dressed are not really of moral significance; but Arthur is right to say that people could take the opposite view without being obviously irrational. Hence, I do not accept Arthur's claim that the weak principle implies little or no duty of benevolence, for it will imply a significant duty of benevolence for those who admit, as I think most nonphilosophers and even off-guard philosophers will admit, that they spend considerable sums on items that by their own standards are of no moral significance. But I do agree that the weak principle is nonetheless too weak, because it makes it too easy for the duty of benevolence to be avoided.

On the other hand, I think the strong principle will stand, 40 whether the notion of moral significance is developed along utilitarian lines, or once again left to the individual reader's own sincere judgment. In either case, I would argue against Arthur's view that we are morally entitled to give greater weight to our own interests and purposes simply because they are our own. This view seems to me contrary to the idea, now widely shared by moral philosophers, that some element of impartiality or universalizability is inherent in the very notion of a moral judgment. Granted, in normal circumstances, it may be better for everyone if we recognize that each of us will be primarily responsible for running our own lives and only secondarily responsible for others. This, however, is not a moral ultimate, but a secondary principle that derives from consideration of how a society may best order its affairs, given the limits of altruism in human beings. Such secondary principles are, I think, swept aside by the extreme evil of people starving to death.

NOTES

1. There was also a third possibility: that India would go to war to enable the refugees to return to their lands. Since I wrote this paper, India has taken this way out. The situation is no longer that described above, but this does not affect my argument, as the next paragraph indicates.

2. In view of the special sense philosophers often give to the term, I should say that I use "obligation" simply as the abstract noun derived from "ought," so that "I have an obligation to" means no more, and no less, than "I ought to." This usage is in accordance with the definition of "ought" given by the *Shorter Oxford English Dictionary*: "the general verb to express duty or obligation." I do not think any issue of substance hangs on the way the term is used; sentences in which I use "obligation" could all be rewritten, although somewhat clumsily, as sentences in which a clause containing "ought" replaces the term "obligation."

The Moral Heart of Capitalism

Michael Novak

1   Thank you, Mr. Secretary.

2   My father-in-law, who was a lawyer in a small town in Iowa, would have been one of the most surprised men in America if he were turning on his television set this morning, and saw that a room full of accomplished practical people like all of you would want to hear anything from a metaphysician. When I was dating his daughter, I was a graduate student in the history and philosophy of religion at Harvard—and he wasn't sure that was going to produce a decent living. He used to refer to me as "my son-in-law, the celestial physicist." He would tell me once a year, "Michael, if you can't do it, teach it." Well, if you can all stand a little metaphysics, I'll do my best to set out the context for our panel, in four brief steps.

The first point is that, of all the important panels today, ours 3
is the most crucial. The reason is simple: The business corporation is the strategically central institution of social justice. If the
business corporation fails to meet its moral responsibilities, the
odds against the rest of society doing so shrink to next to zero.
Take one obvious example: the business corporation is strategically central to the creation of new wealth—and new industries—
and new jobs; no other institution even comes close. The workers
of a corporation depend on its success for their jobs, their career
opportunities, their job training, their pensions, and their health
care—even their friendships. When women and men enjoy their
work, grow as human beings in it, prosper from it, they are
happier in the rest of their lives.

On the other side, when corporations go badly, human misery 4
increases. If human conditions at work are poor, the rest of life
tends to sour with it.

That's why building a good corporation is a noble human 5
calling. It is a calling heavily weighted with moral obligations. In
a set of public opinion polls collected by my colleague Karlyn
Bowman at the American Enterprise Institute, the public holds the
corporation morally responsible for at least *eleven* different moral
tasks. In one book, I list *fourteen* moral responsibilities of business,
but I didn't finish counting. More impressive: In the matter of
corporate responsibility, the stakes are high: the *liberation of the
poor* through jobs and the creation of new wealth; the success of
democracy and human rights [as we learned in Eastern Europe, people are not satisfied with democracy if all it means is voting every
two years, while their daily economic condition does not
improve]; and the project of *building civil society*—that network of
artistic creativity, good works, and medical research that self-
governing citizens choose to initiate by and for themselves. The
corporation is the main creator of the wealth that makes the works
of civil society achievable.

The poor, democracy and human rights, civil society—these 6
are big issues, and all these important projects have now been
injured by corporate scandals. And so my second point: moral
scandals in corporate life—especially by corporate leaders—are
huge evils. They are trebly evil. One disgusting example was
recently reported: A CEO installed a $6,000 shower curtain in his

private home, allegedly at company expense. If that story is true, that was not only an evil harming one man, his reputation, and his company. It was *twice evil* because in the same act he humiliated all the good and decent CEOs in the nation, and dragged them all into ridicule. It was *three times* evil because his stupidity gave ammunition to the classical enemies of the free economy, at a time when the poor of the world depend on the spreading and the growth of the free economy. In his moral carelessness, he did enormous damage to causes far larger than himself.

7   The third point to make is far briefer: Corporate responsibility can be backed up by good law, but it cannot be completed by law alone. The law necessarily rides along behind breakthroughs in technology and invention. The law often arrives—as in this past year—after the damage has been done, in time to put up some monuments. Between the cutting edge of change and the slow course of the law must come something else: character and conscience. "There are many things which the law permits them to do which the religion of the Americans forbids them to do," the great scholar Alexis de Tocqueville wrote in 1835. Things must be so in a free society, which wishes also to be a decent society. Humans must decide how to use their freedom. Conscience has to fill the gap between breakthroughs in technological possibility and the later-arriving decisions of the law. Persons of character know limits; there are things they will not do, no matter what, and no matter what other people are doing.

8   In recent years, too many folk have tried "thinking outside the box," "breaking out of old paradigms," "making new rules." Well, that might be a good thing to do in technological inquiries. But it's a fatal mistake in ethics. For technology may change, but the human need for honesty, trust, and the firm rule never to use other people as means, only as ends, doesn't change. When the American people can't trust a company's financial report, they won't invest in that company. It's as simple as that. You may not be able to see "trust," but it's as real as a huge loss on the stock market. In the daily life of a capitalist system, things of the spirit— like trust—are more real than money. When they are missing, money itself loses its value.

9   All through America, in every organization, in every institution, we need more attention paid to the human spirit, to the

priceless realities, to people whose words, once spoken, can be absolutely relied upon. I have the impression that there were more such persons in our nation's past. But maybe every generation views the past through rosy lenses. Whatever the numbers, every republic needs many such people.

To endure, a republic needs people whose words are rock-   10 solid, reliable, true—until hell freezes over they will not lie, they will not do the dishonest deed. There are such people in America. People with internal North Stars. People who are not saints, but they almost always do the right thing. They are our Mount Rushmores. Fourth, for too many years, economics textbooks and business schools and the public media have been far better at talking about material things—about the bottom line—than about character, and trust, and honesty.

Besides the ecology of the natural world there is also a moral   11 ecology, a moral environment. For 100 years, we have neglected this whole nation's moral ecology. We have used up invaluable resources stored up at great cost in the past.

We need to rebuild this ecology—this moral ecology—all   12 through society. This task is done by emphasizing high morals in every realm, through stories of good and evil, and tales of moral heroes and villains. We need to talk about high morals day-in and day-out, encourage one another, rebuke one another.

As part of this task, many companies these days have drafted   13 moral codes. "In our company," they say, "anybody who does x, y, or z will be fired. Employees who follow paths a, b, or c will be supported all the way up to the Board of Directors. If you act ethically in this company, you will not act alone. The whole organization is with you." Max Weber was partly right, you know, about "the Protestant ethic." You don't have to be Protestant to practice it. But there is an ethic that lies behind capitalism, and in the real world it *has* to be practiced. The system simply will not work without it.

John Stuart Mill and all the classical economists held that   14 economics is a branch of ethics. And they were right. The whole system is based upon trust, honesty, and clarity about the facts— no lies, no illusions, no duplicity. Those are destructive agents in the system.

Finally, although it is not our panel's major focus, we must   15 not lose sight of the corporation's three major responsibilities: to create new wealth; to generate new industries and new jobs; and to inspire new generations who will invest for the future and sacrifice in the present, as well as to nourish workers who have confidence that their business is a noble calling, and that through it they are leading the world into a freer, more prosperous, and more virtuous future.

16   Mr. Secretary, I hope that opens up our discussion.

Why the Rich Are Getting Richer and the Poor, Poorer

Robert Reich

> *The division of labor is limited by the extent of the market.*
> —*Adam Smith,* An Inquiry into the Nature and Causes of the Wealth of Nations *(1776)*

1 Regardless of how your job is officially classified (manufacturing, service, managerial, technical, secretarial, and so on), or the industry in which you work (automotive, steel, computer, advertising, finance, food processing), your real competitive position in the world economy is coming to depend on the function you perform in it. Herein lies the basic reason why incomes are diverging. The fortunes of routine producers are declining. In-person servers are also becoming poorer, although their fates are less clear-cut. But symbolic analysts—who solve, identify, and broker new problems—are, by and large, succeeding in the world economy.

2   All Americans used to be in roughly the same economic boat. Most rose or fell together as the corporations in which they were employed, the industries comprising such corporations, and the national economy as a whole became more productive—or languished. But national borders no longer define our economic fates. We are now in different boats, one sinking rapidly, one sinking more slowly, and the third rising steadily.

The boat containing routine producers is sinking rapidly. 3
Recall that by mid-century routine production workers in the
United States were paid relatively well. The giant pyramid-like
organizations at the core of each major industry coordinated their
prices and investments—avoiding the harsh winds of competition
and thus maintaining healthy earnings. Some of these earnings, in
turn, were reinvested in new plant and equipment (yielding ever-
larger-scale economies); another portion went to top managers and
investors. But a large and increasing portion went to middle managers and production workers. Work stoppages posed such a
threat to high-volume production that organized labor was able to
exact an ever-larger premium for its cooperation. And the pattern
of wages established within the core corporations influenced the
pattern throughout the national economy. Thus the growth of a relatively affluent middle class, able to purchase all the wondrous
things produced in high volume by the core corporations.

But, as has been observed, the core is rapidly breaking down 4
into global webs which earn their largest profits from clever
problem-solving, -identifying, and brokering. As the costs of
transporting standard things and of communicating information
about them continue to drop, profit margins on high-volume,
standardized production are thinning, because there are few barriers to entry. Modern factories and state-of-the-art machinery can
be installed almost anywhere on the globe. Routine producers in
the United States, then, are in direct competition with millions of
routine producers in other nations. Twelve thousand people are
added to the world's population every hour, most of whom,
eventually, will happily work for a small fraction of the wages of
routine producers in America.[1]

The consequence is clearest in older, heavy industries, where 5
high-volume, standardized production continues its ineluctable
move to where labor is cheapest and most accessible around the

---

[1]The reader should note, of course, that lower wages in other areas of the world
are of no particular attraction to global capital unless workers there are sufficiently
productive to make the labor cost of producing *each unit* lower there than in
higher-wage regions. Productivity in many low-wage areas of the world has
improved due to the ease with which state-of-the-art factories and equipment can
be installed there. [This and subsequent notes in the selection are the author's.]

world. Thus, for example, the Maquiladora factories cluttered along the Mexican side of the U.S. border in the sprawling shanty towns of Tijuana, Mexicali, Nogales, Agua Prieta, and Ciudad Juárez— factories owned mostly by Americans, but increasingly by Japanese—in which more than a half million routine producers assemble parts into finished goods to be shipped into the United States.

6   The same story is unfolding worldwide. Until the late 1970s, AT&T had depended on routine producers in Shreveport, Louisiana, to assemble standard telephones. It then discovered that routine producers in Singapore would perform the same tasks at a far lower cost. Facing intense competition from other global webs, AT&T's strategic brokers felt compelled to switch. So in the early 1980s they stopped hiring routine producers in Shreveport and began hiring cheaper routine producers in Singapore. But under this kind of pressure for ever lower high-volume production costs, today's Singaporean can easily end up as yesterday's Louisianan. By the late 1980s, AT&T's strategic brokers found that routine producers in Thailand were eager to assemble telephones for a small fraction of the wages of routine producers in Singapore. Thus, in 1989, AT&T stopped hiring Singaporeans to make telephones and began hiring even cheaper routine producers in Thailand.

7   The search for ever lower wages has not been confined to heavy industry. Routine data processing is equally footloose. Keypunch operators located anywhere around the world can enter data into computers, linked by satellite or transoceanic fiber-optic cable, and take it out again. As the rates charged by satellite networks continue to drop, and as more satellites and fiber-optic cables become available (reducing communication costs still further), routine data processors in the United States find themselves in ever more direct competition with their counterparts abroad, who are often eager to work for far less.

8   By 1990, keypunch operators in the United States were earning, at most, $6.50 per hour. But keypunch operators throughout the rest of the world were willing to work for a fraction of this. Thus, many potential American data-processing jobs were disappearing, and the wages and benefits of the remaining ones were in decline. Typical was Saztec International, a $20-million-a-year data-processing firm headquartered in Kansas City, whose

American strategic brokers contracted with routine data processors in Manila and with American-owned firms that needed such data-processing services. Compared with the average Philippine income of $1,700 per year, data-entry operators working for Saztec earn the princely sum of $2,650. The remainder of Saztec's employees were American problem-solvers and -identifiers, searching for ways to improve the worldwide system and find new uses to which it could be put.[2]

By 1990, American Airlines was employing over 1,000 data   9 processors in Barbados and the Dominican Republic to enter names and flight numbers from used airline tickets (flown daily to Barbados from airports around the United States) into a giant computer bank located in Dallas. Chicago publisher R. R. Donnelley was sending entire manuscripts to Barbados for entry into computers in preparation for printing. The New York Life Insurance Company was dispatching insurance claims to Castleisland, Ireland, where routine producers, guided by simple directions, entered the claims and determined the amounts due, then instantly transmitted the computations back to the United States. (When the firm advertised in Ireland for twenty-five data-processing jobs, it received six hundred applications.) And McGraw-Hill was processing subscription renewal and marketing information for its magazines in nearby Galway. Indeed, literally millions of routine workers around the world were receiving information, converting it into computer-readable form, and then sending it back—at the speed of electronic impulses—whence it came.

The simple coding of computer software has also entered into   10 world commerce. India, with a large English-speaking population of technicians happy to do routine programming cheaply, is proving to be particularly attractive to global webs in need of this service. By 1990, Texas Instruments maintained a software development facility in Bangalore, linking fifty Indian programmers by satellite to TI's Dallas headquarters. Spurred by this and similar ventures, the Indian government was building a teleport in Poona, intended to make it easier and less expensive for many

---

[2]John Maxwell Hamilton, "A Bit Player Buys into the Computer Age," *New York Times Business World*, December 3, 1989, p. 14.

other firms to send their routine software design specifications for coding.[3]

11   This shift of routine production jobs from advanced to developing nations is a great boon to many workers in such nations who otherwise would be jobless or working for much lower wages. These workers, in turn, now have more money with which to purchase symbolic-analytic services from advanced nations (often embedded within all sorts of complex products). The trend is also beneficial to everyone around the world who can now obtain high-volume, standardized products (including information and software) more cheaply than before.

12   But these benefits do not come without certain costs. In particular the burden is borne by those who no longer have good-paying routine production jobs within advanced economies like the United States. Many of these people used to belong to unions or at least benefited from prevailing wage rates established in collective bargaining agreements. But as the old corporate bureaucracies have flattened into global webs, bargaining leverage has been lost. Indeed, the tacit national bargain is no more.

13   Despite the growth in the number of new jobs in the United States, union membership has withered. In 1960, 35 percent of all nonagricultural workers in America belonged to a union. But by 1980 that portion had fallen to just under a quarter, and by 1989 to about 17 percent. Excluding government employees, union membership was down to 13.4 percent.[4] This was a smaller proportion even than in the early 1930s, before the National Labor Relations Act created a legally protected right to labor representation. The drop in membership has been accompanied by a growing number of collective bargaining agreements to freeze wages at current levels, reduce wage levels of entering workers, or reduce wages overall. This is an important reason why the long economic recovery that began in 1982 produced a smaller rise in unit labor costs than any of the eight recoveries since World War II—the low rate of unemployment during its course notwithstanding.

---

[3]Udayan Gupta, "U.S.-Indian Satellite Link Stands to Cut Software Costs," *Wall Street Journal*, March 6, 1989, p. B2.
[4]*Statistical Abstract of the United States* (Washington, D.C.: U.S. Government Printing Office, 1989), p. 416, table 684.

Routine production jobs have vanished fastest in traditional 14 unionized industries (autos, steel, and rubber, for example), where average wages have kept up with inflation. This is because the jobs of older workers in such industries are protected by seniority; the youngest workers are the first to be laid off. Faced with a choice of cutting wages or cutting the number of jobs, a majority of union members (secure in the knowledge that there are many who are junior to them who will be laid off first) often have voted for the latter.

Thus the decline in union membership has been most strik- 15 ing among young men entering the work force without a college education. In the early 1950s, more than 40 percent of this group joined unions; by the late 1980s, less than 20 percent (if public employees are excluded, less than 10 percent).[5] In steelmaking, for example, although many older workers remained employed, almost half of all routine steelmaking jobs in America vanished between 1974 and 1988 (from 480,000 to 260,000). Similarly with automobiles: During the 1980s, the United Auto Workers lost 500,000 members—one-third of their total at the start of the decade. General Motors alone cut 150,000 American production jobs during the 1980s (even as it added employment abroad). Another consequence of the same phenomenon: the gap between the average wages of unionized and nonunionized workers widened dramatically—from 14.6 percent in 1973 to 20.4 percent by end of the 1980s.[6] The lesson is clear. If you drop out of high school or have no more than a high school diploma, do not expect a good routine production job to be awaiting you.

Also vanishing are lower- and middle-level management jobs 16 involving routine production. Between 1981 and 1986, more than 780,000 foremen, supervisors, and section chiefs lost their jobs through plant closings and layoffs.[7] Large numbers of assistant

[5]Calculations from Current Population Surveys by L. Katz and A. Revenga, "Changes in the Structure of Wages: U.S. and Japan," National Bureau of Economic Research, September 1989.
[6]U.S. Department of Commerce, Bureau of Labor Statistics, "Wages of Unionized and Nonunionized Workers," various issues.
[7]U.S. Department of Labor, Bureau of Labor Statistics, "Reemployment Increases among Displaced Workers," BLS News, USDL 86-414, October 14, 1986, table 6.

division heads, assistant directors, assistant managers, and vice presidents also found themselves jobless. GM shed more than 40,000 white-collar employees and planned to eliminate another 25,000 by the mid-1990s.[8] As America's core pyramids metamorphosed into global webs, many middle-level routine producers were as obsolete as routine workers on the line.

17   As has been noted, foreign-owned webs are hiring some Americans to do routine production in the United States. Philips, Sony, and Toyota factories are popping up all over—to the self-congratulatory applause of the nation's governors and mayors, who have lured them with promises of tax abatements and new sewers, among other amenities. But as these ebullient politicians will soon discover, the foreign-owned factories are highly automated and will become far more so in years to come. Routine production jobs account for a small fraction of the cost of producing most items in the United States and other advanced nations, and this fraction will continue to decline sharply as computer-integrated robots take over. In 1977, it took routine producers thirty-five hours to assemble an automobile in the United States; it is estimated that by the mid-1990s, Japanese-owned factories in America will be producing finished automobiles using only eight hours of a routine producer's time.[9]

18   The productivity and resulting wages of American workers who run such robotic machinery may be relatively high, but there may not be many such jobs to go around. A case in point: in the late 1980s, Nippon Steel joined with America's ailing Inland Steel to build a new $400 million cold-rolling mill fifty miles west of Gary, Indiana. The mill was celebrated for its state-of-the-art technology, which cut the time to produce a coil of steel from twelve days to about one hour. In fact, the entire plant could be run by a small team of technicians, which became clear when Inland subsequently closed two of its old cold-rolling mills, laying off hundreds of routine workers. Governors and mayors take note: your much-bally-hooed foreign factories may end up employing distressingly few of your constituents.

---

[8]*Wall Street Journal*, February 16, 1990, p. A5.
[9]Figures from the International Motor Vehicles Program, Massachusetts Institute of Technology, 1989.

Overall, the decline in routine jobs has hurt men more than 19 women. This is because the routine production jobs held by men in high-volume metal bending manufacturing industries had paid higher wages than the routine production jobs held by women in textiles and data processing. As both sets of jobs have been lost, American women in routine production have gained more equal footing with American men—equally poor footing, that is. This is a major reason why the gender gap between male and female wages began to close during the 1980s.

The second of the three boats, carrying in-person servers, is sink- 20 ing as well, but somewhat more slowly and unevenly. Most in-person servers are paid at or just slightly above the minimum wage and many work only part-time, with the result that their take-home pay is modest, to say the least. Nor do they typically receive all the benefits (health care, life insurance, disability, and so forth) garnered by routine producers in large manufacturing corporations or by symbolic analysts affiliated with the more affluent threads of global webs.[10] In-person servers are sheltered from the direct effects of global competition and, like everyone else, benefit from access to lower-cost products from around the world. But they are not immune to its indirect effects.

For one thing, in-person servers increasingly compete with 21 former routine production workers, who, no longer able to find well-paying routine production jobs, have few alternatives but to seek in-person service jobs. The Bureau of Labor Statistics estimates that of the 2.8 million manufacturing workers who lost their jobs during the early 1980s, fully one-third were rehired in service jobs paying at least 20 percent less.[11] In-person servers must also compete with high school graduates and dropouts who years before had moved easily into routine production jobs but no longer can. And if demographic predictions about the American work force in the first decades of the twenty-first century are correct (and they are likely to be, since most of the people who will

---

[10]The growing portion of the American labor force engaged in in-person services, relative to routine production, thus helps explain why the number of Americans lacking health insurance increased by at least 6 million during the 1980s.

[11]U.S. Department of Labor, Bureau of Labor Statistics, "Reemployment Increases among Disabled Workers," October 14, 1986.

comprise the work force are already identifiable), most new entrants into the job market will be black or Hispanic men, or women—groups that in years past have possessed relatively weak technical skills. This will result in an even larger number of people crowding into in-person services. Finally, in-person servers will be competing with growing numbers of immigrants, both legal and illegal, for whom in-person services will comprise the most accessible jobs. (It is estimated that between the mid-1980s and the end of the century, about a quarter of all workers entering the American labor force will be immigrants.[12])

22   Perhaps the fiercest competition that in-person servers face comes from labor-saving machinery (much of it invented, designed, fabricated, or assembled in other nations, of course). Automated tellers, computerized cashiers, automatic car washes, robotized vending machines, self-service gasoline pumps, and all similar gadgets substitute for the human beings that customers once encountered. Even telephone operators are fast disappearing, as electronic sensors and voice simulators become capable of carrying on conversations that are reasonably intelligent and always polite. Retail sales workers—among the largest groups of in-person servers—are similarly imperiled. Through personal computers linked to television screens, tomorrow's consumers will be able to buy furniture, appliances, and all sorts of electronic toys from their living rooms—examining the merchandise from all angles, selecting whatever color, size, special features, and price seem most appealing, and then transmitting the order instantly to warehouses from which the selections will be shipped directly to their homes. So, too, with financial transactions, airline and hotel reservations, rental car agreements, and similar contracts, which will be executed between consumers in their homes and computer banks somewhere else on the globe.[13]

23   Advanced economies like the United States will continue to generate sizable numbers of new in-person service jobs, of course, the automation of older ones notwithstanding. For every bank teller who loses her job to an automated teller, three new jobs

[12]Federal Immigration and Naturalization Service, *Statistical Yearbook* (Washington, D.C.: U.S. Government Printing Office, 1986, 1987).
[13]See Claudia H. Deutsch, "The Powerful Push for Self-Service," *New York Times*, April 9, 1989, section 3, p. 1.

open for aerobics instructors. Human beings, it seems, have an almost insatiable desire for personal attention. But the intense competition nevertheless ensures that the wages of in-person servers will remain relatively low. In-person servers—working on their own, or else dispersed widely amid many small establishments, filling all sorts of personal-care niches—cannot readily organize themselves into labor unions or create powerful lobbies to limit the impact of such competition

In two respects, demographics will work in favor of in-person 24 servers, buoying their collective boat slightly. First, as has been noted, the rate of growth of the American work force is slowing. In particular, the number of young workers is shrinking. Between 1985 and 1995, the number of the eighteen- to twenty-four-year-olds will have declined by 17.5 percent. Thus, employers will have more incentive to hire and train in-person servers whom they might previously have avoided. But this demographic relief from the competitive pressures will be only temporary. The cumulative procreative energies of the postwar baby-boomers (born between 1946 and 1964) will result in a new surge of workers by 2010 or thereabouts.[14] And immigration—both legal and illegal—shows every sign of increasing in years to come.

Next, by the second decade of the twenty-first century, the 25 number of Americans aged sixty-five and over will be rising precipitously, as the baby-boomers reach retirement age and live longer. Their life expectancies will lengthen not just because fewer of them will have smoked their way to their graves and more will have eaten better than their parents, but also because they will receive all sorts of expensive drugs and therapies designed to keep them alive—barely. By 2035, twice as many Americans will be elderly as in 1988, and the number of octogenarians is expected to triple. As these decaying baby-boomers ingest all the chemicals and receive all the treatments, they will need a great deal of personal attention. Millions of deteriorating bodies will require nurses, nursing-home operators, hospital administrators, orderlies, home-care providers, hospice aides, and technicians to operate and maintain all the expensive machinery

[14]U.S. Bureau of the Census, Current Population Reports, Series P-23, no. 138, tables 2-1, 4-6. See W. Johnson, A. Packer, et al., *Workforce 2000: Work and Workers for the 21st Century* (Indianapolis: Hudson Institute, 1987).

that will monitor and temporarily stave off final disintegration. There might even be a booming market for euthanasia specialists. In-person servers catering to the old and ailing will be in strong demand.[15]

26   One small problem: the decaying baby-boomers will not have enough money to pay for these services. They will have used up their personal savings years before. Their Social Security payments will, of course, have been used by the government to pay for the previous generation's retirement and to finance much of the budget deficits of the 1980s. Moreover, with relatively fewer young Americans in the population, the supply of housing will likely exceed the demand, with the result that the boomers' major investments— their homes—will be worth less (in inflation-adjusted dollars) when they retire than they planned for. In consequence, the huge cost of caring for the graying boomers will fall on many of the same people who will be paid to care for them. It will be like a great sump pump: in-person servers of the twenty-first century will have an abundance of health-care jobs, but a large portion of their earnings will be devoted to Social Security payments and income taxes, which will in turn be used to pay their salaries. The net result: no real improvement in their standard of living.

27   The standard of living of in-person servers also depends, indirectly, on the standard of living of the Americans they serve who are engaged in world commerce. To the extent that *these* Americans are richly rewarded by the rest of the world for what they contribute, they will have more money to lavish upon in-person services. Here we find the only form of "trickle-down" economics that has a basis in reality. A waitress in a town whose major factory has just been closed is unlikely to earn a high wage or enjoy much job security; in a swank resort populated by film producers and banking moguls, she is apt to do reasonably well. So, too, with nations. In-person servers in Bangladesh may spend their days performing roughly the same tasks as in-person servers in the United States, but have a far lower standard of living for their efforts. The difference comes in the value that their customers add to the world economy.

---

[15]The Census Bureau estimates that by the year 2000, at least 12 million Americans will work in health services—well over 6 percent of the total work force.

Unlike the boats of routine producers and in-person servers, 28 however, the vessel containing America's symbolic analysts is rising. Worldwide demand for their insights is growing as the ease and speed of communicating them steadily increases. Not every symbolic analyst is rising as quickly or as dramatically as every other, of course; symbolic analysts at the low end are barely holding their own in the world economy. But symbolic analysts at the top are in such great demand worldwide that they have difficulty keeping track of all their earnings. Never before in history has opulence on such a scale been gained by people who have earned it, and done so legally.

Among symbolic analysts in the middle range are American 29 scientists and researchers who are busily selling their discoveries to global enterprise webs. They are not limited to American customers. If the strategic brokers in General Motors' headquarters refuse to pay a high price for a new means of making high-strength ceramic engines dreamed up by a team of engineers affiliated with Carnegie Mellon University in Pittsburgh, the strategic brokers of Honda or Mercedes-Benz are likely to be more than willing.

So, too, with the insights of America's ubiquitous management 30 consultants, which are being sold for large sums to eager entrepreneurs in Europe and Latin America. Also, the insights of America's energy consultants, sold for even larger sums to Arab sheikhs. American design engineers are providing insights to Olivetti, Mazda, Siemens, and other global webs; American marketers, techniques for learning what worldwide consumers will buy; American advertisers, ploys for ensuring that they actually do. American architects are issuing designs and blueprints for opera houses, art galleries, museums, luxury hotels, and residential complexes in the world's major cities; American commercial property developers, marketing these properties to worldwide investors and purchasers.

Americans who specialize in the gentle art of public relations 31 are in demand by corporations, governments, and politicians in virtually every nation. So, too, are American political consultants, some of whom, at this writing, are advising the Hungarian Socialist Party, the remnant of Hungary's ruling Communists, on how to salvage a few parliamentary seats in the nation's first free election in more than forty years. Also at this writing, a team of American agricultural consultants is advising the managers of a Soviet farm collective employing 1,700 Russians eighty miles outside Moscow. As noted, American investment bankers and lawyers specializing in financial circumnavigations are selling their insights to Asians and Europeans who are eager to discover how to make large amounts of money by moving large amounts of money.

32   Developing nations, meanwhile, are hiring American civil engineers to advise on building roads and dams. The present thaw in the Cold War will no doubt expand these opportunities. American engineers from Bechtel (a global firm notable for having employed both Caspar Weinberger and George Shultz for much larger sums than either earned in the Reagan administration) have begun helping the Soviets design and install a new generation of nuclear reactors. Nations also are hiring American bankers and lawyers to help them renegotiate the terms of their loans with global banks, and Washington lobbyists to help them with Congress, the Treasury, the World Bank, the IMF, and other politically sensitive institutions. In fits of obvious desperation, several nations emerging from communism have even hired American economists to teach them about capitalism.

33   Almost everyone around the world is buying the skills and insights of Americans who manipulate oral and visual symbols— musicians, sound engineers, film producers, makeup artists, directors, cinematographers, actors and actresses, boxers, scriptwriters, songwriters, and set designers. Among the wealthiest of symbolic analysts are Steven Spielberg, Bill Cosby, Charles Schulz, Eddie Murphy, Sylvester Stallone, Madonna, and other star directors and performers—who are almost as well known on the streets of Dresden and Tokyo as in the Back Bay of Boston. Less well rewarded but no less renowned are the unctuous anchors on Turner Broadcasting's Cable News, who appear daily, via satellite, in places ranging from Vietnam to Nigeria. Vanna White is the world's most-watched game-show hostess. Behind each of these familiar faces is a collection of American problem-solvers, -identifiers, and brokers who train, coach, advise, promote, amplify, direct, groom, represent, and otherwise add value to their talents.[16]

[16]In 1989, the entertainment business summoned to the United States $5.5 billion in foreign earnings—making it among the nation's largest export industries, just behind aerospace. U.S. Department of Commerce, International Trade Commission, "Composition of U.S. Exports," various issues.

There are also the insights of senior American executives who   34
occupy the world headquarters of global "American" corporations and the national or regional headquarters of global "foreign"
corporations. Their insights are duly exported to the rest of the
world through the webs of global enterprise. IBM does not export
many machines from the United States, for example. Big Blue
makes machines all over the globe and services them on the spot.
Its prime American exports are symbolic and analytic. From IBM's
world headquarters in Armonk, New York, emanate strategic brokerage and related management services bound for the rest of the
world. In return, IBM's top executives are generously rewarded.

The most important reason for this expanding world market and   35
increasing global demand for the symbolic and analytic insights
of Americans has been the dramatic improvement in worldwide
communication and transportation technologies. Designs, instructions, advice, and visual and audio symbols can be communicated
more and more rapidly around the globe, with ever greater precision and at ever-lower cost. Madonna's voice can be transported
to billions of listeners, with perfect clarity, on digital compact
discs. A new invention emanating from engineers in Battelle's laboratory in Columbus, Ohio, can be sent almost anywhere via
modem, in a form that will allow others to examine it in three
dimensions through enhanced computer graphics. When face-to-
face meetings are still required—and videoconferencing will not
suffice—it is relatively easy for designers, consultants, advisers,
artists, and executives to board supersonic jets and, in a matter of
hours, meet directly with their worldwide clients, customers,
audiences, and employees.

With rising demand comes rising compensation. Whether in   36
the form of licensing fees, fees for service, salaries, or shares in final
profits, the economic result is much the same. There are also non-
pecuniary rewards. One of the best-kept secrets among symbolic
analysts is that so many of them enjoy their work. In fact, much of
it does not count as work at all, in the traditional sense. The work
of routine producers and in-person servers is typically monotonous;
it causes muscles to tire or weaken and involves little independence or discretion. The "work" of symbolic analysts, by contrast,
often involves puzzles, experiments, games, a significant amount of

chatter, and substantial discretion over what to do next. Few routine producers or in-person servers would "work" if they did not need to earn the money. Many symbolic analysts would "work" even if money were no object.

37   At mid-century, when America was a national market dominated by core pyramid-shaped corporations, there were constraints on the earnings of people at the highest rungs. First and most obviously, the market for their services was largely limited to the borders of the nation. In addition, whatever conceptual value they might contribute was small relative to the value gleaned from large scale—and it was dependent on large scale for whatever income it was to summon. Most of the problems to be identified and solved had to do with enhancing the efficiency of production and improving the flow of materials, parts, assembly, and distribution. Inventors searched for the rare breakthrough revealing an entirely new product to be made in high volume; management consultants, executives, and engineers thereafter tried to speed and synchronize its manufacture, to better achieve scale efficiencies; advertisers and marketers sought then to whet the public's appetite for the standard item that emerged. Since white-collar earnings increased with larger scale, there was considerable incentive to expand the firm; indeed, many of America's core corporations grew far larger than scale economies would appear to have justified.

38   By the 1990s, in contrast, the earnings of symbolic analysts were limited neither by the size of the national market nor by the volume of production of the firms with which they were affiliated. The marketplace was worldwide, and conceptual value was high relative to value added from scale efficiencies.

39   There had been another constraint on high earnings, which also gave way by the 1990s. At mid-century, the compensation awarded to top executives and advisers of the largest of America's core corporations could not be grossly out of proportion to that of low-level production workers. It would be unseemly for executives who engaged in highly visible rounds of bargaining with labor unions, and who routinely responded to government requests to moderate prices, to take home wages and benefits wildly in excess of what other Americans earned. Unless white-collar executives

restrained themselves, moreover, blue-collar production workers could not be expected to restrain their own demands for higher wages. Unless both groups exercised restraint, the government could not be expected to forbear from imposing direct controls and regulations.

At the same time, the wages of production workers could not be allowed to sink too low, lest there be insufficient purchasing power in the economy. After all, who would buy all the goods flowing out of American factories if not American workers? This, too, was part of the tacit bargain struck between American managers and their workers. 40

Recall the oft-repeated corporate platitude of the era about the chief executive's responsibility to carefully weigh and balance the interests of the corporation's disparate stakeholders. Under the stewardship of the corporate statesman, no set of stakeholders—least of all white-collar executives—was to gain a disproportionately large share of the benefits of corporate activity; nor was any stakeholder—especially the average worker—to be left with a share that was disproportionately small. Banal though it was, this idea helped to maintain the legitimacy of the core American corporation in the eyes of most Americans, and to ensure continued economic growth. 41

But by the 1990s, these informal norms were evaporating, just as (and largely because) the core American corporation was vanishing. The links between top executives and the American production worker were fading: an ever-increasing number of subordinates and contractees were foreign, and a steadily growing number of American routine producers were working for foreign-owned firms. An entire cohort of middle-level managers, who had once been deemed "white collar," had disappeared; and, increasingly, American executives were exporting their insights to global enterprise webs. 42

As the American corporation itself became a global web almost indistinguishable from any other, its stakeholders were turning into a large and diffuse group, spread over the world. Such global stakeholders were less visible, and far less noisy, than national stakeholders. And as the American corporation sold its goods and services all over the world, the purchasing power of American workers became far less relevant to its economic survival. 43

44   Thus have the inhibitions been removed. The salaries and benefits of America's top executives, and many of their advisers and consultants, have soared to what years before would have been unimaginable heights, even as those of other Americans have declined.

Why I Quit the Company

Tomoyuki Iwashita

1   When I tell people that I quit working for the company after only a year, most of them think I'm crazy. They can't understand why I would want to give up a prestigious and secure job. But I think I'd have been crazy to stay, and I'll try to explain why.

2   I started working for the company immediately after graduating from university. It's a big, well-known trading company with about 6,000 employees all over the world. There's a lot of competition to get into this and other similar companies, which promise young people a wealthy and successful future. I was set on course to be a Japanese "yuppie."

3   I'd been used to living independently as a student, looking after myself and organizing my own schedule. As soon as I started working all that changed. I was given a room in the company dormitory, which is like a fancy hotel, with a twenty-four-hour hot bath service and all meals laid on. Most single company employees live in a dormitory like this, and many married employees live in company apartments. The dorm system is actually a great help because living in Tokyo costs more than young people earn—but I found it stifling.

4   My life rapidly became reduced to a shuttle between the dorm and the office. The working day is officially eight hours, but you can never leave the office on time. I used to work from nine in the morning until eight or nine at night, and often until midnight. Drinking with colleagues after work is part of the job; you can't say no. The company building contained cafeterias, shops, a bank, a post office, a doctor's office, a barber's. . . . I never needed to

leave the building. Working, drinking, sleeping, and standing on a horribly crowded commuter train for an hour and a half each way: This was my life. I spent all my time with the same colleagues; when I wasn't involved in entertaining clients on the weekend, I was expected to play golf with my colleagues. I soon lost sight of the world outside the company.

This isolation is part of the brainwashing process. A personnel 5 manager said: "We want excellent students who are active, clever, and tough. Three months is enough to train them to be devoted businessmen." I would hear my colleagues saying: "I'm not making any profit for the company, so I'm not contributing." Very few employees claim all the overtime pay due to them. Keeping an employee costs the company 50 million yen ($400,000) a year, or so the company claims. Many employees put the company's profits before their own mental and physical well-being.

Overtiredness and overwork leave you little energy to ana- 6 lyze or criticize your situation. There are shops full of "health drinks," cocktails of caffeine and other drugs, which will keep you going even when you're exhausted. *Karoshi* (death from overwork) is increasingly common and is always being discussed in the newspapers. I myself collapsed from working too hard. My boss told me: "You should control your health; it's your own fault if you get sick." There is no paid sick leave; I used up half of my fourteen days' annual leave because of sickness.

We had a labor union, but it seemed to have an odd relation- 7 ship with the management. A couple of times a year I was told to go home at five o'clock. The union representatives were coming around to investigate working hours; everyone knew in advance. If it was "discovered" that we were all working overtime in excess of fifty hours a month our boss might have had some problem being promoted; and our prospects would have been affected. So we all pretended to work normal hours that day.

The company also controls its employees' private lives. Many 8 company employees under thirty are single. They are expected to devote all their time to the company and become good workers; they don't have time to find a girlfriend. The company offers scholarships to the most promising young employees to enable them to study abroad for a year or two. But unmarried people who are on these courses are not allowed to get married until they have completed the course! Married employees who are sent to train abroad have to leave their families in Japan for the first year.

9   In fact, the quality of married life is often determined by the husband's work. Men who have just gotten married try to go home early for a while, but soon have to revert to the norm of late-night work. They have little time to spend with their wives and even on the weekend are expected to play golf with colleagues. Fathers cannot find time to communicate with their children and child rearing is largely left to mothers. Married men posted abroad will often leave their family behind in Japan; they fear that their children will fall behind in the fiercely competitive Japanese education system.

10   Why do people put up with this? They believe this to be a normal working life or just cannot see an alternative. Many think that such personal sacrifices are necessary to keep Japan economically successful. Perhaps, saddest of all, Japan's education and socialization processes do not equip people with the intellectual and spiritual resources to question and challenge the status quo. They stamp out even the desire for a different kind of life.

11   However, there are some signs that things are changing. Although many new employees in my company were quickly brainwashed, many others, like myself, complained about life in the company and seriously considered leaving. But most of them were already in fetters—of debt. Pleased with themselves for getting into the company and anticipating a life of executive luxury, these new employees throw their money around. Every night they are out drinking. They buy smart clothes and take a taxi back to the dormitory after the last train has gone. They start borrowing money from the bank and soon they have a debt growing like a snowball rolling down a slope. The banks demand no security for loans; it's enough to be working for a well-known company. Some borrow as much as a year's salary in the first few months. They can't leave the company while they have such debts to pay off.

12   I was one of the few people in my intake of employees who didn't get into debt. I left the company dormitory after three months to share an apartment with a friend. I left the company exactly one year after I entered it. It took me a while to find a new job, but I'm working as a journalist now. My life is still busy, but it's a lot better than it was. I'm lucky because nearly all big

Japanese companies are like the one I worked for, and conditions in many small companies are even worse.

It's not easy to opt out of a life-style that is generally consid- 13 ered to be prestigious and desirable, but more and more young people in Japan are thinking about doing it. You have to give up a lot of superficially attractive material benefits in order to preserve the quality of your life and your sanity. I don't think I was crazy to leave the company. I think I would have gone crazy if I'd stayed.

Ethnicity: If Race Doesn't Exist, Why Is It So Important?

Does Race Exist?

Michael J. Bamshad and Steve E. Olson

1 Look around on the streets of any major city, and you will see a sampling of the outward variety of humanity: skin tones ranging from milk-white to dark brown; hair textures running the gamut from fine and stick-straight to thick and wiry. People often use physical characteristics such as these—along with area of geographic origin and shared culture—to group themselves and others into "races." But how valid is the concept of race from a biological standpoint? Do physical features reliably say anything informative about a person's genetic makeup beyond indicating that the individual has genes for blue eyes or curly hair?

2 The problem is hard in part because the implicit definition of what makes a person a member of a particular race differs from region to region across the globe. Someone classified as "black" in the U.S., for instance, might be considered "white" in Brazil and "colored" (a category distinguished from both "black" and "white") in South Africa.

3 Yet common definitions of race do sometimes work well to divide groups according to genetically determined propensities for certain diseases. Sickle cell disease is usually found among people of largely African or Mediterranean descent, for instance, whereas cystic fibrosis is far more common among those of European ancestry. In addition, although the results have been controversial, a handful of studies have suggested that African-Americans are

406

more likely to respond poorly to some drugs for cardiac disease than are members of other groups.

Over the past few years, scientists have collected data about 4 the genetic constitution of populations around the world in an effort to probe the link between ancestry and patterns of disease. These data are now providing answers to several highly emotional and contentious questions: Can genetic information be used to distinguish human groups having a common heritage and to assign individuals to particular ones? Do such groups correspond well to predefined descriptions now widely used to specify race? And, more practically, does dividing people by familiar racial definitions or by genetic similarities say anything useful about how members of those groups experience disease or respond to drug treatment?

In general, we would answer the first question yes, the sec- 5 ond no, and offer a qualified yes to the third. Our answers rest on several generalizations about race and genetics. Some groups do differ genetically from others, but how groups are divided depends on which genes are examined; simplistically put, you might fit into one group based on your skin-color genes but another based on a different characteristic. Many studies have demonstrated that roughly 90 percent of human genetic variation occurs within a population living on a given continent, whereas about 10 percent of the variation distinguishes continental populations. In other words, individuals from different populations are, on average, just slightly more different from one another than are individuals from the same population. Human populations are very similar, but they often can be distinguished.

CLASSIFYING HUMANS

As a first step to identifying links between social definitions of 6 race and genetic heritage, scientists need a way to divide groups reliably according to their ancestry. Over the past 100,000 years or so, anatomically modern humans have migrated from Africa to other parts of the world, and members of our species have increased dramatically in number. This spread has left a distinct signature in our DNA.

7   To determine the degree of relatedness among groups, geneticists rely on tiny variations, or polymorphisms, in the DNA—specifically in the sequence of base pairs, the building blocks of DNA. Most of these polymorphisms do not occur within genes, the stretches of DNA that encode the information for making proteins (the molecules that constitute much of our bodies and carry out the chemical reactions of life). Accordingly, these common variations are neutral, in that they do not directly affect a particular trait. Some polymorphisms do occur in genes, however; these can contribute to individual variation in traits and to genetic diseases.

8   As scientists have sequenced the human genome (the full set of nuclear DNA), they have also identified millions of polymorphisms. The distribution of these polymorphisms across populations reflects the history of those populations and the effects of natural selection. To distinguish among groups, the ideal genetic polymorphism would be one that is present in all the members of one group and absent in the members of all other groups. But the major human groups have separated from one another too recently and have mixed too much for such differences to exist.

9   Polymorphisms that occur at different frequencies around the world can, however, be used to sort people roughly into groups. One useful class of polymorphisms consists of the Alus, short pieces of DNA that are similar in sequence to one another. Alus replicate occasionally, and the resulting copy splices itself at random into a new position on the original chromosome or on another chromosome, usually in a location that has no effect on the functioning of nearby genes. Each insertion is a unique event. Once an Alu sequence inserts itself, it can remain in place for eons, getting passed from one person to his or her descendants. Therefore, if two people have the same Alu sequence at the same spot in their genome, they must be descended from a common ancestor who gave them that specific segment of DNA.

10   One of us (Bamshad), working with University of Utah scientists Lynn B. Jorde, Stephen Wooding and W. Scott Watkins and with Mark A. Batzer of Louisiana State University, examined 100 different Alu polymorphisms in 565 people born in sub-Saharan Africa, Asia and Europe. First we determined the presence or absence of the 100 Alus in each of the 565 people. Next we removed all the identifying labels (such as place of origin and

ethnic group) from the data and sorted the people into groups using only their genetic information.

Our analysis yielded four different groups. When we added 11 the labels back to see whether each individual's group assignment correlated to common, predefined labels for race or ethnicity, we saw that two of the groups consisted only of individuals from sub-Saharan Africa, with one of those two made up almost entirely of Mbuti Pygmies. The other two groups consisted only of individuals from Europe and East Asia, respectively. We found that we needed 60 Alu polymorphisms to assign individuals to their continent of origin with 90 percent accuracy. To achieve nearly 100 percent accuracy, however, we needed to use about 100 Alus.

Other studies have produced comparable results. Noah A. 12 Rosenberg and Jonathan K. Pritchard, geneticists formerly in the laboratory of Marcus W. Feldman of Stanford University, assayed approximately 375 polymorphisms called short tandem repeats in more than 1,000 people from 52 ethnic groups in Africa, Asia, Europe and the Americas. By looking at the varying frequencies of these polymorphisms, they were able to distinguish five different groups of people whose ancestors were typically isolated by oceans, deserts or mountains: sub-Saharan Africans; Europeans and Asians west of the Himalayas; East Asians; inhabitants of New Guinea and Melanesia; and Native Americans. They were also able to identify subgroups within each region that usually corresponded with each member's self-reported ethnicity.

The results of these studies indicate that genetic analyses can 13 distinguish groups of people according to their geographic origin. But caution is warranted. The groups easiest to resolve were those that were widely separated from one another geographically. Such samples maximize the genetic variation among groups. When Bamshad and his co-workers used their 100 Alu polymorphisms to try to classify a sample of individuals from southern India into a separate group, the Indians instead had more in common with either Europeans or Asians. In other words, because India has been subject to many genetic influences from Europe and Asia, people on the subcontinent did not group into a unique cluster. We concluded that many hundreds—or perhaps thousands—of polymorphisms might have to be examined to distinguish between groups whose ancestors have historically interbred with multiple populations.

THE HUMAN RACE

14 Given that people can be sorted broadly into groups using genetic data, do common notions of race correspond to underlying genetic differences among populations? In some cases they do, but often they do not. For instance, skin color or facial features—traits influenced by natural selection—are routinely used to divide people into races. But groups with similar physical characteristics as a result of selection can be quite different genetically. Individuals from sub-Saharan Africa and Australian Aborigines might have similar skin pigmentation (because of adapting to strong sun), but genetically they are quite dissimilar.

15 In contrast, two groups that are genetically similar to each other might be exposed to different selective forces. In this case, natural selection can exaggerate some of the differences between groups, making them appear more dissimilar on the surface than they are underneath. Because traits such as skin color have been strongly affected by natural selection, they do not necessarily reflect the population processes that have shaped the distribution of neutral polymorphisms such as Alus or short tandem repeats. Therefore, traits or polymorphisms affected by natural selection may be poor predictors of group membership and may imply genetic relatedness where, in fact, little exists.

16 Another example of how difficult it is to categorize people involves populations in the U.S. Most people who describe themselves as African-American have relatively recent ancestors from West Africa, and West Africans generally have polymorphism frequencies that can be distinguished from those of Europeans, Asians and Native Americans. The fraction of gene variations that African-Americans share with West Africans, however, is far from uniform, because over the centuries African-Americans have mixed extensively with groups originating from elsewhere in Africa and beyond.

17 Over the past several years, Mark D. Shriver of Pennsylvania State University and Rick A. Kittles of Howard University have defined a set of polymorphisms that they have used to estimate the fraction of a person's genes originating from each continental region. They found that the West African contribution to the genes of individual African-Americans averages about 80 percent, although it ranges from 20 to 100 percent. Mixing of groups is also apparent in

many individuals who believe they have only European ancestors. According to Shriver's analyses, approximately 30 percent of
Americans who consider themselves "white" have less than 90 percent European ancestry. Thus, self-reported ancestry is not necessarily a good predictor of the genetic composition of a large number
of Americans. Accordingly, common notions of race do not always
reflect a person's genetic background.

MEMBERSHIP HAS ITS PRIVILEGES

Understanding the relation between race and genetic variation has   18
important practical implications. Several of the polymorphisms
that differ in frequency from group to group have specific effects
on health. The mutations responsible for sickle cell disease and
some cases of cystic fibrosis, for instance, result from genetic
changes that appear to have risen in frequency because they were
protective against diseases prevalent in Africa and Europe, respectively. People who inherit one copy of the sickle cell polymorphism
show some resistance to malaria; those with one copy of the cystic fibrosis trait may be less prone to the dehydration resulting
from cholera. The symptoms of these diseases arise only in the
unfortunate individuals who inherit two copies of the mutations.

Genetic variation also plays a role in individual susceptibility   19
to one of the worst scourges of our age: AIDS. Some people have
a small deletion in both their copies of a gene that encodes a particular cell-surface receptor called chemokine receptor 5 (CCR5).
As a result, these individuals fail to produce CCR5 receptors on
the surface of their cells. Most strains of HIV-1, the virus that
causes AIDS, bind to the CCR5 receptor to gain entry to cells, so
people who lack CCR5 receptors are resistant to HIV-1 infection.
This polymorphism in the CCR5 receptor gene is found almost
exclusively in groups from northeastern Europe.

Several polymorphisms in CCR5 do not prevent infection but   20
instead influence the rate at which HIV-1 infection leads to AIDS
and death. Some of these polymorphisms have similar effects in
different populations; others only alter the speed of disease progression in selected groups. One polymorphism, for example,
is associated with delayed disease progression in European-
Americans but accelerated disease in African-Americans.

Researchers can only study such population-specific effects—and use that knowledge to direct therapy—if they can sort people into groups.

21   In these examples—and others like them—a polymorphism has a relatively large effect in a given disease. If genetic screening were inexpensive and efficient, all individuals could be screened for all such disease-related gene variants. But genetic testing remains costly. Perhaps more significantly, genetic screening raises concerns about privacy and consent: some people might not want to know about genetic factors that could increase their risk of developing a particular disease. Until these issues are resolved further, self-reported ancestry will continue to be a potentially useful diagnostic tool for physicians.

22   Ancestry may also be relevant for some diseases that are widespread in particular populations. Most common diseases, such as hypertension and diabetes, are the cumulative results of polymorphisms in several genes, each of which has a small influence on its own. Recent research suggests that polymorphisms that have a particular effect in one group may have a different effect in another group. This kind of complexity would make it much more difficult to use detected polymorphisms as a guide to therapy. Until further studies are done on the genetic and environmental contributions to complex diseases, physicians may have to rely on information about an individual's ancestry to know how best to treat some diseases.

RACE AND MEDICINE

23   But the importance of group membership as it relates to health care has been especially controversial in recent years. Last January the U.S. Food and Drug Administration issued guidelines advocating the collection of race and ethnicity data in all clinical trials. Some investigators contend that the differences between groups are so small and the historical abuses associated with categorizing people by race so extreme that group membership should play little if any role in genetic and medical studies. They assert that the FDA should abandon its recommendation and instead ask researchers conducting clinical trials

to collect genomic data on each individual. Others suggest that only by using group membership, including common definitions of race based on skin color, can we understand how genetic and environmental differences among groups contribute to disease. This debate will be settled only by further research on the validity of race as a scientific variable.

A set of articles in the March 20 issue of the *New England Journal of Medicine* debated both sides of the medical implications of race. The authors of one article—Richard S. Cooper of the Loyola Stritch School of Medicine, Jay S. Kaufman of the University of North Carolina at Chapel Hill and Ryk Ward of the University of Oxford—argued that race is not an adequate criterion for physicians to use in choosing a particular drug for a given patient. They pointed out two findings of racial differences that are both now considered questionable: that a combination of certain blood vessel–dilating drugs was more effective in treating heart failure in people of African ancestry and that specific enzyme inhibitors (angiotensin converting enzyme, or ACE, inhibitors) have little efficacy in such individuals. In the second article, a group led by Neil Risch of Stanford University countered that racial or ethnic groups can differ from one another genetically and that the differences can have medical importance. They cited a study showing that the rate of complications from type 2 diabetes varies according to race, even after adjusting for such factors as disparities in education and income.

The intensity of these arguments reflects both scientific and social factors. Many biomedical studies have not rigorously defined group membership, relying instead on inferred relationships based on racial categories. The dispute over the importance of group membership also illustrates how strongly the perception of race is shaped by different social and political perspectives.

In cases where membership in a geographically or culturally defined group has been correlated with health-related genetic traits, knowing something about an individual's group membership could be important for a physician. And to the extent that human groups live in different environments or have different experiences that affect health, group membership could also reflect nongenetic factors that are medically relevant.

27   Regardless of the medical implications of the genetics of race, the research findings are inherently exciting. For hundreds of years, people have wondered where various human groups came from and how those groups are related to one another. They have speculated about why human populations have different physical appearances and about whether the biological differences between groups are more than skin deep. New genetic data and new methods of analysis are finally allowing us to approach these questions. The result will be a much deeper understanding of both our biological nature and our human interconnectedness.

I Have a Dream

Martin Luther King Jr.

1   I am happy to join with you today in what will go down in history as the greatest demonstration for freedom in the history of our nation.

2   Fivescore years ago, a great American, in whose symbolic shadow we stand today, signed the Emancipation Proclamation. This momentous decree came as a great beacon light of hope to millions of Negro slaves who had been seared in the flames of withering injustice. It came as a joyous daybreak to end the long night of their captivity.

3   But one hundred years later, the Negro still is not free; one hundred years later, the life of the Negro is still sadly crippled by the manacles of segregation and the chains of discrimination; one hundred years later, the Negro lives on a lonely island of poverty in the midst of a vast ocean of material prosperity; one hundred years later, the Negro is still languishing in the corners of American society and finds himself in exile in his own land.

4   So we've come here today to dramatize a shameful condition. In a sense we've come to our nation's capital to cash a check. When the architects of our republic wrote the magnificent words of the Constitution and the Declaration of Independence, they were signing a promissory note to which every American was to fall heir. This note was the promise that all men, yes, black men

as well as white men, would be guaranteed the unalienable rights of life, liberty, and the pursuit of happiness.

It is obvious today that America has defaulted on this prom- 5 issory note in so far as her citizens of color are concerned. Instead of honoring this sacred obligation, America has given the Negro people a bad check; a check which has come back marked "insufficient funds." We refuse to believe that there are insufficient funds in the great vaults of opportunity of this nation. And so we've come to cash this check, a check that will give us upon demand the riches of freedom and the security of justice.

We have also come to this hallowed spot to remind America of 6 the fierce urgency of now. This is no time to engage in the luxury of cooling off or to take the tranquilizing drug of gradualism. Now is the time to make real the promises of democracy; now is the time to rise from the dark and desolate valley of segregation to the sun-lit path of racial justice; now is the time to lift our nation from the quicksands of racial injustice to the solid rock of brotherhood; now is the time to make justice a reality for all God's children. It would be fatal for the nation to overlook the urgency of the moment. This sweltering summer of the Negro's legitimate discontent will not pass until there is an invigorating autumn of freedom and equality.

Nineteen sixty-three is not an end, but a beginning. And those 7 who hope that the Negro needed to blow off steam and will now be content will have a rude awakening if the nation returns to business as usual.

There will be neither rest nor tranquility in America until the 8 Negro is granted his citizenship rights. The whirlwinds of revolt will continue to shake the foundations of our nation until the bright day of justice emerges.

But there is something that I must say to my people who 9 stand on the warm threshold which leads into the palace of justice. In the process of gaining our rightful place we must not be guilty of wrongful deeds.

Let us not seek to satisfy our thirst for freedom by drinking 10 from the cup of bitterness and hatred. We must forever conduct our struggle on the high plane of dignity and discipline. We must not allow our creative protest to degenerate into physical violence. Again and again we must rise to the majestic heights of meeting physical force with soul force.

11   The marvelous new militancy which has engulfed the Negro community must not lead us to a distrust of all white people, for many of our white brothers, as evidenced by their presence here today, have come to realize that their destiny is tied up with our destiny and they have come to realize that their freedom is inextricably bound to our freedom. This offense we share mounted to storm the battlements of injustice must be carried forth by a biracial army. We cannot walk alone.

12   And as we walk, we must make the pledge that we shall always march ahead. We cannot turn back. There are those who are asking the devotees of civil rights, "When will you be satisfied?" We can never be satisfied as long as the Negro is the victim of the unspeakable horrors of police brutality.

13   We can never be satisfied as long as our bodies, heavy with fatigue of travel, cannot gain lodging in the motels of the highways and the hotels of the cities. We cannot be satisfied as long as the Negro's basic mobility is from a smaller ghetto to a larger one.

14   We can never be satisfied as long as our children are stripped of their selfhood and robbed of their dignity by signs stating "for whites only." We cannot be satisfied as long as a Negro in Mississippi cannot vote and a Negro in New York believes he has nothing for which to vote. No, we are not satisfied, and we will not be satisfied until justice rolls down like waters and righteousness like a mighty stream.

15   I am not unmindful that some of you have come here out of excessive trials and tribulation. Some of you have come fresh from narrow jail cells. Some of you have come from areas where your quest for freedom left you battered by the storms of persecution and staggered by the winds of police brutality. You have been the veterans of creative suffering. Continue to work with the faith that unearned suffering is redemptive.

16   Go back to Mississippi; go back to Alabama; go back to South Carolina; go back to Georgia; go back to Louisiana; go back to the slums and ghettos of the northern cities, knowing that somehow this situation can, and will be changed. Let us not wallow in the valley of despair.

17   So I say to you, my friends, that even though we must face the difficulties of today and tomorrow, I still have a dream. It is a dream deeply rooted in the American dream that one day this nation will

rise up and live out the true meaning of its creed—we hold these truths to be self-evident, that all men are created equal.

I have a dream that one day on the red hills of Georgia, sons 18 of former slaves and sons of former slave-owners will be able to sit down together at the table of brotherhood.

I have a dream that one day, even the state of Mississippi, a 19 state sweltering with the heat of injustice, sweltering with the heat of oppression, will be transformed into an oasis of freedom and justice.

I have a dream my four little children will one day live in a 20 nation where they will not be judged by the color of their skin but by the content of their character. I have a dream today!

I have a dream that one day, down in Alabama, with its 21 vicious racists, with its governor having his lips dripping with the words of interposition and nullification, that one day, right there in Alabama, little black boys and black girls will be able to join hands with little white boys and white girls as sisters and brothers. I have a dream today!

I have a dream that one day every valley shall be exalted, every 22 hill and mountain shall be made low, the rough places shall be made plain, and the crooked places shall be made straight and the glory of the Lord will be revealed and all flesh shall see it together.

This is our hope. This is the faith that I go back to the South 23 with.

With this faith we will be able to hear out of the mountain 24 of despair a stone of hope. With this faith we will be able to transform the jangling discords of our nation into a beautiful symphony of brotherhood.

With this faith we will be able to work together, to pray 25 together, to struggle together, to go to jail together, to stand up for freedom together, knowing that we will be free one day. This will be the day when all of God's children will be able to sing with new meaning—"my country 'tis of thee; sweet land of liberty; of thee I sing; land where my fathers died, land of the pilgrims' pride; from every mountain side, let freedom ring"—and if America is to be a great nation, this must become true.

So let freedom ring from the prodigious hilltops of New 26 Hampshire.

Let freedom ring from the mighty mountains of New York. 27

28   Let freedom ring from the heightening Alleghenies of Pennsylvania.

29   Let freedom ring from the snow-capped Rockies of Colorado.

30   Let freedom ring from the curvaceous slopes of California.

31   But not only that.

32   Let freedom ring from Stone Mountain of Georgia.

33   Let freedom ring from Lookout Mountain of Tennessee.

34   Let freedom ring from every hill and molehill of Mississippi, from every mountainside, let freedom ring.

35   And when we allow freedom to ring, when we let it ring from every village and hamlet, from every state and city, we will be able to speed up that day when all of God's children—black men and white men, Jews and Gentiles, Catholics and Protestants—will be able to join hands and to sing in the words of the old Negro spiritual, "Free at last, free at last; thank God Almighty, we are free at last."

Ain't I a Woman?

Sojourner Truth

1 Well, children, where there is so much racket there must be something out of kilter. I think that 'twixt the negroes of the South and the women of the North, all talking about rights, the white men will be in a fix pretty soon. But what's all this here talking about?

2   That man over there says that women need to be helped into carriages, and lifted over ditches, and to have the best place everywhere. Nobody ever helps me into carriages, or over mud-puddles, or gives me any best place! And ain't I a woman? Look at me! Look at my arm! I have ploughed and planted, and gathered into barns, and no man could head me! And ain't I a woman? I could work as much and eat as much as a man—when I could get it—and bear the lash as well! And ain't I a woman? I have borne thirteen children, and seen them most all sold off to slavery, and when I cried out with my mother's grief, none but Jesus heard me! And ain't I a woman?

Then they talk about this thing in the head; what's this they 3
call it? [Intellect, someone whispers.] That's it, honey. What's that
got to do with women's rights or negro's rights? If my cup won't
hold but a pint, and yours holds a quart, wouldn't you be mean
not to let me have my little half-measure full?

Then that little man in black there, he says women can't have 4
as much rights as men, 'cause Christ wasn't a woman! Where did
your Christ come from? Where did your Christ come from? From
God and a woman! Man had nothing to do with Him.

If the first woman God ever made was strong enough to turn 5
the world upside down all alone, these women together ought to
be able to turn it back, and get it right side up again! And now
they is asking to do it, the men better let them.

Obliged to you for hearing me, and now old Sojourner ain't 6
got nothing more to say.

The Harmful Myth of Asian Superiority

Ronald Takaki

Asian Americans have increasingly come to be viewed as a 1
"model minority." But are they as successful as claimed? And for
whom are they supposed to be a model?

Asian Americans have been described in the media as a 2
"excessively, even provocatively" successful in gaining admission
to universities. Asian American shopkeepers have been congratu-
lated, as well as criticized, for their ubiquity and entrepreneurial
effectiveness.

If Asian Americans can make it, many politicians and pundits 3
ask, why can't African Americans? Such comparisons pit minorities against each other and generate African American resentment
toward Asian Americans. The victims are blamed for their plight,
rather than racism and an economy that has made many young
African American workers superfluous.

4   The celebration of Asian Americans has obscured reality. For example, figures on the high earnings of Asian Americans relative to Caucasians are misleading. Most Asian Americans live in California, Hawaii, and New York—states with higher incomes and higher costs of living than the national average.

5   Even Japanese Americans, often touted for their upward mobility, have not reached equality. While Japanese American men in California earned an average income comparable to Caucasian men in 1980, they did so only by acquiring more education and working more hours.

6   Comparing family incomes is even more deceptive. Some Asian American groups do have higher family incomes than Caucasians. But they have more workers per family.

7   The "model minority" image homogenizes Asian Americans and hides their differences. For example, while thousands of Vietnamese American young people attend universities, others are on the streets. They live in motels and hang out in pool halls in places like East Los Angeles; some join gangs.

8   Twenty-five percent of the people in New York City's Chinatown lived below the poverty level in 1980, compared with 17 percent of the city's population. Some 60 percent of the workers in the Chinatowns of Los Angeles and San Francisco are crowded into low-paying jobs in garment factories and restaurants.

9   "Most immigrants coming into Chinatown with a language barrier cannot go outside this confined area into the mainstream of American industry," a Chinese immigrant said. "Before, I was a painter in Hong Kong, but I can't do it here. I got no license, no education. I want a living; so it's dishwasher, janitor, or cook."

10   Hmong and Mien refugees from Laos have unemployment rates that reach as high as 80 percent. A 1987 California study showed that three out of ten Southeast Asian refugee families had been on welfare for four to ten years.

11   Although college-educated Asian Americans are entering the professions and earning good salaries, many hit the "glass ceiling"—the barrier through which high management positions can be seen but not reached. In 1988, only 8 percent of Asian Americans were "officials" and "managers," compared with 12 percent for all groups.

Finally, the triumph of Korean immigrants has been exagger- 12
ated. In 1988, Koreans in the New York metropolitan area earned
only 68 percent of the median income of non-Asians. More than
three-quarters of Korean greengrocers, those so-called paragons of
bootstrap entrepreneurialism, came to America with a college education. Engineers, teachers, or administrators while in Korea, they
became shopkeepers after their arrival. For many of them, the green-
grocery represents dashed dreams, a step downward in status.

For all their hard work and long hours, most Korean shop- 13
keepers do not actually earn very much: $17,000 to $35,000 a year,
usually representing the income from the labor of an entire family.

But most Korean immigrants do not become shopkeepers. 14
Instead, many find themselves trapped as clerks in grocery stores,
service workers in restaurants, seamstresses in garment factories,
and janitors in hotels.

Most Asian Americans know their "success" is largely a myth. 15
They also see how the celebration of Asian Americans as a "model
minority" perpetuates their inequality and exacerbates relations
between them and African Americans.

Just Walk On By: A Black Man Ponders His Power to Alter Public Space

Brent Staples

My first victim was a woman—white, well dressed, probably in her 1
early twenties. I came upon her late one evening on a deserted
street in Hyde Park, a relatively affluent neighborhood in an otherwise mean, impoverished section of Chicago. As I swung onto
the avenue behind her, there seemed to be a discreet, uninflamma-
tory distance between us. Not so. She cast back a worried glance.
To her, the youngish black man—a broad six feet two inches with
a beard and billowing hair, both hands shoved into the pockets of
a bulky military jacket—seemed menacingly close. After a few more

quick glimpses, she picked up her pace and was soon running in earnest. Within seconds she disappeared into a cross street.

2   That was more than a decade ago. I was 22 years old, a graduate student newly arrived at the University of Chicago. It was in the echo of that terrified woman's footfalls that I first began to know the unwieldy inheritance I'd come into—the ability to alter public space in ugly ways. It was clear that she thought herself the quarry of a mugger, a rapist, or worse. Suffering a bout of insomnia, however, I was stalking sleep, not defenseless wayfarers. As a softy who is scarcely able to take a knife to a raw chicken—let alone hold it to a person's throat—I was surprised, embarrassed, and dismayed all at once. Her flight made me feel like an accomplice in tyranny. It also made it clear that I was indistinguishable from the muggers who occasionally seeped into the area from the surrounding ghetto. That first encounter, and those that followed, signified that a vast, unnerving gulf lay between nighttime pedestrians—particularly women—and me. And I soon gathered that being perceived as dangerous is a hazard in itself. I only needed to turn a corner into a dicey situation, or crowd some frightened, armed person in a foyer somewhere, or make an errant move after being pulled over by a policeman. Where fear and weapons meet—and they often do in urban America—there is always the possibility of death.

3   In that first year, my first away from my hometown, I was to become thoroughly familiar with the language of fear. At dark, shadowy intersections in Chicago, I could cross in front of a car stopped at a traffic light and elicit the *thunk, thunk, thunk, thunk* of the driver—black, white, male, or female—hammering down the door locks. On less traveled streets after dark, I grew accustomed to but never comfortable with people who crossed to the other side of the street rather than pass me. Then there were the standard unpleasantries with police, doormen, bouncers, cabdrivers, and others whose business is to screen out troublesome individuals *before* there is any nastiness.

4   I moved to New York nearly two years ago and I have remained an avid night walker. In central Manhattan, the near-constant crowd cover minimizes tense one-on-one street encounters. Elsewhere—visiting friends in SoHo, where sidewalks are narrow and tightly spaced buildings shut out the sky—things can get very taut indeed.

Black men have a firm place in New York mugging litera- 5
ture. Norman Podhoretz in his famed (or infamous) 1963 essay,
"My Negro Problem—And Ours," recalls growing up in terror
of black males; they "were tougher than we were, more ruthless," he writes—and as an adult on the Upper West Side of
Manhattan, he continues, he cannot constrain his nervousness
when he meets black men on certain streets. Similarly, a decade
later, the essayist and novelist Edward Hoagland extols a New
York where once "Negro bitterness bore down mainly on other
Negroes." Where some see mere panhandlers, Hoagland sees "a
mugger who is clearly screwing up his nerve to do more than
just *ask* for money." But Hoagland has "the New Yorker's quick-
hunch posture for broken-field maneuvering," and the bad guy
swerves away.

I often witness that "hunch posture," from women after dark 6
on the warrenlike streets of Brooklyn where I live. They seem to
set their faces on neutral and, with their purse straps strung across
their chests bandolier style, they forge ahead as though bracing
themselves against being tackled. I understand, of course, that the
danger they perceive is not a hallucination. Women are particularly
vulnerable to street violence, and young black males are drastically
overrepresented among the perpetrators of that violence. Yet these
truths are no solace against the kind of alienation that comes of
being ever the suspect, against being set apart, a fearsome entity
with whom pedestrians avoid making eye contact.

It is not altogether clear to me how I reached the ripe old age 7
of 22 without being conscious of the lethality nighttime pedestrians
attributed to me. Perhaps it was because in Chester, Pennsylvania,
the small, angry industrial town where I came of age in the 1960s,
I was scarcely noticeable against a backdrop of gang warfare,
street knifings, and murders. I grew up one of the good boys, had
perhaps a half-dozen fistfights. In retrospect, my shyness of combat has clear sources.

Many things go into the making of a young thug. One of those 8
things is the consummation of the male romance with the power
to intimidate. An infant discovers that random flailings send the
baby bottle flying out of the crib and crashing to the floor.
Delighted, the joyful babe repeats those motions again and again,
seeking to duplicate the feat. Just so, I recall the points at which

some of my boyhood friends were finally seduced by the perception of themselves as tough guys. When a mark cowered and surrendered his money without resistance, myth and reality merged—and paid off. It is, after all, only manly to embrace the power to frighten and intimidate. We, as men, are not supposed to give an inch of our lane on the highway; we are to seize the fighter's edge in work and in play and even in love; we are to be valiant in the face of hostile forces.

9   Unfortunately, poor and powerless young men seem to take all this nonsense literally. As a boy, I saw countless tough guys locked away; I have since buried several, too. They were babies, really—a teenage cousin, a brother of 22, a childhood friend in his mid-twenties—all gone down in episodes of bravado played out in the streets. I came to doubt the virtues of intimidation early on. I chose, perhaps even unconsciously, to remain a shadow—timid, but a survivor.

10   The fearsomeness mistakenly attributed to me in public places often has a perilous flavor. The most frightening of these confusions occurred in the late 1970s and early 1980s when I worked as a journalist in Chicago. One day, rushing into the office of a magazine I was writing for with a deadline story in hand, I was mistaken for a burglar. The office manager called security and, with an ad hoc posse, pursued me through the labyrinthine halls, nearly to my editor's door. I had no way of proving who I was. I could only move briskly toward the company of someone who knew me.

11   Another time I was on assignment for a local paper and killing time before an interview. I entered a jewelry store on the city's affluent Near North Side. The proprietor excused herself and returned with an enormous red Doberman Pinscher straining at the end of a leash. She stood, the dog extended toward me, silent to my questions, her eyes bulging nearly out of her head. I took a cursory look around, nodded, and bade her good night. Relatively speaking, however, I never fared as badly as another black male journalist. He went to nearby Waukegan, Illinois, a couple of summers ago to work on a story about a murderer who was born there. Mistaking the reporter for the killer, police hauled him from his car at gunpoint and but for his press credentials would probably have tried to book him. Such episodes are not uncommon. Black men trade tales like this all the time.

In "My Negro Problem—And Ours," Podhoretz writes that the 12
hatred he feels for blacks makes itself known to him through a variety of avenues—one being his discomfort with that "special brand
of paranoid touchiness" to which he says blacks are prone. No doubt
he is speaking here of black men. In time, I learned to smother the
rage I felt at so often being taken for a criminal. Not to do so would
surely have led to madness—via that special "paranoid touchiness"
that so annoyed Podhoretz at the time he wrote the essay.

I began to take precautions to make myself less threatening. I 13
move about with care, particularly late in the evening. I give a
wide berth to nervous people on subway platforms during the
wee hours, particularly when I have exchanged business clothes
for jeans. If I happen to be entering a building behind some people who appear skittish, I may walk by, letting them clear the
lobby before I return, so as not to seem to be following them. I
have been calm and extremely congenial on those rare occasions
when I've been pulled over by the police.

And on late-evening constitutionals along streets less traveled 14
by, I employ what has proved to be an excellent tension-reducing
measure: I whistle melodies from Beethoven and Vivaldi and the
more popular classical composers. Even steely New Yorkers
hunching toward night-time destinations seem to relax, and occasionally they even join in the tune. Virtually everybody seems to
sense that a mugger wouldn't be warbling bright, sunny selections
from Vivaldi's *Four Seasons*. It is my equivalent of the cowbell that
hikers wear when they know they are in bear country.

Who's White? Who's Hispanic? Who Cares?

Jeff Jacoby

It was big news earlier this year: New census data showed that 1
Hispanics were on the verge of surpassing blacks as the largest
minority group in the nation. This occasioned a good deal of comment, some of it worried, some of it celebratory. At around the
same time came word that in many parts of the country, whites

were dwindling to a minority group themselves—if, indeed, they hadn't become one already.

2   "Boston became a majority minority city in the 1990s for the first time," the *Boston Globe* reported in March, "as Latinos, Asians, and blacks arrived and as tens of thousands of whites left." A continent away, the *Los Angeles Times* put the story on Page 1: "For the first time ever, no racial or ethnic group forms a majority in California."

3 But pull up the Census Bureau data yourself and you discover something interesting about these dramatic changes: They didn't happen.

4   Of the 281 million people enumerated in the 2000 census, 34.7 million gave their race as black. Respondents were allowed to check more than one racial category, and another 1.7 million identified themselves as black and something else. Total black (or partly-black) population: 36.4 million. The comparable number for whites was 217 million; for Asians, 11.9 million; for American Indians, 4.1 million; for native Hawaiians/Pacific Islanders, 0.9 million; and for those choosing "other," 18.5 million.

5   But there is no comparable number for Hispanics, because the Census Bureau doesn't treat "Hispanic" as a race. Last year's questionnaire asked respondents whether they identified themselves as "Spanish/Hispanic/Latino," and 35.3 million said yes. On the separate race question, some of those 35.3 million Hispanics said they were white (48 percent), some said black (2 percent), some marked multiple races (6 percent), and some—presumably those who *do* identify their race as Hispanic—marked the box labeled "other" (42 percent).

6   Hispanics, in other words, come in all colors—just like Catholics, or veterans, or the elderly. Asking whether Hispanics or blacks constitute the nation's largest minority is as meaningless as asking whether the book industry publishes more paperbacks or more mysteries. They are overlapping categories.

7 It is clear that some activists are eager for "Hispanic" to acquire the status of a full-fledged racial category. It's hardly a mystery why: Racial minority status confers political clout and a share of the affirmative action pie. But it is also pretty clear that most Hispanics don't buy into that agenda. More than half, after all, consider themselves white or multiracial.

Which is why you can safely tune out those stories about 8
California and Boston and so many other venues no longer having white majorities. "No racial or ethnic group forms a majority
in California," the *L.A. Times* said, but the Census Bureau begs to
differ. Of California's 33.9 million residents, 20.1 million—59 percent—identified themselves last year as white. Likewise Boston.
In 2000, 589,000 people lived in the city; 321,000 of them—54.5
percent—were white.

The nation as a whole remains overwhelmingly white—75.1 9
percent, the census found. "The suggestion that the white population of America is fast on the way to becoming a minority," writes
Orlando Patterson, the noted sociologist, "is a gross distortion."

So where did the stories about The Incredible Shrinking White 10
Majority come from? From manipulating the data so that white
Hispanics are not counted as white. But whose opinion should we
be relying on? The children and grandchildren of Latin American
immigrants who say they are white? Or the Hispanic journalists
and pressure groups who tell them they aren't?

For 250 years, the American melting pot has been turning eth- 11
nic groups once thought to be racially distinct (and socially indi-
gestible) into undifferentiated—which has usually meant white—
Americans. In 1896, Senator Henry Cabot Lodge bemoaned the
influx of "races with which the English-speaking people have
never hitherto assimilated, and who are most alien to the great
body of the people of the United States." He was talking about
Russians, Poles, and Greeks. Early in the 20th century, Italians,
Jews, and the Irish were classified as separate races by federal
immigration authorities.

Today, it is strange to think that Irish or Russian immigrants 12
were once deemed "nonwhite." Fifty years from now, it will seem
just as odd that Mexicans and Cubans were once regarded the
same way.

But let us hope that by then we will have abandoned the 13
fable that racial categories have concrete meaning in the first
place. How useful is the term "white," after all, if its definition
is so mutable? Isn't race, as the confusion over "Hispanic" suggests, ultimately a matter of personal choice? In a nation where
millions of people fall in love and raise children without regard
to the color line, isn't it time the government stopped counting
by race altogether?

Within, Between, and Beyond Race

Maria P. P. Root

1 The "biracial baby boom" in the United States started about 25 years ago, around the time the last laws against miscegenation (race mixing) were repealed in 1967. The presence of racially mixed persons defies the social order predicated upon race, blurs racial and ethnic group boundaries, and challenges generally accepted proscriptions and prescriptions regarding intergroup relations. Furthermore, and perhaps most threatening, the existence of racially mixed persons challenges long-held notions about the biological, moral, and social meaning of race.

2 The emergence of a racially mixed population is transforming the "face" of the United States. The increasing presence of multiracial[1] people necessitates that we as a nation ask ourselves questions about our identity: Who are we? How do we see ourselves? Who are we in relation to one another? These questions arise in the context of a country that has held particular views of race—a country that has subscribed to race as an immutable construct, perceived itself as White, and been dedicated to preserving racial lines. Thus such questions of race and identity can only precipitate a full-scale "identity crisis" that this country is ill equipped to resolve. Resolving the identity crisis may force us to reexamine our construction of race and the hierarchical social order it supports.

3 The "racial ecology" is complex in a phenotypically heterogeneous society that has imbued physical differences with significant meaning in a convention that benefits selective segments of the society. At a personal level, race is very much in the eye of the beholder; at a political level, race is in the service of economic and social privilege. Similarly, ethnic identity is relevant only in an ethnically heterogeneous environment. Whereas race can contribute to ethnicity, it is neither a sufficient nor necessary condition for assuming one's ethnicity, particularly with multiracial populations. Our confusion of race and ethnicity indicates that it will be difficult to abandon the smoke screen that hides our "caste system" surrounding theory, politics, health care, education, and other resources.

Our tendency to think simplistically about complex relation- 4
ships has resulted in dichotomous, hierarchical classification
systems that have become vehicles of oppression. The way in
which we have utilized the construction of race has placed the
multiracial person "betwixt and between" in the racial ecology
since colonial times. The publication of this volume suggests that
the emerging critical mass of multiracial persons, catalyzing a
national identity crisis, might enable us to disassemble the vehicle of oppression.

Although oppression takes different forms, it is consistently 5
characterized by the hierarchical interpretation of differences.
Sandoval provides an insightful four-tier model for examining
the development of social oppression by gender and racial group
social status, which affect and order economic power:

> Most definitions of "freedom" in the U.S. are activated in rela-
> tion to a primary category most easily embodied by the white,
> capitalist and male reality. White males who move into this
> power nodule do so by defining themselves in opposition to
> white women and to third world women and men who are
> cast as "others." White women inhabit the second category in
> this hierarchy through the very definition of a primary white
> male position. Interestingly, even though white women expe-
> rience the pain of oppression they also experience the will-to-
> power. For while white women are "othered" by men and feel
> the pain of objectification, within this secondary category they
> can only construct a solid sense of "self" through the objecti-
> fication of people of color. Within the dialectic of this power
> construct no one can deny the oppression of third world men.
> However, men of color can call upon the circuits which charge
> the primary category with the gendered aspect of its privileges
> and powers, even without the benefit of race or class privi-
> leges. This kind of identification with the powerful stra-
> tum/caste of "male" for the construction of a solid sense of
> self has been utilized as an effective weapon for confronting
> the oppressions they experience. Ironically, however, women
> of color are cast into the critical category against which third
> world "male" subjectivity becomes constituted. The final and
> fourth category belongs to women of color who become sur-
> vivors in a dynamic which places them as the final "other" in
> a complex of power moves.

6   Extending this model, racially mixed men and women would occupy the fifth and sixth tiers in this model, respectively, because of the rigidity of the dichotomy between White and non-White. Subsequently, multiracial people experience a "squeeze" of oppression *as* people of color and *by* people of color. People of color who have internalized the vehicle of oppression in turn apply rigid rules of belonging or establishing "legitimate" membership. The internalization of either/or systems of thinking operates even between communities of color, such as Asian American and African American communities. As Paulo Freirè suggests, marginal status is created by the society and structures and rules that order it. Anzaldua challengingly observes:

> The internalization of negative images of ourselves, our self-hatred, poor self-esteem, makes our own people the *Other.* We shun the white-looking Indian, the "high yellow" Black woman, the Asian with the white lover, the Native woman who brings her white girl friend to the Pow Wow, the Chicana who doesn't speak Spanish, the academic, the uneducated. Her difference makes her a person we can't trust. Para que sea "legal," she must pass the ethnic legitimacy test we have devised. And it is exactly your internalized whiteness that desperately wants boundary lines (this part of me is Mexican, this Indian) marked out and woe to any sister or any part of us that steps out of our assigned places.

7   The mechanisms that have historically evolved to suppress multiple heritage identification have largely benefited White society. The rules of hypodescent enlist simplistic, dichotomous rules of classification (e.g., White versus non-White) and have been obviously employed in our historical amnesia. These strategies have fueled the oppression of America's people of color and definitely that of the multiracial people of our country. In fact, attempts by racially mixed persons to move back and forth between color lines have been viewed pejoratively rather than as creative strategies in a multiracial reality. Furthermore, persons of color mixing with other persons of color—such as American Indians and Blacks, Filipinos and Native Americans, Latinos and Blacks—has been given little attention in the literature. This mixing does not conventionally threaten the border between White and non-White. The racial mixes over which there has been the

most concern are those between groups that are most distant culturally and socially—Blacks and Whites, Japanese and Blacks, and
Japanese and Whites. Furthermore, this concern has involved
groups that are most convinced of the immutability of race and
most wedded to preserving "purity" of race: Whites and Asians.

The simplicity and irrationality of our basis for conceptualiz- 8
ing race affects how we subsequently think about social identity.
Linear models of social relations have provided the basis for many
social psychological theories about racially mixed persons. The
monoracial and monocultural bias of these theories is evident in
constructions of assimilation and acculturation models (see Phinney,
1990) and many early theories addressing identity issues for persons with mixed heritages (Park, 1928; Stonequist, 1937). The theories, like our racial classification system, are characterized by
dichotomous or bipolar schemes and as such can only marginal-
ize the status of racially or ethnically mixed persons.

The recent consideration of multidimensional models has 9
allowed the possibility that an individual can have simultaneous
membership and multiple, fluid identities with different groups.
These models abolish either/or classifications systems that create
marginality. Multidimensional models of identity will not be per-
plexed that phenotype, "genotype," and ethnicity do not necessarily coincide with or reliably predict identity. Several studies
illustrate this phenomenon. A person of Black-Japanese heritage
may look Filipino and may identify as both African American and
Asian American. Similarly, a person of White-Asian background
may phenotypically appear more similar to someone of European
than Asian descent but may identify as a first-generation Japanese
American. It is confusing to our linear models of identity to consider that a multiracial Black-Indian-European person who looks
African American self-identifies as multiracial, when someone of a
similar heritage identifies as a monoracial African American. Moreover, the difference is more likely to be pathologized in a linear
model. Many persons will be challenged to consider that the mul-
tiracially identified person is liberated from oppressive rules of
classification rather than confined by them if they do not fit his or
her experience.

Why has the United States suppressed the historical reality 10
that a significant proportion of its citizenry has multigenerational

multiracial roots? On one hand, it might be suggested that we have manufactured a media image. Winterson observes: "Very often history is a means of denying the past. Denying the past is to refuse to recognize its integrity. To fit it, force it, function it, to suck out the spirit until it looks the way you think it should." On the other hand, this tendency may be seen as simply consistent with social models of assimilation that encourage a casting off of cultural ties and roots to blend into the mythical "melting pot." It is more likely, however, that this tendency is largely tied to economic motives and class privileges and to ideas of supremacy that guide rules of hypodescent (assignment to the racial group with lower status). An ethnic past remains relevant to the extent that it is physically visible, such as with people of color and multiracial people.

11   The silence on the topic of multiraciality must be understood in context. In the not-so-distant past—in the lifetimes of almost all the contributors to this volume—antimiscegenist sentiments were profound. These attitudes were supported by legislation in most states, ruling these interracial unions and marriages illegal until a U.S. Supreme Court ruling in 1967. The history of antimiscegenist laws and attitudes combined with rules of hypodescent, a pseudoscientific literature on race mixing, and the internalized oppression still evident in communities of color have unquestionably contributed to the silence on this topic.

12   Whereas one of the breakthroughs of the civil rights movement was empowerment of American racial minority groups by self-naming, this process is just beginning among multiracial persons. In essence, to name oneself is to validate one's existence and declare visibility. This seemingly simple process is a significant step in the liberation of multiracial persons from the oppressive structure of the racial classification system that has relegated them to the land of "in between." A confluence of factors has prevented this form of empowerment until now:

(1)   The social understanding of race has allowed only one category of racial identification (a practice supported by the U.S. Census Bureau).

(2)   Recent pride in being a person of color has demanded full-fledged commitment to the racial and ethnic minority group in order to pass "legitimacy tests."

(3) Epithets, which have been multiracial persons' only "universal" labels, have discouraged pride in self-identification.

(4) Isolation of interracial families, in part because of antimiscegenist legislation, has kept many multiracial families and individuals from meeting and accumulating a critical mass, a catalyst for empowerment.

(5) Race and ethnicity have been confused such that many multiracial people may identify monoculturally, as in the case of many Latinos, American Indians, and African Americans.

The biracial baby boom forces us to confront the meaning of race and the social order predicated upon it. *Race,* as constructed by social Darwinism and government construction by *blood quantum,* is more an artifice of the mind than a biological fact. Cooper and David observe that although the scientific construction of race was intended to provide a means of understanding and interpreting human variation, uncritical acceptance of the biological concept of race and lack of consistent definition by phenotypical markers is a problem even in biological arenas. Furthermore, a significant number of people around the world are not classifiable by such a system, including multiracial people. Unfortunately, this problematic taxonomy has been transformed into a sociopolitical system that has been deeply imprinted in our psyches. Subsequently, race has become insidiously enmeshed with our social structure, determining the distribution of resources among social groups and even influencing the methodologies and theories of social science research.

Nowhere is the validity or reliability of race more questionable than in government policies. For example, blood quantum, used to operationalize the definition of race biologically, has been used liberally to justify the dislocation of American Indians and Native Hawaiians off their native lands, to intern Japanese Americans during World War II, to determine immigration quotas, and to determine African Americans' racial identity and subsequent limits of access to resources. Generally, small blood quantum have been used to deprive people of color of their civil rights. Conversely, in more recent years conservatives have used blood quantum— that is, proportions of heritage—to determine allocations of lands to Native Americans (including Native Hawaiians) or qualification for government funding. Race cannot be a scientific construct if it has changing boundaries mitigated by laws, history, emotions, or politics.

15   Despite the significant number of people of all colors who have questioned the validity of race and the way it is abused in this country, taxonomies and institutions, like attitudes, are slow to change. Nowhere is this illustrated better than in how the U.S. Census Bureau has insisted on distinct monoracial categories. When Hawaii became the fiftieth state, the U.S. Census Bureau imposed its categories on a population that up until then had recorded its population according to categories and mixtures that reflected its multiracial reality (Lind, 1980). The Census Bureau does not acknowledge multiple heritages, despite the following facts: Currently, it is estimated that 30–70% of African Americans by multigenerational history are multiracial, virtually all Latinos and Filipinos are multiracial, as are the majority of American Indians and Native Hawaiians. Even a significant proportion of White identified persons are of multiracial origins. The way in which the Census Bureau records data on race makes it very difficult to estimate the number of biracial people, let alone multiracial persons, in the United States. Any estimates that have been made are conservative.

16   Now that we have almost 25 years' distance from the 1967 Supreme Court ruling that required the last 14 states holding antimiscegenist laws to repeal them, perhaps we can reconsider the subject of racially mixed persons in a less biased and less hostile context. It is likely that in the next decade, many persons previously identified as monoracial will begin to identify as multiracial, as they experience the dynamic nature of identity. As time evolves we will have more and more difficulty "judging the book by its cover." If we are truly to attempt constructive answers to the questions offered earlier (Who are we? How do we see ourselves? Who are we as a nation in relation to one another?), we will need to perform several social, political, and psychological "surgeries" to remove the deeply embedded, insidious, pseudoscientific construct of race from our social structure.

17   Initially, I thought my interest in exploring this topic was too personal. However, after a decade of contemplation, reading, writing, doing therapy, teaching, and finally a year of living in Honolulu, Hawaii, I think there is much to say. The topic of racially mixed persons provides us with a vehicle for examining

ideologies surrounding race, race relations, and the role of the social sciences in the deconstruction of race. It is suggested that the multiracial person's understanding of her- or himself can enhance society's understanding of intra- and intergroup relations, identity, and resilience.

Confusion may be a necessary element in the deconstruction and subsequent reconstruction of our social relationships in a qualitatively different way.   18

We go full circle, beginning with the questions that have been posed to racially mixed persons for decades: What are you? Which one are you? With which group do you identify most? How do you see yourself? Then, questions are posed that we must attempt to answer as a nation in order to resolve a developing national identity crisis: Who are we? How do we see ourselves? Who are we as a nation in relation to one another? The answers are not likely to be found in a new system of classification, but in deconstruction, synthesis, and evolution.   19

NOTE

[1]In this essay the terms *biracial* and *multiracial* are sometimes used interchangeably. *Biracial* refers to someone with two socially and phenotypically distinct racial heritages—one from each parent. However, this term can also refer to a multigenerational history of prior racial blending. For example, someone may have a parent or grandparent who was biracial and may acknowledge this heritage through self-identification as biracial. In this "looser" definition, one moves away from the notion of "halves"—half Black, half White. *Multiracial* includes the case of the biracial person and persons synthesizing two or more diverse heritages, such as the person with African, Indian, and European heritages. It also is a term that acknowledges that the suppression of multiracial heritage in this country may limit people's knowledge about their "racial" roots; subsequently, *multiracial* may be a more accurate term than *biracial*. This term is inclusive of all racially mixed persons.

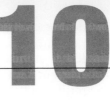

Nature and Its Resources: To Sustain or To Exploit?

Natural Selection

Charles Darwin

1 How will the struggle for existence, act in regard to variation? Can the principle of selection, which we have seen is so potent in the hands of man, apply in nature? I think we shall see that it can act most effectually. Let it be borne in mind in what an endless number of strange peculiarities our domestic productions, and, in a lesser degree, those under nature, vary; and how strong the hereditary tendency is. Under domestication, it may be truly said that the whole organisation becomes in some degree plastic. Let it be borne in mind how infinitely complex and close-fitting are the mutual relations of all organic beings to each other and to their physical conditions of life. Can it, then, be thought improbable, seeing that variations useful to man have undoubtedly occurred, that other variations useful in some way to each being in the great and complex battle of life, should sometimes occur in the course of thousands of generations? If such do occur, can we doubt (remembering that many more individuals are born than can possibly survive) that individuals having any advantage, however slight, over others, would have the best chance of surviving and of procreating their kind? On the other hand, we may feel sure that any variation in the least degree injurious would be rigidly destroyed. This preservation of favourable variations and the

436

rejection of injurious variations, I call Natural Selection. Variations neither useful nor injurious would not be affected by natural selection, and would be left a fluctuating element, as perhaps we see in the species called polymorphic.

We shall best understand the probable course of natural selection by taking the case of a country undergoing some physical change, for instance, of climate. The proportional numbers of its inhabitants would almost immediately undergo a change, and some species might become extinct. We may conclude, from what we have seen of the intimate and complex manner in which the inhabitants of each country are bound together, that any change in the numerical proportions of some of the inhabitants, independently of the change of climate itself, would most seriously affect many of the others. If the country were open on its borders, new forms would certainly immigrate, and this also would seriously disturb the relations of some of the former inhabitants. Let it be remembered how powerful the influence of a single introduced tree or mammal has been shown to be. But in the case of an island, or of a country partly surrounded by barriers, into which new and better adapted forms could not freely enter, we should then have places in the economy of nature which would assuredly be better filled up, if some of the original inhabitants were in some manner modified; for, had the area been open to immigration, these same places would have been seized on by intruders. In such case, every slight modification, which in the course of ages chanced to arise, and which in any way favoured the individuals of any of the species, by better adapting them to their altered conditions, would tend to be preserved; and natural selection would thus have free scope for the work of improvement.

We have reason to believe that a change in the conditions of life, by specially acting on the reproductive system, causes or increases variability; and in the foregoing case the conditions of life are supposed to have undergone a change, and this would manifestly be favourable to natural selection, by giving a better chance of profitable variations occurring; and unless profitable variations do occur, natural selection can do nothing. Not that, as I believe, any extreme amount of variability is necessary; as man can certainly produce great results by adding up in any given direction mere individual differences, so could Nature, but far more easily, from having incomparably longer time at her disposal. Nor do I believe that any great physical change, as of climate, or any unusual degree of isolation to check immigration, is actually necessary to produce new and unoccupied places for natural selection to fill up by modifying and improving some of the varying inhabitants. For as all the inhabitants of each country are struggling together with nicely balanced forces, extremely slight modifications in the structure or habits of one inhabitant would often give it an advantage over others; and still further modifications of the same kind would often still further increase the advantage. No country can be named in which all the native inhabitants are now so perfectly adapted to each other and to the physical conditions under which they live, that none of them could anyhow be improved; for in all countries, the natives have been so far conquered by naturalised productions, that they have allowed foreigners to take firm possession of the land. And as foreigners have thus everywhere beaten some of the natives, we may safely conclude that the natives might have been modified with advantage, so as to have better resisted such intruders.

4   As man can produce and certainly has produced a great result by his methodical and unconscious means of selection, what may not nature effect? Man can act only on external and visible characters: nature cares nothing for appearances, except in so far as they may be useful to any being. She can act on every internal organ, on every shade of constitutional difference, on the whole machinery of life. Man selects only for his own good; Nature only for that of the being which she tends. Every selected character is fully exercised by her; and the being is placed under well-suited conditions of life. Man keeps the natives of many climates in the same country; he seldom exercises each selected character in some peculiar and fitting manner; he feeds a long and a short beaked pigeon on the same food; he does not exercise a long-backed or long-legged quadruped in any peculiar manner; he exposes sheep with long and short wool to the same climate. He does not allow the most vigorous males to struggle for the females. He does not rigidly destroy all inferior animals, but protects during each varying season, as far as lies in his

power, all his productions. He often begins his selection by some half-monstrous form; or at least by some modification prominent enough to catch his eye, or to be plainly useful to him. Under nature, the slightest difference of structure or constitution may well turn the nicely-balanced scale in the struggle for life, and so be preserved. How fleeting are the wishes and efforts of man! how short his time! and consequently how poor will his products be, compared with those accumulated by nature during whole geological periods. Can we wonder, then, that nature's productions should be far "truer" in character than man's productions; that they should be infinitely better adapted to the most complex conditions of life, and should plainly bear the stamp of far higher workmanship?

It may be said that natural selection is daily and hourly 5 scrutinising, throughout the world, every variation, even the slightest; rejecting that which is bad, preserving and adding up all that is good; silently and insensibly working, whenever and wherever opportunity offers, at the improvement of each organic being in relation to its organic and inorganic conditions of life. We see nothing of these slow changes in progress, until the hand of time has marked the long lapses of ages, and then so imperfect is our view into long past geological ages, that we only see that the forms of life are now different from what they formerly were.

Although natural selection can act only through and for the 6 good of each being, yet characters and structures, which we are apt to consider as of very trifling importance, may thus be acted on. When we see leaf-eating insects green, and bark-feeders mottled-grey; the alpine ptarmigan white in winter, the red-grouse the colour of heather, and the black-grouse that of peaty earth, we must believe that these tints are of service to these birds and insects in preserving them from danger. Grouse, if not destroyed at some period of their lives, would increase in countless numbers; they are known to suffer largely from birds of prey; and hawks are guided by eyesight to their prey, so much so, that on parts of the Continent, persons are warned not to keep white pigeons, as being the most liable to destruction. Hence I can see no reason to doubt that natural selection might be most effective in giving the proper colour to each kind of grouse, and in keeping that colour, when once acquired, true and constant. Nor ought we to think that the occasional destruction of an animal of any particular colour would produce little effect: we should remember how essential it is in a flock of white sheep to destroy every lamb with the faintest trace of black. In plants the down on the fruit and the colour of the flesh are considered by botanists as characters of the most trifling importance: yet we hear from an excellent horticulturist, Downing, that in the United States smooth-skinned fruits suffer far more from a beetle, a curculio, than those with down; that purple plums suffer far more from a certain disease than yellow plums; whereas another disease attacks yellow-fleshed peaches far more than those with other coloured flesh. If, with all the aids of art, these slight differences make a great difference in cultivating the several varieties, assuredly, in a state of nature, where the trees would have to struggle with other trees and with a host of enemies, such differences would effectually settle which variety, whether a smooth or downy, a yellow or purple fleshed fruit, should succeed.

7   In looking at many small points of difference between species, which, as far as our ignorance permits us to judge, seem to be quite unimportant, we must not forget that climate, food, etc., probably produce some slight and direct effect. It is, however, far more necessary to bear in mind that there are many unknown laws of correlation of growth, which, when one part of the organisation is modified through variation, and the modifications are accumulated by natural selection for the good of the being, will cause other modifications, often of the most unexpected nature.

8   As we see that those variations which under domestication appear at any particular period of life, tend to reappear in the offspring at the same period; for instance, in the seeds of the many varieties of our culinary and agricultural plants; in the caterpillar and cocoon stages of the varieties of the silkworm; in the eggs of poultry, and in the colour of the down of their chickens; in the horns of our sheep and cattle when nearly adult; so in a state of nature, natural selection will be enabled to act on and modify organic beings at any age, by the accumulation of profitable variations at that age, and by their inheritance at a corresponding age. If it profit a plant to have its seeds more and more

widely disseminated by the wind, I can see no greater difficulty in this being effected through natural selection, than in the
cotton-planter increasing and improving by selection the down
in the pods on his cotton-trees. Natural selection may modify
and adapt the larva of an insect to a score of contingencies,
wholly different from those which concern the mature insect.
These modifications will no doubt affect, through the laws of
correlation, the structure of the adult; and probably in the case
of those insects which live only for a few hours, and which never
feed, a large part of their structure is merely the correlated result
of successive changes in the structure of their larvae. So, conversely, modifications in the adult will probably often affect the
structure of the larva; but in all cases natural selection will
ensure that modifications consequent on other modifications at
a different period of life, shall not be in the least degree injurious: for if they became so, they would cause the extinction of
the species.

Natural selection will modify the structure of the young in 9
relation to the parent, and of the parent in relation to the young.
In social animals it will adapt the structure of each individual
for the benefit of the community; if each in consequence profits
by the selected change. What natural selection cannot do, is to
modify the structure of one species, without giving it any
advantage, for the good of another species; and though statements to this effect may be found in works of natural history, I
cannot find one case which will bear investigation. A structure
used only once in an animal's whole life, if of high importance
to it, might be modified to any extent by natural selection; for
instance, the great jaws possessed by certain insects, and used
exclusively for opening the cocoon or the hard tip to the beak
of nestling birds, used for breaking the egg. It has been asserted,
that of the best short-beaked tumbler-pigeons more perish in the
egg than are able to get out of it; so that fanciers assist in the
act of hatching. Now, if nature had to make the beak of a full-
grown pigeon very short for the bird's own advantage, the
process of modification would be very slow, and there would
be simultaneously the most rigorous selection of the young
birds within the egg, which had the most powerful and hardest
beaks, for all with weak beaks would inevitably perish: or, more

delicate and more easily broken shells might be selected, the thickness of the shell being known to vary like every other structure.

The Obligation to Endure

Rachel Carson

1 The history of life on earth has been a history of interaction between living things and their surroundings. To a large extent, the physical form and the habits of the earth's vegetation and its animal life have been molded by the environment. Considering the whole span of earthly time, the opposite effect, in which life actually modifies its surroundings, has been relatively slight. Only within the moment of time represented by the present century has one species—man— acquired significant power to alter the nature of his world.

2   During the past quarter century this power has not only increased to one of disturbing magnitude but it has changed in character. The most alarming of all man's assaults upon the environment is the contamination of air, earth, rivers, and sea with dangerous and even lethal materials. This pollution is for the most part irrecoverable; the chain of evil it initiates not only in the world that must support life but in living tissues is for the most part irreversible. In this now universal contamination of the environment, chemicals are the sinister and little-recognized partners of radiation in changing the very nature of the world—the very nature of its life. Strontium 90, released through nuclear explosions into the air, comes to earth in rain or drifts down as fallout, lodges in soil, enters into the grass or corn or wheat grown there, and in time takes up its abode in the bones of a human being, there to remain until his death. Similarly, chemicals sprayed on croplands or forests or gardens lie long in soil, entering into living organisms, passing from one to another in a chain of poisoning and death. Or they pass mysteriously by underground streams until they emerge and, through the alchemy of air and sunlight, combine into new forms that kill vegetation, sicken cattle, and work unknown harm on those who drink from once

pure wells. As Albert Schweitzer has said, "Man can hardly even recognize the devils of his own creation."

It took hundreds of millions of years to produce the life that now inhabits the earth—eons of time in which that developing and evolving and diversifying life reached a state of adjustment and balance with its surroundings. The environment, rigorously shaping and directing the life it supported, contained elements that were hostile as well as supporting. Certain rocks gave out dangerous radiation; even within the light of the sun, from which all life draws its energy, there were shortwave radiations with power to injure. Given time—time not in years but in millennia—life adjusts, and a balance has been reached. For time is the essential ingredient; but in the modern world there is no time.

The rapidity of change and the speed with which new situations are created follow the impetuous and heedless pace of man rather than the deliberate pace of nature. Radiation is no longer merely the background radiation of rocks, the bombardment of cosmic rays, the ultraviolet of the sun that have existed before there was any life on earth; radiation is now the unnatural creation of man's tampering with the atom. The chemicals to which life is asked to make its adjustment are no longer merely the calcium and silica and copper and all the rest of the minerals washed out of the rocks and carried in rivers to the sea; they are the synthetic creations of man's inventive mind, brewed in his laboratories, and having no counterparts in nature.

To adjust to these chemicals would require time on the scale that is nature's; it would require not merely the years of a man's life but the life of generations. And even this, were it by some miracle possible, would be futile, for the new chemicals come from our laboratories in an endless stream; almost five hundred annually find their way into actual use in the United States alone. The figure is staggering and its implications are not easily grasped— 500 new chemicals to which the bodies of men and animals are required somehow to adapt each year, chemicals totally outside the limits of biologic experience.

Among them are many that are used in man's war against nature. Since the mid-1940s over 200 basic chemicals have been created for use in killing insects, weeds, rodents, and other organisms described in the modern vernacular as "pests"; and they are sold under several thousand different brand names.

7   These sprays, dusts, and aerosols are now applied almost universally to farms, gardens, forests, and homes—nonselective chemicals that have the power to kill every insect, the "good" and the "bad," to still the song of birds and the leaping of fish in the streams, to coat the leaves with a deadly film, and to linger on in soil—all this though the intended target may be only a few weeds or insects. Can anyone believe it is possible to lay down such a barrage of poisons on the surface of the earth without making it unfit for all life? They should not be called "insecticides," but "biocides."

8   The whole process of spraying seems caught up in an endless spiral. Since DDT was released for civilian use, a process of escalation has been going on in which ever more toxic materials must be found. This has happened because insects, in a triumphant vindication of Darwin's principle of the survival of the fittest, have evolved super races immune to the particular insecticide used, hence a deadlier one has always to be developed—and then a deadlier one than that. It has happened also because, for reasons to be described later, destructive insects often undergo a "flareback," or resurgence, after spraying in numbers greater than before. Thus the chemical war is never won, and all life is caught in its violent crossfire.

9   Along with the possibility of the extinction of mankind by nuclear war, the central problem of our age has therefore become the contamination of man's total environment with such substances of incredible potential for harm—substances that accumulate in the tissues of plants and animals and even penetrate the germ cells to shatter or alter the very material of heredity upon which the shape of the future depends.

10   Some would-be architects of our future look toward a time when it will be possible to alter the human germ plasm by design. But we may easily be doing so now by inadvertence, for many chemicals, like radiation, bring about gene mutations. It is ironic to think that man might determine his own future by something so seemingly trivial as the choice of an insect spray.

11   All this has been risked—for what? Future historians may well be amazed by our distorted sense of proportion. How could

intelligent beings seek to control a few unwanted species by a method that contaminated the entire environment and brought the threat of disease and death even to their own kind? Yet this is precisely what we have done. We have done it, moreover, for reasons that collapse the moment we examine them. We are told that the enormous and expanding use of pesticides is necessary to maintain farm production. Yet is our real problem not one of *overproduction?* Our farms, despite measures to remove acreages from production and to pay farmers *not* to produce, have yielded such a staggering excess of crops that the American taxpayer in 1962 is paying out more than one billion dollars a year as the total carrying cost of the surplus-food storage program. And is the situation helped when one branch of the Agriculture Department tries to reduce production while another states, as it did in 1958, "It is believed generally that reduction of crop acreages under provisions of the Soil Bank will stimulate interest in use of chemicals to obtain maximum production on the land retained in crops."

All this is not to say there is no insect problem and no need 12 of control. I am saying, rather, that control must be geared to realities, not to mythical situations, and that the methods employed must be such that they do not destroy us along with the insects.

The problem whose attempted solution has brought such a train 13 of disaster in its wake is an accompaniment of our modern way of life. Long before the age of man, insects inhabited the earth— a group of extraordinarily varied and adaptable beings. Over the course of time since man's advent, a small percentage of the more than half a million species of insects have come into conflict with human welfare in two principal ways: as competitors for the food supply and as carriers of human disease.

Disease-carrying insects become important where human 14 beings are crowded together, especially under conditions where sanitation is poor, as in times of natural disaster or war or in situations of extreme poverty and deprivation. Then control of some sort becomes necessary. It is a sobering fact, however, as we shall presently see, that the method of massive chemical control has had only limited success, and also threatens to worsen the very conditions it is intended to curb.

15 Under primitive agricultural conditions the farmer had few insect problems. These arose with the intensification of agriculture—the devotion of immense acreages to a single crop. Such a system set the stage for explosive increases in specific insect populations. Single-crop farming does not take advantage of the principles by which nature works; it is agriculture as an engineer might conceive it to be. Nature has introduced great variety into the landscape, but man has displayed a passion for simplifying it. Thus he undoes the built-in checks and balances by which nature holds the species within bounds. One important natural check is a limit on the amount of suitable habitat for each species. Obviously then, an insect that lives on wheat can build up its population to much higher levels on a farm devoted to wheat than on one in which wheat is intermingled with other crops to which the insect is not adapted.

16 The same thing happens in other situations. A generation or more ago, the towns of large areas of the United States lined their streets with the noble elm tree. Now the beauty they hopefully created is threatened with complete destruction as disease sweeps through the elms, carried by a beetle that would have only limited chance to build up large populations and to spread from tree to tree if the elms were only occasional trees in a richly diversified planting.

17 Another factor in the modern insect problem is one that must be viewed against a background of geologic and human history: the spreading of thousands of different kinds of organisms from their native homes to invade new territories. This worldwide migration has been studied and graphically described by the British ecologist Charles Elton in his recent book *The Ecology of Invasions.* During the Cretaceous Period, some hundred million years ago, flooding seas cut many land bridges between continents and living things found themselves confined in what Elton calls "colossal separate nature reserves." There, isolated from others of their kind, they developed many new species. When some of the land masses were joined again, about 15 million years ago, these species began to move out into new territories—a movement that is not only still in progress but is now receiving considerable assistance from man.

18 The importation of plants is the primary agent in the modern spread of species, for animals have almost invariably gone along

with the plants, quarantine being a comparatively recent and not completely effective innovation. The United States Office of Plant Introduction alone has introduced almost 200,000 species and varieties of plants from all over the world. Nearly half of the 180 or so major insect enemies of plants in the United States are accidental imports from abroad, and most of them have come as hitchhikers on plants.

In new territory, out of reach of the restraining hand of the natural enemies that kept down its numbers in its native land, an invading plant or animal is able to become enormously abundant. Thus it is no accident that our most troublesome insects are introduced species. [19]

These invasions, both the naturally occurring and those dependent on human assistance, are likely to continue indefinitely. Quarantine and massive chemical campaigns are only extremely expensive ways of buying time. We are faced, according to Dr. Elton, "with a life-and-death need not just to find new technological means of suppressing this plant or that animal"; instead we need the basic knowledge of animal populations and their relations to their surroundings that will "promote an even balance and damp down the explosive power of outbreaks and new invasions." [20]

Much of the necessary knowledge is now available but we do not use it. We train ecologists in our universities and even employ them in our governmental agencies but we seldom take their advice. We allow the chemical death rain to fall as though there were no alternative, whereas in fact there are many, and our ingenuity could soon discover many more if given opportunity. [21]

Have we fallen into a mesmerized state that makes us accept as inevitable that which is inferior or detrimental, as though having lost the will or the vision to demand that which is good? Such thinking, in the words of the ecologist Paul Shepard, "idealizes life with only its head out of water, inches above the limits of toleration of the corruption of its own environment. . . . Why should we tolerate a diet of weak poisons, a home in insipid surroundings, a circle of acquaintances who are not quite our enemies, the noise of motors with just enough relief to prevent insanity? Who would want to live in a world which is just not quite fatal?" [22]

Yet such a world is pressed upon us. The crusade to create a chemically sterile, insect-free world seems to have engendered [23] a fanatic zeal on the part of many specialists and most of the so-called control agencies. On every hand there is evidence that those engaged in spraying operations exercise a ruthless power. "The regulatory entomologists . . . function as prosecutor, judge and jury, tax assessor and collector and sheriff to enforce their own orders," said Connecticut entomologist Neely Turner. The most flagrant abuses go unchecked in both state and federal agencies.

24   It is not my contention that chemical insecticides must never be used. I do contend that we have put poisonous and biologically potent chemicals indiscriminately into the hands of persons largely or wholly ignorant of their potentials for harm. We have subjected enormous numbers of people to contact with these poisons, without their consent and often without their knowledge. If the Bill of Rights contains no guarantee that a citizen shall be secure against lethal poisons distributed either by private individuals or by public officials, it is surely only because our forefathers, despite their considerable wisdom and foresight, could conceive of no such problem.

25   I contend, furthermore, that we have allowed these chemicals to be used with little or no advance investigation of their effect on soil, water, wildlife, and man himself. Future generations are unlikely to condone our lack of prudent concern for the integrity of the natural world that supports all life.

26   There is still very limited awareness of the nature of the threat. This is an era of specialists, each of whom sees his own problem and is unaware of or intolerant of the larger frame into which it fits. It is also an era dominated by industry, in which the right to make a dollar at whatever cost is seldom challenged. When the public protests, confronted with some obvious evidence of damaging results of pesticide applications, it is fed little tranquilizing pills of half truth. We urgently need an end to these false assurances, to the sugar coating of unpalatable facts. It is the public that is being asked to assume the risks that the insect controllers calculate. The public must decide whether it wishes to continue on the present road, and it can do so only when in full possession of the facts. In the words of Jean Rostand, "The obligation to endure gives us the right to know."

Touching the Earth

bell hooks

> *I wish to live because life has within it that*
> *which is good, that which is beautiful, and that*
> *which is love. Therefore, since I have known all*
> *these things, I have found them to be reason*
> *enough and—I wish to live. Moreover, because*
> *this is so, I wish others to live for generations*
> *and generations and generations and generations.*
> —Lorraine Hansberry,
> *To Be Young, Gifted, and Black*

When we love the earth, we are able to love ourselves more
fully. I believe this. The ancestors taught me it was so. As a child
I loved playing in dirt, in that rich Kentucky soil, that was a
source of life. Before I understood anything about the pain and
exploitation of the southern system of sharecropping, I understood that grown-up black folks loved the land. I could stand
with my grandfather Daddy Jerry and look out at fields of growing vegetables, tomatoes, corn, collards, and know that this was
his handiwork. I could see the look of pride on his face as I
expressed wonder and awe at the magic of growing things. I
knew that my grandmother Baba's backyard garden would yield
beans, sweet potatoes, cabbage, and yellow squash, that she
would walk with pride among the rows and rows of growing
vegetables showing us what the earth will give when tended
lovingly.

From the moment of their first meeting, Native American and
African people shared with one another a respect for the life-
giving forces of nature, of the earth. African settlers in Florida
taught the Creek Nation runaways, the "Seminoles," methods for
rice cultivation. Native peoples taught recently arrived black folks
all about the many uses of corn. (The hotwater cornbread we grew
up eating came to our black southern diet from the world of the
Indian.) Sharing the reverence for the earth, black and red people
helped one another remember that, despite the white man's ways,

the land belonged to everyone. Listen to these words attributed to Chief Seattle in 1854:

> How can you buy or sell the sky, the warmth of the land? The idea is strange to us. If we do not own the freshness of the air and the sparkle of the water, how can you buy them? Every part of this earth is sacred to my people. Every shining pine needle, every sandy shore, every mist in the dark woods, every clearing and humming insect is holy in the memory and experience of my people . . . We are part of the earth and it is part of us. The perfumed flowers are our sisters; the deer, the horse, the great eagle, these are our brothers. The rocky crests, the juices in the meadows, the body heat of the pony, and man—all belong to the same family.

3   The sense of union and harmony with nature expressed here is echoed in testimony by black people who found that even though life in the new world was "harsh, harsh," in relationship to the earth one could be at peace. In the oral autobiography of granny midwife Onnie Lee Logan, who lived all her life in Alabama, she talks about the richness of farm life—growing vegetables, raising chickens, and smoking meat. She reports:

> We lived a happy, comfortable life to be right outa slavery times. I didn't know nothin else but the farm so it was happy and we was happy . . . We couldn't do anything else but be happy. We accept the days as they come and as they were. Day by day until you couldn't say there was any great hard time. We overlooked it. We didn't think nothing about it. We just went along. We had what it takes to make a good livin and go about it.

Living in modern society, without a sense of history, it has been easy for folks to forget that black people were first and foremost a people of the land, farmers. It is easy for folks to forget that at the first part of the 20th century, the vast majority of black folks in the United States lived in the agrarian south.

4   Living close to nature, black folks were able to cultivate a spirit of wonder and reverence for life. Growing food to sustain life and flowers to please the soul, they were able to make a connection with the earth that was ongoing and life-affirming. They were witnesses to beauty. In Wendell Berry's important discussion of the relationship between agriculture and human spiritual

well-being, *The Unsettling of America*, he reminds us that working the land provides a location where folks can experience a sense of personal power and well-being:

> We are working well when we use ourselves as the fellow creature of the plants, animals, material, and other people we are working with. Such work is unifying, healing. It brings us home from pride and despair, and places us responsibly within the human estate. It defines us as we are: not too good to work without our bodies, but too good to work poorly or joylessly or selfishly or alone.

There has been little or no work done on the psychological 5 impact of the "great migration" of black people from the agrarian south to the industrialized north. Toni Morrison's novel *The Bluest Eye* attempts to fictively document the way moving from the agrarian south to the industrialized north wounded the psyches of black folk. Estranged from a natural world, where there was time for silence and contemplation, one of the "displaced" black folks in Morrison's novel, Miss Pauline, loses her capacity to experience the sensual world around her when she leaves southern soil to live in a northern city. The south is associated in her mind with a world of sensual beauty most deeply expressed in the world of nature. Indeed, when she falls in love for the first time she can name that experience only by evoking images from nature, from an agrarian world and near wilderness of natural splendor:

> When I first seed Cholly, I want you to know it was like all the bits of color from that time down home when all us chil'ren went berry picking after a funeral and I put some in the pocket of my Sunday dress, and they mashed up and stained my hips. My whole dress was messed with purple, and it never did wash out. Not the dress nor me. I could feel that purple deep inside me. And that lemonade Mama used to make when Pap came out of the fields. It be cool and yellowish, with seeds floating near the bottom. And that streak of green them june bugs made on the tress that night we left from down home. All of them colors was in me. Just sitting there.

Certainly, it must have been a profound blow to the collective psyche of black people to find themselves struggling to make a

living in the industrial north away from the land. Industrial capitalism was not simply changing the nature of black work life, it
altered the communal practices that were so central to survival in
the agrarian south. And it fundamentally altered black people's
relationship to the body. It is the loss of any capacity to appreciate her body, despite its flaws, Miss Pauline suffers when she
moves north.

6   The motivation for black folks to leave the south and move
north was both material and psychological. Black folks wanted to
be free of the overt racial harassment that was a constant in southern life and they wanted access to material goods—to a level of
material well-being that was not available in the agrarian south
where white folks limited access to the spheres of economic
power. Of course, they found that life in the north had its own
perverse hardships, that racism was just as virulent there, that it
was much harder for black people to become landowners. Without the space to grow food, to commune with nature, or to medi-
ate the starkness of poverty with the splendor of nature, black
people experienced profound depression. Working in conditions
where the body was regarded solely as a tool (as in slavery), a
profound estrangement occurred between mind and body. The
way the body was represented became more important than the
body itself. It did not matter if the body was well, only that it
appeared well.

7   Estrangement from nature and engagement in mind/body
splits made it all the more possible for black people to internalize
white-supremacist assumptions about black identity. Learning
contempt for blackness, southerners transplanted in the north suffered both culture shock and soul loss. Contrasting the harshness
of city life with an agrarian world, the poet Waring Cuney wrote
this popular poem in the 1920s, testifying to lost connection:

> She does not know her beauty
> She thinks her brown body
> has no glory.
> If she could dance naked,
> Under palm trees
> And see her image in the river
> She would know.

But there are no palm trees on the street,
And dishwater gives back no images.

For many years, and even now, generations of black folks 8
who migrated north to escape life in the south, returned down
home in search of a spiritual nourishment, a healing, that was
fundamentally connected to reaffirming one's connection to
nature, to a contemplative life where one could take time, sit on
the porch, walk, fish, and catch lightning bugs. If we think of
urban life as a location where black folks learned to accept a
mind/body split that made it possible to abuse the body, we can
better understand the growth of nihilism and despair in the
black psyche. And we can know that when we talk about healing that psyche we must also speak about restoring our connection to the natural world.

Wherever black folks live we can restore our relationship to 9
the natural world by taking the time to commune with nature, to
appreciate the other creatures who share this planet with humans.
Even in my small New York City apartment I can pause to listen
to birds sing, find a tree and watch it. We can grow plants—herbs,
flowers, vegetables. Those novels by African-American writers
(women and men) that talk about black migration from the agrarian south to the industrialized north describe in detail the way
folks created space to grow flowers and vegetables. Although I
come from country people with serious green thumbs, I have
always felt that I could not garden. In the past few years, I have
found that I can do it—that many gardens will grow, that I feel
connected to my ancestors when I can put a meal on the table of
food I grew. I especially love to plant collard greens. They are
hardy, and easy to grow.

In modern society, there is also a tendency to see no correlation 10
between the struggle for collective black self-recovery and ecological movements that seek to restore balance to the planet by changing our relationship to nature and to natural resources. Unmindful
of our history of living harmoniously on the land, many contemporary black folks see no value in supporting ecological movements, or see ecology and the struggle to end racism as competing
concerns. Recalling the legacy of our ancestors who knew that the
way we regard land and nature will determine the level of our

self-regard, black people must reclaim a spiritual legacy where we connect our well-being to the well-being of the earth. This is a necessary dimension of healing. As Berry reminds us:

> Only by restoring the broken connections can we be healed. Connection is health. And what our society does its best to disguise from us is how ordinary, how commonly attainable, health is. We lose our health—and create profitable diseases and dependencies—by failing to see the direct connections between living and eating, eating and working, working and loving. In gardening, for instance, one works with the body to feed the body. The work, if it is knowledgeable, makes for excellent food. And it makes one hungry. The work thus makes eating both nourishing and joyful, not consumptive, and keeps the eater from getting fat and weak. This health, wholeness, is a source of delight.

Collective black self-recovery takes place when we begin to renew our relationship to the earth, when we remember the way of our ancestors. When the earth is sacred to us, our bodies can also be sacred to us.

Against Nature

Joyce Carol Oates

> *We soon get through with Nature. She excites an expectation which she cannot satisfy.*
> —Thoreau, Journal, 1854

> *Sir, if a man has experienced the inexpressible, he is under no obligation to attempt to express it.*
> —Samuel Johnson

1 *The writer's resistance to Nature.*

2   It has no sense of humor: in its beauty, as in its ugliness, or its neutrality, there is no laughter.

3   It lacks a moral purpose.

4   It lacks a satiric dimension, registers no irony.

Its pleasures lack resonance, being accidental; its horrors, even 5
when premeditated, are equally perfunctory, "red in tooth and
claw" et cetera.

It lacks a symbolic subtext—excepting that provided by man. 6

It has no (verbal) language. 7

It has no interest in ours. 8

It inspires a painfully limited set of responses in "nature- 9
writers"—REVERENCE, AWE, PIETY, MYSTICAL ONENESS.

It eludes us even as it prepares to swallow us up, books and all. 10

I was lying on my back in the dirt-gravel of the towpath beside 11
the Delaware-Raritan Canal, Titusville, New Jersey, staring up at
the sky and trying, with no success, to overcome a sudden attack
of tachycardia that had come upon me out of nowhere—such
attacks are always "out of nowhere," that's their charm—and all
around me Nature thrummed with life, the air smelling of mois-
ture and sunlight, the canal reflecting the sky, red-winged black-
birds testing their spring calls—the usual. I'd become the jar in
Tennessee, a fictitious center, or parenthesis, aware beyond my
erratic heartbeat of the numberless heartbeats of the earth, its
pulsing pumping life, sheer life, incalculable. Struck down in the
midst of motion—I'd been jogging a minute before—I was "out
of time" like a fallen, stunned boxer, privileged (in an abstract
manner of speaking) to be an involuntary witness to the random,
wayward, nameless motion on all sides of me.

Paroxysmal tachycardia is rarely fatal, but if the heartbeat accel- 12
erates to 250–270 beats a minute you're in trouble. The average
attack is about 100–150 beats and mine seemed so far to be about
average; the trick now was to prevent it from getting worse. Brainy
people try brainy strategies, such as thinking calming thoughts,
pseudo-mystic thoughts, *If I die now it's a good death,* that sort of
thing, *if I die this is a good place and a good time,* the idea is to deceive
the frenzied heartbeat that, really, you don't care: you hadn't any
other plans for the afternoon. The important thing with tachycardia
is to prevent panic! you must prevent panic! otherwise you'll have
to be taken by ambulance to the closest emergency room, which is
not so very nice a way to spend the afternoon, really. So I contemplated the blue sky overhead. The earth beneath my head. Nature
surrounding me on all sides, I couldn't quite see it but I could hear

it, smell it, sense it—there is something *there,* no mistake about it. Completely oblivious to the predicament of the individual but that's only "natural" after all, one hardly expects otherwise.

13   When you discover yourself lying on the ground, limp and unresisting, head in the dirt, and helpless, the earth seems to shift forward as a presence; hard, emphatic, not mere surface but a genuine force—there is no other word for it but *presence.* To keep in motion is to keep in time and to be stopped, stilled, is to be abruptly out of time, in another time-dimension perhaps, an alien one, where human language has no resonance. Nothing to be said about it expresses it, nothing touches it, it's an absolute against which nothing human can be measured. . . . Moving through space and time by way of your own volition you inhabit an interior consciousness, a hallucinatory consciousness, it might be said, so long as breath, heartbeat, the body's autonomy hold; when motion is stopped you are jarred out of it. The interior is invaded by the exterior. The outside wants to come in, and only the self's fragile membrane prevents it.

14   The fly buzzing at Emily's death.

15   Still, the earth *is* your place. A tidy grave-site measured to your size. Or, from another angle of vision, one vast democratic grave.

16   Let's contemplate the sky. Forget the crazy hammering heartbeat, don't listen to it, don't start counting, remember that there is a clever way of breathing that conserves oxygen as if you're lying below the surface of a body of water breathing through a very thin straw but you *can* breathe through it if you're careful, if you don't panic, one breath and then another and then another, isn't that the story of all lives? careers? Just a matter of breathing. Of course it is. But contemplate the sky, it's there to be contemplated. A mild shock to see it so blank, blue, a thin airy ghostly blue, no clouds to disguise its emptiness. You are beginning to feel not only weightless but near-bodiless, lying on the earth like a scrap of paper about to be blown off. Two dimensions and you'd imagined you were three! And there's the sky rolling away forever, into infinity—if "infinity" can be "rolled into"—and the forlorn truth is, that's where you're going too. And the lovely blue isn't even blue, is it? isn't even there, is it? a mere optical illusion, isn't it? no matter what art has urged you to believe.

Early Nature memories. Which it's best not to suppress.   17

. . . Wading, as a small child, in Tonawanda Creek near our   18
house, and afterward trying to tear off, in a frenzy of terror and
revulsion, the sticky fat black bloodsuckers that had attached
themselves to my feet, particularly between my toes.

. . . Coming upon a friend's dog in a drainage ditch, dead for   19
several days, evidently the poor creature had been shot by a hunter
and left to die, bleeding to death, and we're stupefied with grief and
horror but can't resist sliding down to where he's lying on his belly,
and we can't resist squatting over him, turning the body over . . .

. . . The raccoon, mad with rabies, frothing at the mouth and   20
tearing at his own belly with his teeth, so that his intestines spilled
out onto the ground . . . a sight I seem to remember though in fact
I did not see. I've been told I did not see.

Consequently, my chronic uneasiness with Nature-mysticism;   21
Nature-adoration; Nature-as-(moral)-instruction-for-mankind. My
doubt that one can, with philosophical validity, address "Nature" as
a single coherent noun, anything other than a Platonic, hence discredited, is-ness. My resistance to "Nature-writing" as a genre,
except when it is brilliantly fictionalized in the service of a writer's
individual vision—Throeau's books and *Journal,* of course—but also,
less known in this country, the miniaturist prose-poems of Colette
(*Flowers and Fruit*) and Ponge (*Taking the Side of Things*)—in which
case it becomes yet another, and ingenious, form of storytelling. The
subject is *there* only by the grace of the author's language.

Nature has no instructions for mankind except that our poor   22
beleaguered humanist-democratic way of life, our fantasies of the
individual's high worth, our sense that the weak, no less than the
strong, have a right to survive, are absurd.

In any case, where *is* Nature? one might (skeptically) inquire. 23
Who has looked upon her/its face and survived?

But isn't this all exaggeration, in the spirit of rhetorical con- 24
tentiousness? Surely Nature is, for you, as for most reasonably
intelligent people, a "perennial" source of beauty, comfort, peace,
escape from the delirium of civilized life; a respite from the ego's
ever-frantic strategies of self-promotion, as a way of insuring (at
least in fantasy) some small measure of immortality? Surely

Nature, as it is understood in the usual slapdash way, as human, if not dilettante, *experience* (hiking in a national park, jogging on the beach at dawn, even tending, with the usual comical frustrations, a suburban garden), is wonderfully consoling; a place where, when you go there, it has to take you in?—a palimpsest of sorts you choose to read, layer by layer, always with care, always cautiously, in proportion to your psychological strength?

25   Nature: as in Thoreau's upbeat Transcendentalist mode ("The indescribable innocence and beneficence of Nature,—such health, such cheer, they afford forever! and such sympathy have they ever with our race, that all Nature would be affected . . . if any man should ever for a just cause grieve"), and not in Thoreau's grim mode ("Nature is hard to be overcome but she must be overcome").

26   Another way of saying, not *Nature-in-itself* but *Nature-as-experience.*

27   The former, Nature-in-itself, is, to allude slantwise to Melville, a blankness ten times blank; the latter is what we commonly, or perhaps always, mean when we speak of Nature as a noun, a single entity—something of *ours.* Most of the time it's just an activity, a sort of hobby, a weekend, a few days, perhaps a few hours, staring out the window at the mind-dazzling autumn foliage of, say, Northern Michigan, being rendered speechless—temporarily—at the sight of Mt. Shasta, the Grand Canyon, Ansel Adams's West. Or Nature writ small, contained in the back yard. Nature filtered through our optical nerves, our "senses," our fiercely romantic expectations. Nature that pleases us because it mirrors our souls, or gives the comforting illusion of doing so. As in our first mother's awakening to the self's fatal beauty—

>   I thither went
> With unexperienc't thought, and laid me down
> On the green bank, to look into the clear
> Smooth Lake, that to me seem'd another Sky.
> As I bent down to look, just opposite,
> A Shape within the watr'y gleam appear'd
> Bending to look on me, I started back,
> It started back, but pleas'd I soon return'd,
> Pleas'd it return'd as soon with answering looks
> Of sympathy and love; there I had fixt
> Mine eyes till now, and pin'd with vain desire.

—in these surpassingly beautiful lines from Book IV of Milton's
Paradise Lost.

Nature as the self's (flattering) mirror, but not ever, no, never,   28
Nature-in-itself.

Nature is mouths, or maybe a single mouth. Why glamorize it,   29
romanticize it, well yes but we must, we're writers, poets, mystics
(of a sort) aren't we, precisely what else are we to do but glamorize and romanticize and generally exaggerate the significance of
anything we focus the white heat of our "creativity" upon . . . ? And
why not Nature, since it's there, common property, mute, can't talk
back, allows us the possibility of transcending the human condition
for a while, writing prettily of mountain ranges, white-tailed deer,
the purple crocuses outside this very window, the thrumming dazzling "life-force" we imagine we all support. Why not.

Nature *is* more than a mouth—it's a dazzling variety of   30
mouths. And it pleases the senses, in any case, as the physicists'
chill universe of numbers certainly does not.

Oscar Wilde, on our subject: "Nature is no great mother who has   31
borne us. She is our creation. It is in our brain that she quickens
to life. Things are because we see them, and what we see, and how
we see it, depends on the Arts that have influenced us. To look at
a thing is very different from seeing a thing. . . . At present, people
see fogs, not because there are fogs, but because poets and painters
have taught them the mysterious loveliness of such effects. There
may have been fogs for centuries in London. I dare say there were.
But no one saw them. They did not exist until Art had invented
them. . . . Yesterday evening Mrs. Arundel insisted on my going to
the window and looking at the glorious sky, as she called it. And
so I had to look at it. . . . And what was it? It was simply a very
second-rate Turner, a Turner of a bad period, with all the painter's
worst faults exaggerated and over-emphasized."

(If we were to put it to Oscar Wilde that he exaggerates, his   32
reply might well be: "Exaggeration? I don't know the meaning of
the word.")

Walden, that most artfully composed of prose fictions, concludes,   33
in the rhapsodic chapter "Spring," with Henry David Thoreau's
contemplation of death, decay, and regeneration as it is suggested

to him, or to his protagonist, by the spectacle of vultures feeding off carrion. There is a dead horse close by his cabin and the stench of its decomposition, in certain winds, is daunting. Yet: "... the assurance it gave me of the strong appetite and inviolable health of Nature was my compensation. I love to see that Nature is so rife with life that myriads can be afforded to be sacrificed and suffered to prey upon one another; that tender organizations can be so serenely squashed out of existence like pulp,—tadpoles which herons gobble up, and tortoises and toads run over in the road; and that sometimes it has rained flesh and blood!... The impression made on a wise man is that of universal innocence."

34   Come off it, Henry David. You've grieved these many years for your elder brother John, who died a ghastly death of lockjaw; you've never wholly recovered from the experience of watching him die. And you know, or must know, that you're fated too to die young of consumption.... But this doctrinaire Transcendentalist passage ends *Walden* on just the right note. It's as impersonal, as coolly detached, as the Oversoul itself: a "wise man" filters his emotions through his brain.

35   Or through his prose.

36 Nietzsche: "We all pretend to ourselves that we are more simple-minded than we are: that is how we get a rest from our fellow men."

> Once out of nature I shall never take
> My bodily form from any natural thing,
> But such a form as Grecian goldsmiths make
> Of hammered gold and gold enamelling
> To keep a drowsy Emperor awake;
> Or set upon a golden bough to sing
> To lords and ladies of Byzantium
> Of what is past, passing, or to come.
> —*William Butler Yeats, "Sailing to
> Byzantium"*

Yet even the golden bird is a "bodily form taken from (a) natural thing." No, it's impossible to escape!

37 *The writer's resistance to Nature.*

Wallace Stevens: "In the presence of extraordinary actuality, con- 38
sciousness takes the place of imagination."

Once, years ago, in 1972 to be precise, when I seemed to have been 39
another person, related to the person I am now as one is related,
tangentially, sometimes embarrassingly, to cousins not seen for
decades,—once, when we were living in London, and I was very
sick, I had a mystical vision. That is, I "had" a "mystical vision"—
the heart sinks: such pretension—or something resembling one. A
fever-dream, let's call it. It impressed me enormously and
impresses me still, though I've long since lost the capacity to see
it with my mind's eye, or even, I suppose, to believe in it. There
is a statute of limitations on "mystical visions" as on romantic love.

I was very sick; and I imagined my life as a thread, a thread 40
of breath, or heartbeat, or pulse, or light, yes it was light, radiant
light, I was burning with fever and I ascended to that plane of
serenity that might be mistaken for (or *is*, in fact) Nirvana, where
I had a waking dream of uncanny lucidity—

My body is a tall column of light and heat.   41
My body is not "I" but "it."   42
My body is not one but many.   43
My body, which "I" inhabit, is inhabited as well by other crea- 44
tures, unknown to me, imperceptible—the smallest of them mere
sparks of light.

My body, which I perceive as substance, is in fact an organ- 45
ization of infinitely complex, overlapping, imbricated structures,
radiant light their manifestation, the "body" a tall column of light
and blood-heat, a temporary agreement among atoms, like a
high-rise building with numberless rooms, corridors, corners, ele-
vator shafts, windows. . . . In this fantastical structure the "I" is
deluded as to its sovereignty, let alone its autonomy in the (outside) world; the most astonishing secret is that the "I" doesn't
exist!—but it behaves as if it does, as if it were one and not many.

In any case, without the "I" the tall column of light and heat 46
would die, and the microscopic life-particles would die with
it . . . will die with it. The "I," which doesn't exist, is everything.

But Dr. Johnson is right, the inexpressible need not be expressed.
And what resistance, finally? There is none.

47 This morning, an invasion of tiny black ants. One by one they appear, out of nowhere—that's their charm too!—moving single file across the white Parsons table where I am sitting, trying without much success to write a poem. A poem of only three or four lines is what I want, something short, tight, mean, I want it to hurt like a white-hot wire up the nostrils, small and compact and turned in upon itself with the density of a hunk of rock from the planet Jupiter. . . .

48 But here come the black ants: harbingers, you might say, of spring. One by one by one they appear on the dazzling white table and one by one I kill them with a forefinger, my deft right forefinger, mashing each against the surface of the table and then dropping it into a wastebasket at my side. Idle labor, mesmerizing, effortless, and I'm curious as to how long I can do it, sit here in the brilliant March sunshine killing ants with my right forefinger, how long I, and the ants, can keep it up.

49 After a while I realize that I can do it a long time. And that I've written my poem.

Save the Whales, Screw the Shrimp

Joy Williams

1 I don't want to talk about *me*, of course, but it seems as though far too much attention has been lavished on *you* lately—that your greed and vanities and quest for self-fulfillment have been catered to far too much. You just want and want and want. You haven't had a mandala dream since the eighties began. To have a mandala dream you'd have to instinctively know that it was an attempt at self-healing on the part of Nature, and you don't believe in Nature anymore. It's too isolated from you. You've abstracted it. It's so messy and damaged and sad. Your eyes glaze as you travel life's highway past all the crushed animals and the Big Gulp cups. You don't even take pleasure in looking at nature photographs these days. Oh, they can be just as pretty, as always, but don't they make you feel increasingly . . . anxious? Filled with more trepidation than peace? So what's the point? You see

the picture of the baby condor or the panda munching on a bamboo shoot, and your heart just sinks, doesn't it? A picture of a poor old sea turtle with barnacles on her back, all ancient and exhausted, depositing her five gallons of doomed eggs in the sand hardly fills you with joy, because you realize, quite rightly, that just outside the frame falls the shadow of the condo. What's cropped from the shot of ocean waves crashing on a pristine shore is the plastics plant, and just beyond the dunes lies a parking lot. Hidden from immediate view in the butterfly-bright meadow, in the dusky thicket, in the oak and holly wood, are the surveyors' stakes, for someone wants to build a mall exactly there—some gas stations and supermarkets, some pizza and video shops, a health club, maybe a bulimia treatment center. Those lovely pictures of leopards and herons and wild rivers, well, you just know they're going to be accompanied by a text that will serve only to bring you down. You don't want to think about it! It's all so uncool. And you don't want to feel guilty either. Guilt is uncool. Regret maybe you'll consider. *Maybe.* Regret is a possibility, but don't push me, you say. Nature photographs have become something of a problem, along with almost everything else. Even though they leave the bad stuff out—maybe because you *know* they're leaving all the bad stuff out—such pictures are making you increasingly aware that you're a little too late for Nature. Do you feel that? Twenty years too late, maybe only ten? Not *way* too late, just a little too late? Well, it appears that you are. And since you are, you've decided you're just not going to attend this particular party.

Pascal said that it is easier to endure death without thinking about it than to endure the thought of death without dying. This is how you manage to dance the strange dance with that grim partner, nuclear annihilation. When the U.S. Army notified Winston Churchill that the first atom bomb had been detonated in New Mexico, it chose the code phrase BABIES SATISFACTORILY BORN. So you entered the age of irony, and the strange double life you've been leading with the world ever since. Joyce Carol Oates suggests that the reason writers—*real* writers, one assumes—don't write about Nature is that it lacks a sense of humor and registers no irony. It just doesn't seem to be of the times—these slick, sleek, knowing, objective, indulgent times. And the word *Environment*. Such a bloodless word. A flat-footed word with a shrunken heart. A word increasingly disengaged from its association with the natural world. Urban planners, industrialists, economists, and developers use it. It's a lost word, really. A cold word, mechanistic, suited strangely to the coldness generally felt toward Nature. It's their word now. You don't mind giving it up. As for *Environmentalist,* that's one that can really bring on the yawns, for you've tamed and tidied it, neutered it quite nicely. An environmentalist must be calm, rational, reasonable, and willing to compromise, otherwise you won't listen to him. Still, his beliefs are *opinions* only, for this is the age of radical subjectivism. Not long ago, Barry Commoner spoke to the Environmental Protection Agency. He scolded them. They loved it. The way they protect the environment these days is apparently to find an "acceptable level of harm from a pollutant and then issue rules allowing industry to pollute to that level." Commoner suggested that this was inappropriate. An EPA employee suggested that any other approach would place limits on economic growth and implied that Commoner was advocating this. Limits on economic growth! Commoner vigorously denied this. Oh, it was a healthy exchange of ideas, healthier certainly than our air and water. We needed that little spanking, the EPA felt. It was refreshing. The agency has recently lumbered into action in its campaign to ban dinoseb. You seem to have liked your dinoseb. It's been a popular weed killer, even though it has been directly linked with birth defects. You must hate weeds a lot. Although the EPA appears successful in banning the poison, it will still have to pay the disposal costs and compensate the manufacturers for the market value of the chemicals they still have in stock.

3   That's ironic, you say, but farmers will suffer losses, too, oh dreadful financial losses, if herbicide and pesticide use is restricted.

4   Farmers grow way too much stuff anyway. They grow surplus crops with subsidized water created by turning rivers great and small into a plumbing system of dams and canals. Rivers have become *systems*. Wetlands are increasingly being referred to as *filtering systems*—things deigned *useful* because of their ability to absorb urban run-off, oil from roads, et cetera.

We know that. We've known that for years about farmers. We   5
know a lot these days. We're very well informed. If farmers aren't
allowed to make a profit by growing surplus crops, they'll have
to sell their land to developers, who'll turn all that *arable land* into
office parks. Arable land isn't Nature anyway, and besides, we like
those office parks and shopping plazas, with their monster supermarkets open twenty-four hours a day with aisle after aisle after
aisle of *products.* It's fun. Products are fun.

Farmers like their poisons, but ranchers like them even more.   6
There are well-funded predominantly federal and cooperative
programs like the Agriculture Department's Animal Damage
Control Unit that poison, shoot, and trap several thousand animals each year. This unit loves to kill things. It was created to
kill things—bobcats, foxes, black bears, mountain lions, rabbits,
badgers, countless birds—all to make this great land safe for the
string bean and the corn, the sheep and the cow, even though
you're not consuming as much cow these days. A burger now
and then, but burgers are hardly cows at all, you feel. They're
not all *our* cows in any case, for some burger matter is imported.
There's a bit of Central American burger matter in your bun.
Which is contributing to the conversion of tropical rain forest
into cow pasture. Even so, you're getting away from meat these
days. You're eschewing cow. It's seafood you love, shrimp most
of all. And when you love something, it had better watch out,
because you have a tendency to love it to death. Shrimp, shrimp,
shrimp. It's more common on menus than chicken. In the wilds
of Ohio, far, far from watery shores, four out of the six entrées
on a menu will be shrimp, for some modest sum. Everywhere,
it's all the shrimp you can eat or all you *care* to eat, for sometimes you just don't feel like eating all you *can.* You are inten-
sively *harvesting* shrimp. Soon there won't be any left and then
you can stop. It takes that, often, to make you stop. Shrimpers
shrimp, of course. That's their *business.* They put out these big
nets and in these nets, for each pound of shrimp, they catch
more than ten times that amount of fish, turtles, and dolphins.
These, quite the worse for wear, they dump back in. There is an
object called TED (Turtle Excluder Device), which would save
thousands of turtles and some dolphins from dying in the nets,

but the shrimpers are loath to use TEDs, as they say it would cut the size of their shrimp catch.

7   We've heard about TED, you say.

8   They want you, all of you, to have all the shrimp you can eat and more. At Kiawah Island, off the coast of South Carolina, visitors go out on Jeep "safaris" through the part of the island that hasn't been developed yet. ("Wherever you see trees," the guide says, "really, that's a lot.") The safari comprises six Jeeps, and these days they go out at least four times a day, with more trips promised soon. The tourists drive their own Jeeps and the guide talks to them by radio. Kiawah has nice beaches, and the guide talks about turtles. When he mentions the shrimpers' role in the decline of the turtle, the shrimpers, who share the same frequency, scream at him. Shrimpers and most commercial fishermen (many of them working with drift and gill nets anywhere from six to thirty miles long) think of themselves as an *endangered species*. A recent newspaper headline said, "Shrimpers Spared Anti-Turtle Devices." Even so with the continuing wanton depletion of shrimp beds, they will undoubtedly have to find some other means of employment soon. They might, for instance, become part of that vast throng laboring in the *tourist industry*.

9 Tourism has become an industry as destructive as any other. You are no longer benign in your traveling somewhere to look at the scenery. You never thought there was much gain in just looking anyway, you've always preferred to *use* the scenery in some manner. In your desire to get away from what you've got, you've caused there to be no place to get away *to*. You're just all bumpered up out there. Sewage and dumps have become prime indicators of America's lifestyle. In resort towns in New England and the Adirondacks, measuring the flow into the sewage plant serves as a business barometer. Tourism is a growth industry. You believe in growth. *Controlled* growth, of course. Controlled exponential growth is what you'd really like to see. You certainly don't want to put a moratorium or a cap on anything. That's illegal, isn't it? Retro you're not. You don't want to go back or anything. Forward. Maybe ask directions later. Growth is *desirable* as well as being *inevitable*. Growth is the one thing you seem to be powerless before, so you try to be realistic about it. Growth is—it's weird—it's like cancer or something.

Recently you, as tourist, have discovered your national parks 10
and are quickly *overburdening* them. Spare land and it belongs to
you! It's exotic land too, not looking like all the stuff around it
that looks like everything else. You want to take advantage of
this land, of course, and use it in every way you can. Thus the
managers—or *stewards,* as they like to be called—have developed
wise and *multiple-use* plans, keeping in mind exploiters' interests
(for they have their needs, too) as well as the desires of the back-
packers. Thus mining, timbering, and ranching activities take
place in the national forests, where the Forest Service maintains a
system of logging roads eight times larger than the interstate highway system. The national parks are more of a public playground
and are becoming increasingly Europeanized in their look and
management. Lots of concessions and motels. You deserve a clean
bed and a hot meal when you go into the wilderness. At least your
stewards think that you do. You keep your stewards busy. Not
only must they cater to your multiple and conflicting desires, they
have to manage your wildlife *resources.* They have managed wild-
fowl to such an extent that the reasoning has become, If it weren't
for hunters, ducks would disappear. Duck stamps and licensing
fees support the whole rickety duck-management system. Yes! If
it weren't for the people who killed them, wild ducks wouldn't
exist! Managers are managing all wild creatures, not just those
that fly. They track and tape and tag and band. They relocate,
restock, and reintroduce. They cull and control. It's hard to keep
it all straight. Protect or poison? Extirpate or just mostly eliminate? Sometimes even the stewards get mixed up.

This is the time of machines and models, hands-on management 11
and master plans. Don't you ever wonder as you pass that bill-
board advertising another MASTER-PLANNED COMMUNITY just
what master they are actually talking about? Not the Big Master,
certainly. Something brought to you by one of the tiny masters,
of which there are many. But you like these tiny masters and have
even come to expect and require them. In Florida they've just
started a ten-thousand-acre city in the Everglades. It's a *megaproject,*
one of the largest ever in the state. Yes, they must have thought
you wanted it. No, what you thought of as the Everglades, the
Park, is only a little bitty part of the Everglades. Developers have

been gnawing at this irreplaceable, strange land for years. It's like they just *hate* this ancient sea of grass. Maybe you could ask them about this sometime. Roy Rogers is the senior vice president of strategic planning, and the old cowboy says that every tree and bush and inch of sidewalk in the project has been planned. Nevertheless, because the whole thing will take twenty-five years to complete, the plan is going to be constantly changed. You can understand this. The important thing is that there be a blueprint. You trust a blueprint. The tiny masters know what you like. You like *a secure landscape* and *access to services.* You like grass—that is, lawns. The ultimate lawn is the golf course, which you've been told has "some ecological value." You believe this! Not that it really matters, you just like to play golf. These golf courses require a lot of watering. So much that the more inspired of the masters have taken to watering them with effluent, *treated* effluent, but yours, from all the condos and villas built around the stocked artificial lakes you fancy.

12   I really don't want to think about sewage, you say, but it sounds like progress.

13   It is true that the masters are struggling with the problems of your incessant flushing. Cuisine is also one of their concerns. Advances in sorbets—sorbet intermezzos—in their clubs and fine restaurants. They know what you want. You want A HAVEN FROM THE ORDINARY WORLD. If you're A NATURE LOVER in the West you want to live in a $200,000 home in A WILD ANIMAL HABITAT. If you're eastern and consider yourself more hip, you want to live in new towns—brand-new reconstructed-from-scratch towns—in a house of NINETEENTH-CENTURY DESIGN. But in these new towns the masters are building, getting around can be confusing. There is an abundance of curves and an infrequency of through streets. It's the new wilderness without any trees. You can get lost, even with all the "mental bread crumbs" the masters scatter about as visual landmarks—the windmill, the water views, the various groupings of landscape "material." You *are* lost, you know. But you trust a Realtor will show you the way. There are many more Realtors than tiny masters, and many of them have to make do with less than a loaf—that is, trying to sell stuff that's already been built in an environment already "enhanced" rather than something being planned—but they're everywhere, willing to

show you the path. If Dante returned to Hell today, he'd probably be escorted down by a Realtor, talking all the while about how
it was just another level of Paradise.

When have you last watched a sunset? Do you remember where you 14
were? With whom? At Loews Ventana Canyon Resort, the Grand Foyer
will provide you with that opportunity through lighting which is com-
puterized to diminish with the approaching sunset!

The tiny masters are willing to arrange Nature for you. They will 15
compose it into a picture that you can look at, at your leisure,
when you're not doing work or something like that. Nature
becomes scenery, a prop. At some golf courses in the Southwest,
the saguaro cacti are reported to be repaired with green paste
when balls blast into their skin. The saguaro can attempt to heal
themselves by growing over the balls, but this takes time, and the
effect can be somewhat . . . baroque. It's better to get out the
pastepot. Nature has become simply a visual form of entertainment,
and it had better look snappy.

Listen, you say, we've been at Ventana Canyon. It's in the 16
desert, right? It's very, very nice, a world-class resort. A totally
self-contained environment with everything that a person could
possibly want, on more than a thousand acres in the middle of
zip. It sprawls but nestles, like. And they've maintained the
integrity of as much of the desert ecosystem as possible. Give
them credit for that. *Great* restaurant, too. We had baby bay scal-
lops there. Coming into the lobby there are these two big hand-
carved coyotes, mutely howling. And that's the way we like them,
mute. God, why do those things howl like that?

Wildlife is a personal matter, you think. The attitude is up to you. 17
You can prefer to see it dead or not dead. You might want to let
it mosey about its business or blow it away. Wild things exist only
if you have the graciousness to allow them to. Just outside Tucson, Arizona, there is a brand-new structure modeled after a
French foreign legion outpost. It's the *International Wildlife
Museum,* and it's full of dead animals. Three hundred species are
there, at least a third of them—the rarest ones—killed and collected by one C. J. McElroy, who enjoyed doing it and now shares

what's left with you. The museum claims to be educational because you can watch a taxidermist at work or touch a lion's tooth. You can get real close to these dead animals, closer than you can in a zoo. Some of you prefer zoos, however, which are becoming bigger, better, and bioclimatic. New-age zoo designers want the animals to *flow right out into your space.* In Dallas there will soon be a Wilds of Africa exhibit; in San Diego there's a simulated rain forest, where you can thread your way "down the side of a lush canyon, the air filled with a fine mist from 300 high-pressure nozzles"; in New Orleans you've constructed a swamp, the real swamp not far away on the verge of disappearing. Animals in these places are abstractions—wandering relics of their true selves, but that doesn't matter. Animal behavior in a zoo is nothing like natural behavior, but that doesn't really matter, either. Zoos are pretty, contained, and accessible. These new habitats can contain one hundred different species—not more than one or two of each thing, of course—on seven acres, three, one. You don't want to see *too much* of anything, certainly. An *example* will suffice. Sort of like a biological Crabtree & Evelyn basket selected with *you* in mind. You like things reduced, simplified. It's easier to take it all in, park it in your mind. You like things inside better than outside anyway. You are increasingly looking at and living in proxy environments created by substitution and simulation. *Resource economists* are a wee branch in the tree of tiny masters, and one, Martin Krieger, wrote, "Artificial prairies and wildernesses have been created, and there is no reason to believe that these artificial environments need be unsatisfactory for those who experience them. . . . We will have to realize that the way in which we experience nature is conditioned by our society—which more and more is seen to be receptive to responsible intervention."

18   Nature has become a world of appearances, a mere source of materials. You've been editing it for quite some time; now you're in the process of deleting it. Earth is beginning to look like not much more than a launching pad. Back near Tucson, on the opposite side of the mountain from the dead-animal habitat, you're building Biosphere II (as compared with or opposed to Biosphere I, more commonly known as Earth)—a 2½-acre terrarium, an artificial ecosystem that will include a rain forest, a desert, a thirty-five-foot ocean, and several thousand species of life (lots of microbes),

including eight human beings, who will cultivate a bit of farm-
land. You think it would be nice to colonize other worlds after
you've made it necessary to leave this one.

Hey, that's pretty good, you say, all that stuff packed into just   19
2½ acres. That's only about three times bigger than my entire
house.

It's small all right, but still not small enough to be, apparently,   20
useful. For the purposes of NASA, say, it would have to be
smaller, oh much smaller, and energy-efficient too. Fiddle, fiddle,
fiddle. You support fiddling, as well as meddling. This is how you
learn. Though it's quite apparent the environment has been
grossly polluted and the natural world abused and defiled, you
seem to prefer to continue pondering effects rather than preventing causes. You want proof, you insist on proof. A Dr. Lave from
Carnegie-Mellon—and he's an expert, an economist, and an environmental *expert*—says that scientists will have to prove to you
that you will suffer if you don't become less of a "throw-away
society." *If you really want me to give up my car or my air conditioner,
you'd better prove to me first that the earth would otherwise be uninhabitable,* Dr. Lave says. *Me is you,* I presume, whereas *you* refers
to them. You as in me—that is, *me, me, me*—certainly strike a hard
bargain. Uninhabitable the world has to get before you rein in
your requirements. You're a consumer after all, *the* consumer
upon whom so much attention is lavished, the ultimate user of a
commodity that has become, these days, everything. To try to
appease your appetite for proof, for example, scientists have been
leasing for experimentation forty-six pristine lakes in Canada.

They don't want to *keep* them, they just want to *borrow* them.   21

They've been intentionally contaminating many of the lakes   22
with a variety of pollutants dribbled into the propeller wash of
research boats. It's *one of the boldest experiments in lake ecology ever
conducted.* They've turned these remote lakes into huge *real-world
test tubes.* They've been doing this since 1976! And what they've
found so far in these *preliminary* studies is that pollutants are
really destructive. The lakes get gross. Life in them ceases. It took
about eight years to make this happen in one of them, everything
carefully measured and controlled all the while. Now the scientists are slowly reversing the process. But it will take hundreds of
years for the lakes to recover. They think.

23   Remember when you used to like rain, the sound of it, the feel of it, the way it made the plants and trees all glisten. We needed that rain, you would say. It looked pretty too, you thought, particularly in the movies. Now it rains and you go, Oh-oh. A nice walloping rain these days means *overtaxing our sewage treatment plants*. It means *untreated waste discharged directly into our waterways*. It means . . .

24   Okay. Okay.

25   *Acid rain!* And we all know what this is. Or most of us do. People of power in government and industry still don't seem to know what it is. Whatever it is, they say, they don't want to curb it, but they're willing to study it some more. Economists call air and water pollution "externalities" anyway. Oh, acid rain. You do get so sick of hearing about it. The words have already become a white-noise kind of thing. But you think in terms of *mitigating* it maybe. As for *the greenhouse effect*, you think in terms of *countering* that. One way that's been discussed recently is the planting of new forests, not for the sake of the forests alone, oh my heavens, no. Not for the sake of majesty and mystery or of Thumper and Bambi, are you kidding me, but because, as every schoolchild knows, trees absorb carbon dioxide. They just soak it up and store it. They just love it. So this is the plan: you plant millions of acres of trees, and you can go on doing pretty much whatever you're doing—driving around, using staggering amounts of energy, keeping those power plants fired to the max. Isn't Nature remarkable? So willing to serve? You wouldn't think it had anything more to offer, but it seems it does. Of course these "forests" wouldn't exactly be forests. They would be more like trees. *Managed* trees. The Forest Service, which now manages our forests by cutting them down, might be called upon to evolve in their thinking and allow these trees to grow. They would probably be patented trees after a time. Fast-growing, uniform, genetically-created-to-be-toxin-eating *machines*. They would be *new-age* trees, because the problem with planting the old-fashioned variety to *combat* the greenhouse effect, which is caused by pollution, is that they're already dying from it. All along the crest of the Appalachians from Maine to Georgia, forests struggle to survive in a toxic soup of poisons. They can't *help* us if we've killed them, now can they?

All right, you say, wow, lighten up will you? Relax. Tell about 26 yourself.

Well, I say, I live in Florida . . .   27

Oh my God, you say. Florida! Florida is a joke! How do you 28 expect us to take you seriously if you still live there! Florida is crazy, it's pink concrete. It's paved, it's over. And a little girl just got eaten by an alligator down there. It came out of some swamp next to a subdivision and just carried her off. That set your Endangered Species Act back fifty years, you can bet.

I . . .   29

Listen, we don't want to hear any more about Florida. We 30 don't want to hear about Phoenix or Hilton Head or California's Central Valley. If our wetlands—our *vanishing* wetlands—are mentioned one more time, we'll scream. And the talk about condors and grizzlies and wolves is becoming too *de trop*. We had just managed to get whales out of our minds when those three showed up under the ice in Alaska. They even had *names*. Bone is the dead one, right? It's almost the twenty-first century! Those last condors are *pathetic*. Can't we just get this over with?

Aristotle said that all living beings are ensouled and striving 31 to participate in eternity.

Oh, I just bet he said that, you say. That doesn't sound like 32 Aristotle. He was a humanist. We're all humanists here. This is the age of humanism. And it has been for a long time.

You are driving with a stranger in the car, and it is the stranger 33 behind the wheel. In the back seat are your pals for many years now—DO WHAT YOU LIKE and his swilling sidekick, WHY NOT. A deer, or some emblematic animal, something from that myriad natural world you've come from that you treat with such indifference and scorn—steps from the dimming woods and tentatively upon the highway. The stranger does not decelerate or brake, not yet, maybe not at all. The feeling is that whatever it is *will get out of the way*. Oh, it's a fine car you've got, a fine machine, and oddly you don't mind the stranger driving it, because in a way, everything has gotten too complicated, way, way out of your control. You've given the wheel to the masters, the managers, the comptrollers. Something is wrong, *maybe*, you feel a little sick, *actually,* but the car is luxurious and fast and you're *moving,* which is the most important thing by far.

34   Why make a fuss when you're so comfortable? Don't make a fuss, make a baby. Go out and get something to eat, build something. Make *another* baby. Babies are cute. Babies show you have faith in the future. Although faith is perhaps too strong a word. They're everywhere these days, in all the crowds and traffic jams, there are the babies too. You don't seem to associate them with the problems of population increase. They're just babies! And you've come to believe in them again. They're a lot more tangible than the afterlife, which, of course, you haven't believed in in ages. At least not for yourself. The afterlife now belongs to plastics and poisons. Yes, plastics and poisons will have a far more extensive afterlife than you, that's known. A disposable diaper, for example, which is all plastic and wood pulp—you like them for all those babies, so easy to use and toss—will take around four centuries to degrade. Almost all plastics do, centuries and centuries. In the sea, many marine animals die from ingesting or being entangled in discarded plastic. In the dumps, plastic squats on more than 25 percent of dump space. But your heart is disposed toward plastic. Someone, no doubt the plastics industry, told you it was convenient. This same industry is now looking into recycling in an attempt to get the critics of their nefarious, multifarious products off their backs. That should make you feel better, because *recycling* has become an honorable word, no longer merely the hobby of Volvo owners. The fact is that people in plastics are born obscurants. Recycling (practically impossible) won't solve the plastic glut, only reduction of production will, and the plastics industry isn't looking into that, you can be sure. Waste is not just the stuff you throw away, of course, it's the stuff you use to excess. With the exception of *hazardous waste,* which you do worry about from time to time, it's even thought you have a declining sense of emergency about the problem. Builders are building bigger houses because you want bigger. You're trading up. Utility companies are beginning to worry about your constantly rising consumption. Utility companies! You haven't entered a new age at all but one of upscale nihilism, deluxe nihilism.

In the summer, particularly in *the industrial Northeast,* you did ₃₅ get a little excited. The filth cut into your fun time. Dead stuff floating around. Sludge and bloody vials. Hygienic devices— "appearing not quite so hygienic out of context—all coming in on the tide. The air smelled funny, too. You tolerate a great deal, but the summer of '88 was truly creepy. It was even thought for a moment that the environment would become a political issue. But it didn't. You didn't want it to be, preferring instead to continue in your politics of subsidizing and advancing avarice. The issues were the same as always—jobs, defense, the economy, maintaining and improving the standard of living in this greedy, selfish, expansionistic, industrialized society.

You're getting a little shrill here, you say.   ₃₆

You're pretty well off. You expect to be better off soon. You do. ₃₇ What does this mean? More software, more scampi, more square footage? You have created an ecological crisis. The earth is infinitely variable and alive, and you are killing it. It seems safer this way. But you are not safe. You want to find wholeness and happiness in a land increasingly damaged and betrayed, and you never will. More than material matters. You must change your ways.

What is this? *Sinners in the Hands of an Angry God?*   ₃₈

The ecological crisis cannot be resolved by politics. It cannot ₃₉ be solved by science or technology. It is a crisis caused by culture and character, and a deep change in personal consciousness is needed. Your fundamental attitudes toward the earth have become twisted. You have made only brutal contact with Nature, you cannot comprehend its grace. You must change. Have few desires and simple pleasures. Honor nonhuman life. Control yourself, become more authentic. Live lightly upon the earth and treat it with respect. Redefine the word *progress* and dismiss the managers and masters. Grow inwardly and with knowledge become truly wiser. Make connections. Think differently, behave differently. For this is essentially a moral issue we face and moral decisions must be made.

A *moral issue!* Okay, this discussion is now toast. A *moral* ₄₀ issue . . . And who's this *we* now? Who are *you* is what I'd like to know. You're not me, anyway. I admit, someone's to blame and something should be done. But I've got to go. It's getting late.

That's dusk out there. That is dusk, isn't it? It certainly doesn't look like any dawn I've ever seen. Well, take care.

The Clan of One-Breasted Women

Terry Tempest Williams

1 I belong to a Clan of One-Breasted Women. My mother, my grand-mothers, and six aunts have all had mastectomies. Seven are dead. The two who survive have just completed rounds of chemotherapy and radiation.

2   I've had my own problems: two biopsies for breast cancer and a small tumor between my ribs diagnosed as "a border-line malignancy."

3   This is my family history.

4   Most statistics tell us breast cancer is genetic, hereditary, with rising percentages attached to fatty diets, childlessness, or becoming pregnant after thirty. What they don't say is living in Utah may be the greatest hazard of all.

5   We are a Mormon family with roots in Utah since 1847. The word-of-wisdom, a religious doctrine of health, kept the women in my family aligned with good foods: no coffee, no tea, tobacco, or alcohol. For the most part, these women were finished having their babies by the time they were thirty. And only one faced breast cancer prior to 1960. Traditionally, as a group of people, Mormons have a low rate of cancer.

6   Is our family a cultural anomaly? The truth is we didn't think about it. Those who did, usually the men, simply said, "bad genes." The women's attitude was stoic. Cancer was part of life. On February 16, 1971, the eve before my mother's surgery, I accidentally picked up the telephone and overheard her ask my grandmother what she could expect.

7   "Diane, it is one of the most spiritual experiences you will ever encounter."

8   I quietly put down the receiver.

9   Two days later, my father took my three brothers and me to the hospital to visit her. She met us in the lobby in a wheelchair. No bandages were visible. I'll never forget her radiance, the way

she held herself in a purple veloer robe and how she gathered us around her.

"Children, I am fine. I want you to know I felt the arms of God around me." 10

We believed her. My father cried. Our mother, his wife, was thirty-eight years old. 11

Two years ago, after my mother's death from cancer, my father and I were having dinner together. He had just returned from St. George where his construction company was putting in natural gas lines for towns in southern Utah. He spoke of his love for the country: the sandstoned landscape, bare-boned and beautiful. He had just finished hiking the Kolob trail in Zion National Park. We got caught up in reminiscing, recalling with fondness our walk up Angel's Landing on his fiftieth birthday and the years our family had vacationed there. This was a remembered landscape where we had been raised. 12

Over dessert, I shared a recurring dream of mine. I told my father that for years, as long as I could remember, I saw this flash of light in the night in the desert. That this image had so permeated my being, I could not venture south without seeing it again, on the horizon, illuminating buttes and mesas. 13

"You did see it," he said. 14

"Saw what?" I asked, a bit tentative. 15

"The bomb. The cloud. We were driving home from Riverside, California. You were sitting on your mother's lap. She was pregnant. In fact, I remember the date, September 7, 1957. We had just gotten out of the Service. We were driving north, past Las Vegas. It was an hour or so before dawn, when this explosion went off. We not only heard it, but felt it. I thought the oil tanker in front of us had blown up. We pulled over and suddenly, rising from the desert floor, we saw it, clearly, this golden-stemmed cloud, the mushroom. The sky seemed to vibrate with an eerie pink glow. Within a few minutes, a light ash was raining on the car." 16

I stared at my father. This was new information to me. 17

"I thought you knew that," my father said. "It was a common occurrence in the fifties." 18

It was at this moment I realized the deceit I had been living under. Children growing up in the American Southwest, drinking 19

contaminated milk from contaminated cows, even from the contaminated breasts of their mother, my mother—members, years
later, of the Clan of One-Breasted Women.

20   It is a well-known story in the Desert West, "The Day We
Bombed Utah," or perhaps, "The Years We Bombed Utah."[1] Above
ground atomic testing in Nevada took place from January 27,
1951, through July 11, 1962. Not only were the winds blowing
north, covering "low use segments of the population" with fallout and leaving sheep dead in their tracks, but the climate was
right.[2] The United States of the 1950s was red, white, and blue.
The Korean War was raging. McCarthyism was rampant. Ike was
in and the Cold War was hot. If you were against nuclear testing,
you were for a communist regime.

21   Much has been written about this "American nuclear tragedy."
Public health was secondary to national security. The Atomic
Energy Commissioner, Thomas Murray said, "Gentlemen, we
must not let anything interfere with this series of tests, nothing."[3]

22   Again and again, the American public was told by its government, in spite of burns, blisters, and nausea, "It has been
found that the tests may be conducted with adequate assurance
of safety under conditions prevailing at the bombing reservations."[4] Assuaging public fears was simply a matter of public
relations. "Your best action," an Atomic Energy Commission
booklet read, "is not to be worried about fallout." A news
release typical of the times stated, "We find no basis for con-
cluding that harm to any individual has resulted from radioactive fallout."[5]

23   In August 30, 1979, during Jimmy Carter's presidency, a suit
was filed entitled "Irene Allen vs. the United States of America."
Mrs. Allen's was the first to be alphabetically listed with twenty-

[1]Fuller, John G., *The Day We Bombed Utah* (New York: New American Library,
1984). [This and subsequent notes in the selection are the author's.]
[2]Discussion on March 14, 1988, with Carole Gallagher, photographer and author,
Nuclear Towns: The Secret War in the American Southwest, published by Doubleday,
Spring, 1990.
[3]Szasz, Ferenc M., "Downwind from the Bomb," *Nevada Historical Society Quarterly,*
Fall, 1987 Vol. xxx, No. 3, p. 185.
[4]Fradkin, Philip L., *Fallout* (Tucson: University of Arizona Press, 1989), 98.
[5]Ibid., 109.

four test cases, representative of nearly 1200 plaintiffs seeking compensation from the United States government for cancers caused from nuclear testing in Nevada.

Irene Allen lived in Hurricane, Utah. She was the mother of five children and had been widowed twice. Her first husband with their two oldest boys had watched the tests from the roof of the local high school. He died of leukemia in 1956. Her second husband dies of pancreatic cancer in 1978.

In a town meeting conducted by Utah Senator Orrin Hatch, shortly before the suit was filed, Mrs. Allen said, "I am not blaming the government, I want you to know that, Senator Hatch. But I thought if my testimony could help in any way so this wouldn't happen again to any of the generations coming up after us . . . I am really happy to be here this day to bear testimony of this."[6]

God-fearing people. This is just one story in an anthology of thousands.

On May 10, 1984, Judge Bruce S. Jenkins handed down his opinion. Ten of the plaintiffs were awarded damages. It was the first time a federal court had determined that nuclear tests had been the cause of cancers. For the remaining fourteen test cases, the proof of causation was not sufficient. In spite of the split decision, it was considered a landmark ruling.[7] It was not to remain so for long.

In April 1987, the 10th Circuit Court of Appeals overturned Judge Jenkins' ruling on the basis that the United States was protected from suit by the legal doctrine of sovereign immunity, the centuries-old idea from England in the days of absolute monarchs.[8]

In January 1988, the Supreme Court refused to review the Appeals Court decision. To our court system, it does not matter whether the United States Government was irresponsible, whether it lied to its citizens, or even that citizens died from the fallout of

[6]Town meeting held by Senator Orrin Hatch in St. George, Utah, April 17, 1979, transcript, 26–28.
[7]Fradkin, Op. Cit., 228.
[8]U.S. vs. Allen, 816 Federal Reporter, 2d/1417 (10th Circuit Court 1987), cert. denied, 108 S. CT. 694 (1988).

nuclear testing. What matters is that our government is immune. "The King can do no wrong."

30 In Mormon culture, authority is respected, obedience is revered, and independent thinking is not. I was taught as a young girl not to "make waves" or "rock the boat."

31   "Just let it go—" my mother would say. "You know how you feel, that's what counts."

32   For many years, I did just that—listened, observed, and quietly formed my own opinions within a culture that rarely asked questions because they had all the answers. But one by one, I watched the women in my family die common, heroic deaths. We sat in waiting rooms hoping for good news, always receiving the bad. I cared for them, bathed their scarred bodies and kept their secrets. I watched beautiful women become bald as cytoxan, cisplatin and adriamycin were injected into their veins. I held their foreheads as they vomited green-black bile and I shot them with morphine when the pain became inhuman. In the end, I witnessed their last peaceful breaths, becoming a midwife to the rebirth of their souls. But the price of obedience became too high.

33   The fear and inability to question authority that ultimately killed rural communities in Utah during atmospheric testing of atomic weapons was the same fear I saw being held in my mother's body. Sheep. Dead sheep. The evidence is buried.

34   I cannot prove that my mother, Diane Dixon Tempest, or my grandmothers, Lettie Romney Dixon and Kathryn Blackett Tempest, along with my aunts contracted cancer from nuclear fallout in Utah. But I can't prove they didn't.

35   My father's memory was correct, the September blast we drove through in 1957 was part of Operation Plumbbob, one of the most intensive series of bomb tests to be initiated. The flash of light in the night in the desert I had always thought was a dream developed into a family nightmare. It took fourteen years, from 1957 to 1971, for cancer to show up in my mother—the same time, Howard L. Andrews, an authority in radioactive fallout at the National Institutes of Health, says radiation cancer requires to become evident.[9] The more I learn about what it means to be a "downwinder," the more questions I drown in.

[9]Fradkin, Op. cit. 116.

What I do know, however, is that as a Mormon woman of the fifth 36
generation of "Latter-day Saints," I must question everything, even
if it means losing my faith, even if it means becoming a member of
a border tribe among my own people. Tolerating blind obedience
in the name of patriotism or religion ultimately takes our lives.

When the Atomic Energy Commission described the country 37
north of the Nevada Test Site as "virtually uninhabited desert
terrain," my family members were some of the "virtual uninhab-
itants."

One night, I dreamed women from all over the world circling a 38
blazing fire in the desert. They spoke of change, of how they hold
the moon in their bellies and wax and wane with its phases. They
mocked at the presumption of even-tempered beings and made
promises that they would never fear the witch inside themselves.
The women danced wildly as sparks broke away from the flames
and entered the night sky as stars.

And they sang a song given to them by Shoshoni grand- 39
mothers:

> Ah ne nah, nah
> nin nah nah—
> Ah ne nah, nah
> nin nah nah—
> Nyaga mutzi
> oh ne nay—
> Nyaga mutzi
> oh ne nay—[10]

The women danced and drummed and sang for weeks, 40
preparing themselves for what was to come. They would reclaim
the desert for the sake of their children, for the sake of the land.

A few miles downwind from the fire circle, bombs were being 41
tested. Rabbits felt the tremors. Their soft leather pads on paws

---

[10]This song was sung by the Western Shoshone women as they crossed the line at
the Nevada Test Site on March 18, 1988, as part of their "Reclaim the Land" action.
The translation they gave was: "Consider the rabbits how gently they walk on the
earth. Consider the rabbits how gently they walk on the earth. We remember them.
We can walk gently also. We remember them. We can walk gently also."

and feet recognized the shaking sands, while the roots of mesquite and sage were smoldering. Rocks were hot from the inside out and dust devils hummed unnaturally. And each time there was another nuclear test, ravens watched the desert heave. Stretch marks appeared. The land was losing its muscle.

42   The women couldn't bear it any longer. They were mothers. They had suffered labor pains but always under the promise of birth. The red hot pains beneath the desert promised death only as each bomb became a stillborn. A contract had been broken between human beings and the land. A new contract was being drawn by the women who understood the fate of the earth as their own.

43   Under the cover of darkness, ten women slipped under the barbed-wire fence and entered the contaminated country. They were trespassing. They walked toward the town of Mercury in moonlight, taking their cues from coyote, kit fox, antelope squirrel, and quail. They moved quietly and deliberately through the maze of Joshua trees. When a hint of daylight appeared they rested, drinking tea and sharing their rations of food. The women closed their eyes. The time had come to protest with the heart, that to deny one's genealogy with the earth was to commit treason against one's soul.

44   At dawn, the women draped themselves in mylar, wrapping long streamers of silver plastic around their arms to blow in the breeze. They wore clear masks, that became the faces of humanity. And when they arrived on the edge of Mercury, they carried all the butterflies of a summer day in their wombs. They paused to allow their courage to settle.

45   The town which forbids pregnant women and children to enter because of radiation risks to their health was asleep. The women moved through the streets as winged messengers, twirling around each other in slow motion, peeking inside homes and watching the easy sleep of men and women. They were astonished by such stillness and periodically would utter a shrill note or low cry just to verify life.

46   The residents finally awoke to what appeared as strange apparitions. Some simply stared. Others called authorities, and in time, the women were apprehended by wary soldiers dressed in desert fatigues. They were taken to a white, square building on

the other edge of Mercury. When asked who they were and why they were there, the women replied, "We are mothers and we have come to reclaim the desert for our children."

The soldiers arrested them. As the ten women were blind- 47 folded and handcuffed, they began singing.

> You can't forbid us everything
> You can't forbid us to think—
> You can't forbid our tears to flow
> And you can't stop the songs that we sing.

The women continued to sing louder and louder, until they 48 heard the voices of their sisters moving across the mesa.

> Ah ne nah, nah
> nin nah nah—
> Ah ne nah, nah
> nin nah nah—
> Nyaga mutzi
> oh ne nay—
> Nyaga mutzi
> oh ne nay—

"Call for re-enforcement," one soldier said. 49

"We have," interrupted one woman. "We have—and you have 50 no idea of our numbers."

On March 18, 1988, I crossed the line at the Nevada Test Site and 51 was arrested with nine other Utahns for trespassing on military lands. They are still conducting nuclear tests in the desert. Ours was an act of civil disobedience. But as I walked toward the town of Mercury, it was more than a gesture of peace. It was a gesture on behalf of the Clan of One-Breasted Women.

As one officer cinched the handcuffs around my wrists, 52 another frisked my body. She found a pen and a pad of paper tucked inside my left boot.

"And these?" she asked sternly. 53

"Weapons," I replied. 54

Our eyes met. I smiled. She pulled the leg of my trousers back 55 over my boot.

56   "Step forward, please," she said as she took my arm.

57   We were booked under an afternoon sun and bussed to Tonopah, Nevada. It was a two-hour ride. This was familiar country to me. The Joshua trees standing their ground had been named by my ancestors who believed they looked like prophets pointing west to the Promised Land. These were the same trees that bloomed each spring, flowers appearing like white flames in the Mojave. And I recalled a full moon in May when my Mother and I had walked among them, flushing out mourning doves and owls.

58   The bus stopped short of town. We were released. The officials thought it was a cruel joke to leave us stranded in the desert with no way to get home. What they didn't realize is that we were home, soul-centered and strong, women who recognized the sweet smell of sage as fuel for our spirits.

Chapter 11

Technology: Do We Control Machines or Do They Control Us?

The Tyranny of the Clock

George Woodcock

In no characteristic is existing society in the West so sharply dis-   1
tinguished from the earlier societies, whether of Europe or the
East, than in its conception of time. To the ancient Chinese or
Greek, to the Arab herdsman or Mexican peon of today, time is represented in the cyclic processes of nature, the alternation of day
and night, the passage from season to season. The nomads and
farmers measured and still measure their day from sunrise to sunset, and their year in terms of the seedtime and harvest, of the
falling leaf and the ice thawing on the lakes and rivers. The farmer
worked according to the elements, the craftsman for so long as he
felt it necessary to perfect his product. Time was seen in a process
of natural change, and men were not concerned in its exact mea-
surement. For this reason civilisations highly developed in other
respects had the most primitive means of measuring time, the
hour glass with it's trickling sand or dripping water, the sundial,
useless on a dull day, and the candle or lamp whose unburnt remnant of oil or wax indicated the hours. All these devices were
approximate and inexact, and were often rendered unreliable by
the weather or the personal laziness of the tender. Nowhere in the
ancient or medieval world were more than a tiny minority of men
concerned with time in the terms of mathematical exactitude.

485

2   Modern, Western man, however, lives in a world which runs according to the mechanical and mathematical symbols of clock time. The clock dictates his movements and inhibits his actions. The clock turns time from a process of nature into a commodity that can be measured and bought and sold like soap or sultanas. And because, without some means of exact time keeping, industrial capitalism could never have developed and could not continue to exploit the workers, the clock represents an element of mechanical tyranny in the lives of modern men more potent than any individual exploiter or any other machine. It is valuable to trace the historical process by which the clock influenced the social development of modern European civilisation.

3   It is a frequent circumstance of history that a culture or civilisation develops the device which will later be used for its destruction. The ancient Chinese, for example, invented gunpowder, which was developed by the military experts of the West and eventually led to the Chinese civilisation itself being destroyed by the high explosives of modern warfare. Similarly, the supreme achievement of the ingenuity of the craftsmen in the medieval cities of Europe was the invention of the mechanical clock, which, with its revolutionary alteration of the concept of time, materially assisted the growth of exploiting capitalism and the destruction of medieval culture.

4   There is a tradition that the clock appeared in the eleventh century, as a device for ringing bells at regular intervals in the monasteries which, with the regimented life they imposed on their inmates, were the closest social approximation in the middle ages to the factory of today. The first authenticated clock, however, appeared in the thirteenth century, and it was not until the fourteenth century that clocks became common ornaments of the public buildings in the German cities.

5   These early clocks, operated by weights, were not particularly accurate, and it was not until the sixteenth century that any great reliability was obtained. In England, for instance, the clock at Hampton Court, made in 1540, is said to have been the first accurate clock in the country. And even the accuracy of the sixteenth century clocks are relative, for they were only equipped with hour hands. The idea of measuring time in minutes and seconds had been thought out by the early mathematicians as

far back as the fourteenth century, but it was not until the invention of the pendulum in 1657 that sufficient accuracy was attained to permit the addition of a minute hand, and the second hand did not appear until the eighteenth century. These two centuries, it should be observed, were those in which capitalism grew to such an extent that it was able to take advantage of the industrial revolution in technique in order to establish its domination over society.

The clock, as Lewis Mumford has pointed out, represents the 6 key machine of the machine age, both for its influence on technology and its influence on the habits of men. Technically, the clock was the first really automatic machine that attained any importance in the life of men. Previous to its invention, the common machines were of such a nature that their operation depended on some external and unreliable force, such as human or animal muscles, water or wind. It is true that the Greeks had invented a number of primitive automatic machines, but these where used, like Hero's steam engine, for obtaining "supernatural" effects in the temples or for amusing the tyrants of Levantine cities. But the clock was the first automatic machine that attained a public importance and a social function. Clock-making became the industry from which men learnt the elements of machine making and gained the technical skill that was to produce the complicated machinery of the industrial revolution.

Socially the clock had a more radical influence than any other 7 machine, in that it was the means by which the regularisation and regimentation of life necessary for an exploiting system of industry could best be attained. The clock provided the means by which time—a category so elusive that no philosophy has yet determined its nature—could be measured concretely in more tangible forms of space provided by the circumference of a clock dial. Time as duration became disregarded, and men began to talk and think always of "lengths" of time, just as if they were talking of lengths of calico. And time, being now measurable in mathematical symbols, became regarded as a commodity that could be bought and sold in the same way as any other commodity.

The new capitalists, in particular, became rabidly time- 8 conscious. Time, here symbolising the labour of workers, was regarded by them almost as if it were the chief raw material of industry. "Time is money" became one of the key slogans of capitalist ideology, and the timekeeper was the most significant of the new types of official introduced by the capitalist dispensation.

9   In the early factories the employers went so far as to manipulate their clocks or sound their factory whistles at the wrong times in order to defraud their workers a little of this valuable new commodity. Later such practices became less frequent, but the influence of the clock imposed a regularity on the lives of the majority of men which had previously been known only in the monastery. Men actually became like clocks, acting with a repetitive regularity which had no resemblance to the rhythmic life of a natural being. They became, as the Victorian phrase put it, "as regular as clockwork". Only in the country districts where the natural lives of animals and plants and the elements still dominated life, did any large proportion of the population fail to succumb to the deadly tick of monotony.

10   At first this new attitude to time, this new regularity of life, was imposed by the clock-owning masters on the unwilling poor. The factory slave reacted in his spare time by living with a chaotic irregularity which characterised the gin-sodden slums of early nineteenth century industrialism. Men fled to the timeless world of drink or Methodist inspiration. But gradually the idea of regularity spread downwards among the workers. Nineteenth century religion and morality played their part by proclaiming the sin of "wasting time". The introduction of mass-produced watches and clocks in the 1850s spread time-consciousness among those who had previously merely reacted to the stimulus of the knocker-up or the factory whistle. In the church and in the school, in the office and the workshop, punctuality was held up as the greatest of the virtues.

11   Out of this slavish dependence on mechanical time which spread insidiously into every class in the nineteenth century there grew up the demoralising regimentation of life which characterises factory work today. The man who fails to conform faces social disapproval and economic ruin. If he is late at the factory the worker will lose his job or even, at the present day [1944—while wartime regulations were in force], find himself in prison. Hurried meals, the regular morning and evening scramble for trains or buses,

the strain of having to work to time schedules, all contribute to digestive and nervous disorders, to ruin health and shorten life.

Nor does the financial imposition of regularity tend, in the long run, to greater efficiency. Indeed, the quality of the product is usually much poorer, because the employer, regarding time as a commodity which he has to pay for, forces the operative to maintain such a speed that his work must necessarily be skimped. Quantity rather than quality becomes the criterion, the enjoyment is taken out of work itself, and the worker in his turn becomes a "clock-watcher", concerned only when he will be able to escape to the scanty and monotonous leisure of industrial society, in which he "kills time" by cramming in as much time-scheduled and mechanised enjoyment of cinema, radio and newspapers as his wage packet and his tiredness allow. Only if he is willing to accept of the hazards of living by his faith or his wits can the man without money avoid living as a slave to the clock.

The problem of the clock is, in general, similar to that of the machine. Mechanical time is valuable as a means of co-ordination of activities in a highly developed society, just as the machine is valuable as a means of reducing unnecessary labour to the minimum. Both are valuable for the contribution they make to the smooth running of society, and should be used insofar as they assist men to co-operate efficiently and to eliminate monotonous toil and social confusion. But neither should be allowed to dominate men's lives as they do today.

Now the movement of the clock sets the tempo of men's lives—they become the servant of the concept of time which they themselves have made, and are held in fear, like Frankenstein by his own monster. In a sane and free society such an arbitrary domination of man's functions by either clock or machine would obviously be out of the question. The domination of man by the creation of man is even more ridiculous than the domination of man by man. Mechanical time would be relegated to its true function of a means of reference and co-ordination, and men would return again to a balanced view of life no longer dominated by the worship of the clock. Complete liberty implies freedom from the tyranny of abstractions as well as from the rule of men.

The Virtual Community

Howard Rheingold

1   In the summer of 1986, my then-two-year-old daughter picked up a tick. There was this blood-bloated *thing* sucking on our baby's scalp, and we weren't quite sure how to go about getting it off. My wife, Judy, called the pediatrician. It was eleven o'clock in the evening. I logged onto the WELL. I got my answer online within minutes from a fellow with the improbable but genuine name of Flash Gordon, M.D. I had removed the tick by the time Judy got the callback from the pediatrician's office.

2   What amazed me wasn't just the speed with which we obtained precisely the information we needed to know, right when we needed to know it. It was also the immense inner sense of security that comes with discovering that real people—most of them parents, some of them nurses, doctors, and midwives—are available, around the clock, if you need them. There is a magic protective circle around the atmosphere of this particular conference. We're talking about our sons and daughters in this forum, not about our computers or our opinions about philosophy, and many of us feel that this tacit understanding sanctifies the virtual space.

3   The atmosphere of the Parenting conference—the attitudes people exhibit to each other in the tone of what they say in public—is part of what continues to attract me. People who never have much to contribute in political debate, technical argument, or intellectual gamesmanship turn out to have a lot to say about raising children. People you knew as fierce, even nasty, intellectual opponents in other contexts give you emotional support on a deeper level, parent to parent, within the boundaries of Parenting, a small but warmly human corner of cyberspace.

4   Here is a short list of examples from the hundreds of separate topics available for discussion in the Parenting conference. Each of these entries is the name of a conversation that includes scores or hundreds of individual contributions spread over a period of days or years, like a long, topical cocktail party you can rewind back to the beginning to find out who said what before you got there.

Great Expectations: You're Pregnant: Now What? Part III
What's Bad About Children's TV?

Movies: The Good, the Bad, and the Ugly

Initiations and Rites of Passage

Brand New Well Baby!!

How Does Being a Parent Change Your Life?

Tall Teenage Tales (cont.)

Guilt

MOTHERS

Vasectomy—Did It Hurt?

Introductions! Who Are We?

Fathers (Continued)

Books for Kids, Section Two

Gay and Lesbian Teenagers

Children and Spirituality

Great Parks for Kids

Quality Toys

Parenting in an Often-Violent World

Children's Radio Programming

New WELL Baby

Home Schooling

Newly Separated/Divorced Fathers

Another Well Baby—Carson Arrives in Seattle!

Single Parenting

Uncle Philcat's Back Fence: Gossip Here!

Embarrassing Moments

Kids and Death

All the Poop on Diapers

Pediatric Problems—Little Sicknesses and Sick Little Ones

Talking with Kids About the Prospect of War

Dealing with Incest and Abuse

Other People's Children

When They're Crying

Pets for Kids

5   People who talk about a shared interest, albeit a deep one such as being a parent, don't often disclose enough about themselves as whole individuals online to inspire real trust in others. In the case of the subcommunity of the Parenting conference, a few dozen of us, scattered across the country, few of whom rarely if ever saw the others face-to-face, had a few years of minor crises to knit us together and prepare us for serious business when it came our way. Another several dozen read the conference regularly but contribute only when they have something important to add. Hundreds more every week read the conference without comment, except when something extraordinary happens. . . .

6   Many people are alarmed by the very idea of a virtual community, fearing that is another step in the wrong direction, substituting more technological ersatz for yet another natural resource or human freedom. These critics often voice their sadness at what people have been reduced to doing in a civilization that worships technology, decrying the circumstances that lead some people into such pathetically disconnected lives that they prefer to find their companions on the other side of a computer screen. There is a seed of truth in this fear, for virtual communities require more than words on a screen at some point if they intend to be other than ersatz.

7   Some people—many people—don't do well in spontaneous spoken interaction, but turn out to have valuable contributions to make in a conversation in which they have time to think about what to say. These people, who might constitute a significant proportion of the population, can find written communication more authentic than the face-to-face kind. Who is to say that this preference for one mode of communication—informal written text—is somehow less authentically human than audible speech? Those who critique CMC because some people use it obsessively hit an important target, but miss a great deal more when they don't take into consideration people who use the medium for genuine human interaction. Those who find virtual communities cold places point at the limits of the technology, its most dangerous pitfalls, and we need to pay attention to those boundaries. But these critiques don't tell us how Philcat and Lhary and the Allisons and my own family could have found the community of support and information we found in the WELL when we needed it. And those of us who do find communion in cyberspace

might do well to pay attention to the way the medium we love can be abused. . . .

Because we cannot see one another in cyberspace, gender, age, 8 national origin, and physical appearance are not apparent unless a person wants to make such characteristics public. People whose physical handicaps make it difficult to form new friendships find that virtual communities treat them as they always wanted to be treated—as thinkers and transmitters of ideas and feeling beings, not carnal vessels with a certain appearance and way of walking and talking (or not walking and not talking).

One of the few things that enthusiastic members of virtual 9 communities in Japan, England, France, and the United States all agree on is that expanding their circle of friends is one of the most important advantages of computer conferencing. CMC is a way to *meet* people, whether or not you feel the need to affiliate with them on a community level. It's a way of both making contact with and maintaining a distance from others. The way you meet people in cyberspace puts a different spin on affiliation: in traditional kinds of communities, we are accustomed to meeting people, then getting to know them; in virtual communities, you can get to know people and then choose to meet them. Affiliation also can be far more ephemeral in cyberspace because you can get to know people you might never meet on the physical plane.

How does anybody find friends? In the traditional commu- 10 nity, we search through our pool of neighbors and professional colleagues, of acquaintances and acquaintances of acquaintances, in order to find people who share our values and interests. We then exchange information about one another, disclose and discuss our mutual interests, and sometimes we become friends. In a virtual community we can go directly to the place where our favorite subjects are being discussed, then get acquainted with people who share our passions or who use words in a way we find attractive. In this sense, the topic is the address: you can't simply pick up a phone and ask to be connected with someone who wants to talk about Islamic art or California wine, or someone with a three-year-old daughter or a forty-year-old Hudson; you can, however, join a computer conference on any of those topics, then open a public or private correspondence with the previously unknown people you find there. Your chances of making friends are magnified by orders of magnitude over the old methods of finding a peer group.

11   You can be fooled about people in cyberspace, behind the cloak of words. But that can be said about telephones or face-to-face communication as well; computer-mediated communications provide new ways to fool people, and the most obvious identity swindles will die out only when enough people learn to use the medium critically. In some ways, the medium will, by its nature, be forever biased toward certain kinds of obfuscation. It will also be a place that people often end up revealing themselves far more intimately than they would be inclined to do without the intermediation of screens and pseudonyms. . . .

12   Three different kinds of social criticisms of technology are relevant to claims of CMC as a means of enhancing democracy. One school of criticism emerges from the longer-term history of communications media, and focuses on the way electronic communications media already have preempted public discussions by turning more and more of the content of the media into advertisements for various commodities—a process these critics call commodification. Even the political process, according to this school of critics, has been turned into a commodity. The formal name for this criticism is "the commodification of the public sphere." The public sphere is what these social critics claim we used to have as citizens of a democracy, but have lost to the tide of commodization. The public sphere is also the focus of the hopes of online activists, who see CMC as a way of revitalizing the open and widespread discussions among citizens that feed the roots of democratic societies.

13   The second school of criticism focuses on the fact that high-bandwidth interactive networks could be used in conjunction with other technologies as a means of surveillance, control, and disinformation as well as a conduit for useful information. This direct assault on personal liberty is compounded by a more diffuse erosion of old social values due to the capabilities of new technologies; the most problematic example is the way traditional notions of privacy are challenged on several fronts by the ease of collecting and disseminating detailed information about individuals via cyberspace technologies. When people use the convenience of electronic communication or transaction, we leave invisible digital trails; now that technologies for tracking those

trails are maturing, there is cause to worry. The spreading use of computer matching to piece together the digital trails we all leave in cyberspace is one indication of privacy problems to come.

Along with all the person-to-person communications exchanged 14 on the world's telecommunications networks are vast flows of other kinds of personal information—credit information, transaction processing, health information. Most people take it for granted that no one can search through all the electronic transactions that move through the world's networks in order to pin down an individual for marketing—or political—motives. Remember the "knowbots" that would act as personal servants, swimming in the info-tides, fishing for information to suit your interests? What if people could turn loose knowbots to collect all the information digitally linked to *you*? What if the Net and cheap, powerful computers give that power not only to governments and large corporations but to everyone?

Every time we travel or shop or communicate, citizens of the 15 credit-card society contribute to streams of information that travel between point of purchase, remote credit bureaus, municipal and federal information systems, crime information databases, central transaction databases. And all these other forms of cyberspace interaction take place via the same packet-switched, high-bandwidth network technology—those packets can contain transactions as well as video clips and text files. When these streams of information begin to connect together, the unscrupulous or would-be tyrants can use the Net to catch citizens in a more ominous kind of net.

The same channels of communication that enable citizens 16 around the world to communicate with one another also allow government and private interests to gather information about them. This school of criticism is known as Panoptic in reference to the perfect prison proposed in the eighteenth century by Jeremy Bentham—a theoretical model that happens to fit the real capabilities of today's technologies.

Another category of critical claim deserves mention, despite the 17 rather bizarre and incredible imagery used by its most well known spokesmen—the hyper-realist school. These critics believe that information technologies have already changed what used to pass for reality into a slicked-up electronic simulation. Twenty years before the United States elected a Hollywood actor as president, the first hyper-realists pointed out how politics had become a movie, a spectacle that raised the old Roman tactic of bread and circuses to the level of mass hypnotism. We live in a hyper-reality that was carefully constructed to mimic the real world and extract money from the pockets of consumers: the forests around the Matterhorn might be dying, but the Disneyland version continues to rake in the dollars. The television programs, movie stars, and theme parks work together to create global industry devoted to maintaining a web of illusion that grows more lifelike as more people buy into it and as technologies grow more powerful.

18   Many other social scientists have intellectual suspicions of the hyper-realist critiques, because so many are abstract and theoretical, based on little or no direct knowledge of technology itself. Nevertheless, this perspective does capture something about the way the effects of communications technologies have changed our modes of thought. One good reason for paying attention to the claims of the hyper-realists is that the society they predicted decades ago bears a disturbingly closer resemblance to real life than do the forecasts of the rosier-visioned technological utopians. While McLuhan's image of the global village has taken on a certain irony in light of what has happened since his predictions of the 1960s, "the society of the spectacle"—another prediction from the 1960s, based on the advent of electronic media—offered a far less rosy and, as events have proved, more realistic portrayal of the way information technologies have changed social customs. . . .

19   What should those of us who believe in the democratizing potential of virtual communities do about the technological critics? I believe we should invite them to the table and help them see the flaws in our dreams, the bugs in our designs. I believe we should study what the historians and social scientists have to say about the illusions and power shifts that accompanied the diffusion of previous technologies. CMC and technology in general have real limits; it's best to continue to listen to those who understand the limits, even as we continue to explore the technologies' positive capabilities. Failing to fall under the spell of the "rhetoric of the technological sublime," actively questioning and examining social assumptions about the effects of new technologies, reminding ourselves that electronic communication has powerful illusory capabilities, are all good steps to take to prevent disasters.

If electronic democracy is to succeed, however, in the face of 20
all the obstacles, activists must do more than avoid mistakes. Those
who would use computer networks as political tools must go forward and actively apply their theories to more and different kinds
of communities. If there is a last good hope, a bulwark against the
hyper-reality of Baudrillard or Forster, it will come from a new way
of looking at technology. Instead of falling under the spell of a sales
pitch, or rejecting new technologies as instruments of illusion, we
need to look closely at new technologies and ask how they can help
build stronger, more humane communities—and ask how they
might be obstacles to that goal. The late 1990s may eventually be
seen in retrospect as a narrow window of historical opportunity,
when people either acted or failed to act effectively to regain control over communications technologies. Armed with knowledge,
guided by a clear, human-centered vision, governed by a commitment to civil discourse, we the citizens hold the key levers at a
pivotal time. What happens next is largely up to us.

Cyberspace and Identity

Sherry Turkle

We come to see ourselves differently as we catch sight of our 1
images in the mirror of the machine. Over a decade ago, when I
first called the computer a "second self" (1984), these identity-
transforming relationships were most usually one-on-one, a person alone with a machine. This is no longer the case. A rapidly
expanding system of networks, collectively known as the Internet,
links millions of people together in new spaces that are changing
the way we think, the nature of our sexuality, the form of our communities, our very identities. In cyberspace, we are learning to live
in virtual worlds. We may find ourselves alone as we navigate virtual oceans, unravel virtual mysteries, and engineer virtual sky-
scrapers. But increasingly, when we step through the looking
glass, other people are there as well.

Over the past decade, I have been engaged in the ethnographic 2
and clinical study of how people negotiate the virtual and the
"real" as they represent themselves on computer screens linked

through the Internet. For many people, such experiences challenge what they have traditionally called "identity," which they are moved to recast in terms of multiple windows and parallel lives. Online life is not the only factor that is pushing them in this direction; there is no simple sense in which computers are causing a shift in notions of identity. It is, rather, that today's life on the screen dramatizes and concretizes a range of cultural trends that encourage us to think of identity in terms of multiplicity and flexibility.

VIRTUAL PERSONAE

3   In this essay, I focus on one key element of online life and its impact on identity: the creation and projection of constructed personae into virtual space. In cyberspace, it is well known, one's body can be represented by one's own textual description: The obese can be slender, the beautiful plain. The fact that self-presentation is written in text means that there is time to reflect upon and edit one's "composition," which makes it easier for the shy to be outgoing, the "nerdy" sophisticated. The relative anonymity of life on the screen—one has the choice of being known only by one's chosen "handle" or online name—gives people the chance to express often unexplored aspects of the self. Additionally, multiple aspects of self can be explored in parallel. Online services offer their users the opportunity to be known by several different names. For example, it is not unusual for someone to be BroncoBill in one online community, ArmaniBoy in another, and MrSensitive in a third.

4   The online exercise of playing with identity and trying out new identities is perhaps most explicit in "role playing" virtual communities (such as Multi-User Domains, or MUDs) where participation literally begins with the creation of a persona (or several); but it is by no means confined to these somewhat exotic locations. In bulletin boards, newsgroups, and chat rooms, the creation of personae may be less explicit than on MUDs, but it is no less psychologically real. One IRC (Internet Relay Chat) participant describes her experience of online talk: "I go from channel to channel depending on my mood. . . . I actually feel a part of several of the channels, several conversations. . . . I'm different in the different chats. They bring out different things in me." Identity play can happen by changing names and by changing places.

For many people, joining online communities means crossing 5 a boundary into highly charged territory. Some feel an uncomfortable sense of fragmentation, some a sense of relief. Some sense the possibilities for self-discovery. A 26-year-old graduate student in history says, "When I log on to a new community and I create a character and know I have to start typing my description, I always feel a sense of panic. Like I could find out something I don't want to know." A woman in her late thirties who just got an account with America Online used the fact that she could create five "names" for herself on her account as a chance to "lay out all the moods I'm in—all the ways I want to be in different places on the system."

The creation of site-specific online personae depends not only 6 on adopting a new name. Shifting of personae happens with a change of virtual place. Cycling through virtual environments is made possible by the existence of what have come to be called "windows" in modern computing environments. Windows are a way to work with a computer that makes it possible for the machine to place you in several contexts at the same time. As a user, you are attentive to just one of windows on your screen at any given moment, but in a certain sense, you are a presence in all of them at all times. You might be writing a paper in bacteriology and using your computer in several ways to help you: You are "present" to a word processing program on which you are taking notes and collecting thoughts, you are "present" to communications software that is in touch with a distant computer for collecting reference materials, you are "present" to a simulation program that is charting the growth of bacterial colonies when a new organism enters their ecology, and you are "present" to an online chat session where participants are discussing recent research in the field. Each of these activities takes place in a "window," and your identity on the computer is the sum of your distributed presence.

The development of the windows metaphor for computer 7 interfaces was a technical innovation motivated by the desire to get people working more efficiently by "cycling through" different applications, much as time-sharing computers cycle through the computing needs of different people. But in practice, windows have become a potent metaphor for thinking about the self as a multiple, distributed, "time-sharing" system.

8   The self no longer simply plays different roles in different settings—something that people experience when, for example, one wakes up as a lover; makes breakfast as a mother; and drives to work as a lawyer. The windows metaphor suggests a distributed self that exists in many worlds and plays many roles at the same time. The "windows" enabled by a computer operating system support the metaphor, and cyberspace raises the experience to a higher power by translating the metaphor into a life experience of "cycling through."

IDENTITY, MORATORIA, AND PLAY

9   Cyberspace, like all complex phenomena, has a range of psychological effects. For some people, it is a place to "act out" unresolved conflicts, to play and replay characterological difficulties on a new and exotic stage. For others, it provides an opportunity to "work through" significant personal issues, to use the new materials of cybersociality to reach for new resolutions. These more positive identity effects follow from the fact that for some, cyberspace provides what Erik Erikson would have called a "psychosocial moratorium," a central element in how he thought about identity development in adolescence. Although the term moratorium implies a "time out," what Erikson had in mind was not withdrawal. On the contrary, the adolescent moratorium is a time of intense interaction with people and ideas. It is a time of passionate friendships and experimentation. The adolescent falls in and out of love with people and ideas. Erikson's notion of the moratorium was not a "hold" on significant experiences but on their consequences. It is a time during which one's actions are, in a certain sense, not counted as they will be later in life. They are not given as much weight, not given the force of full judgment. In this context, experimentation can become the norm rather than a brave departure. Relatively consequence-free experimentation facilitates the development of a "core self," a personal sense of what gives life meaning that Erikson called "identity."

10   Erikson developed these ideas about the importance of a moratorium during the late 1950s and early 1960s. At that time, the notion corresponded to a common understanding of what

"the college years" were about. Today, 30 years later, the idea
of the college years as a consequence-free "time out" seems of
another era. College is pre-professional, and AIDS has made
consequence-free sexual experimentation an impossibility. The
years associated with adolescence no longer seem a "time out."
But if our culture no longer offers an adolescent moratorium, virtual communities often do. It is part of what makes them seem so
attractive.

Erikson's ideas about stages did not suggest rigid sequences. 11
His stages describe what people need to achieve before they can
move ahead easily to another developmental task. For example, Erikson pointed out that successful intimacy in young
adulthood is difficult if one does not come to it with a sense
of who one is, the challenge of adolescent identity building. In
real life, however, people frequently move on with serious
deficits. With incompletely resolved "stages," they simply do
the best they can. They use whatever materials they have at
hand to get as much as they can of what they have missed.
Now virtual social life can play a role in these dramas of self-
reparation. Time in cyberspace reworks the notion of the
moratorium because it may now exist on an always-available
"window."

EXPANDING ONE'S RANGE IN THE REAL

Case, a 34-year-old industrial designer happily married to a 12
female co-worker, describes his real-life (RL) persona as a "nice
guy," a "Jimmy Stewart type like my father." He describes his
outgoing, assertive mother as a "Katharine Hepburn type." For
Case, who views assertiveness through the prism of this Jimmy
Stewart/Katharine Hepburn dichotomy, an assertive man is
quickly perceived as "being a bastard." An assertive woman, in
contrast, is perceived as being "modern and together." Case
says that although he is comfortable with his temperament and
loves and respects his father, he feels he pays a high price for
his own low-key ways. In particular, he feels at a loss when it
comes to confrontation, both at home and at work. Online, in a
wide range of virtual communities, Case presents himself as

females whom he calls his "Katharine Hepburn types." These are strong, dynamic, "out there" women who remind Case of his mother, who "says exactly what's on her mind." He tells me that presenting himself as a woman online has brought him to a point where he is more comfortable with confrontation in his RL as a man.

13   Case describes his Katharine Hepburn personae as "externalizations of a part of myself." In one interview with him, I used the expression "aspects of the self," and he picked it up eagerly, for his online life reminds him of how Hindu gods could have different aspects or subpersonalities, all the while being a whole self. In response to my question "Do you feel that you call upon your personae in real life?" Case responded:

> Yes, an aspect sort of clears its throat and says, "I can do this. You are being so amazingly conflicted over this and I know exactly what to do. Why don't you just let me do it?" . . . In real life, I tend to be extremely diplomatic, non-confrontational. I don't like to ram my ideas down anyone's throat. [Online] I can be, "Take it or leave it." All of my Hepburn characters are that way. That's probably why I play them. Because they are smart-mouthed, they will not sugarcoat their words.

In some ways, Case's description of his inner world of actors who address him and are able to take over negotiations is reminiscent of the language of people with multiple-personality disorder. But the contrast is significant: Case's inner actors are not split off from each other or from his sense of "himself." He experiences himself very much as a collective self, not feeling that he must goad or repress this or that aspect of himself into conformity. He is at ease, cycling through from Katharine Hepburn to Jimmy Stewart. To use analyst Philip Bromberg's language, online life has helped Case learn how to "stand in the spaces between selves and still feel one, to see the multiplicity and still feel a unity." To use computer scientist Marvin Minsky's phrase, Case feels at ease cycling through his "society of mind," a notion of identity as distributed and heterogeneous. Identity, from the Latin *idem*, has been used habitually to refer to the sameness between two qualities. On the Internet, however, one can be many, and one usually is.

AN OBJECT TO THINK WITH FOR THINKING ABOUT IDENTITY

In the late 1960s and early 1970s, I was first exposed to notions of   14
identity and multiplicity. These ideas—most notably that there is
no such thing as "the ego," that each of us is a multiplicity of
parts, fragments, and desiring connections—surfaced in the intellectual hothouse of Paris; they presented the world according to
such authors as Jacques Lacan, Gilles Deleuze, and Felix Guattari.
But despite such ideal conditions for absorbing theory, my
"French lessons" remained abstract exercises. These theorists of
poststructuralism spoke words that addressed the relationship
between mind and body, but from my point of view had little to
do with my own.

In my lack of personal connection with these ideas, I was not   15
alone. To take one example, for many people it is hard to accept
any challenge to the idea of an autonomous ego. While in recent
years, many psychologists, social theorists, psychoanalysts, and
philosophers have argued that the self should be thought of as
essentially decentered, the normal requirements of everyday life
exert strong pressure on people to take responsibility for their
actions and to see themselves as unitary actors. This disjuncture
between theory (the unitary self is an illusion) and lived experience (the unitary self is the most basic reality) is one of the main
reasons why multiple and decentered theories have been slow to
catch on—or when they do, why we tend to settle back quickly
into older, centralized ways of looking at things.

When, 20 years later, I used my personal computer and   16
modem to join online communities, I had an experience of this
theoretical perspective which brought it shockingly down to
earth. I used language to create several characters. My textual
actions are my actions—my words make things happen. I created
selves that were made and transformed by language. And different personae were exploring different aspects of the self. The
notion of a decentered identity was concretized by experiences on
a computer screen. In this way, cyberspace becomes an object to
think with for thinking about identity—an element of cultural
bricolage.

Appropriable theories—ideas that capture the imagination   17
of the culture at large—tend to be those with which people can

become actively involved. They tend to be theories that can be "played" with. So one way to think about the social appropriability of a given theory is to ask whether it is accompanied by its own objects-to-think-with that can help it move out beyond intellectual circles.

18   For example, the popular appropriation of Freudian ideas had little to do with scientific demonstrations of their validity. Freudian ideas passed into the popular culture because they offered robust and down-to-earth objects to think with. The objects were not physical but almost-tangible ideas, such as dreams and slips of the tongue. People were able to play with such Freudian "objects." They became used to looking for them and manipulating them, both seriously and not so seriously. And as they did so, the idea that slips and dreams betray an unconscious began to feel natural.

19   In Freud's work, dreams and slips of the tongue carried the theory. Today, life on the computer screen carries theory. People decide that they want to interact with others on a computer network. They get an account on a commercial service. They think that this will provide them with new access to people and information, and of course it does. But it does more. When they log on, they may find themselves playing multiple roles; they may find themselves playing characters of the opposite sex. In this way, they are swept up by experiences that enable them to explore previously unexamined aspects of their sexuality or that challenge their ideas about a unitary self. The instrumental computer, the computer that does things for us, has revealed another side: a subjective computer that does things *to* us as people, to our view of ourselves and our relationships, to our ways of looking at our minds. In simulation, identity can be fluid and multiple, a signifier no longer clearly points to a thing that is signified, and understanding is less likely to proceed through analysis than by navigation through virtual space.

20   Within the psychoanalytic tradition, many "schools" have departed from a unitary view of identity, among these the Jungian, object-relations, and Lacanian. In different ways, each of these groups of analysts was banished from the ranks of orthodox Freudians for such suggestions, or somehow relegated to the margins. As the United States became the center of psychoanalytic

politics in the mid-twentieth century, ideas about a robust executive ego began to constitute the psychoanalytic mainstream.

But today, the pendulum has swung away from that complacent view of a unitary self. Through the fragmented selves presented by patients and through theories that stress the decentered subject, contemporary social and psychological thinkers are confronting what has been left out of theories of the unitary self. It is asking such questions as, What is the self when it functions as a society? What is the self when it divides its labors among its constituent "alters"? Those burdened by posttraumatic dissociative disorders suffer these questions; I am suggesting that inhabitants of virtual communities play with them. In our lives on the screen, people are developing ideas about identity as multiplicity through new social *practices* of identity as multiplicity.

With these remarks, I am not implying that chat rooms or MUDs or the option to declare multiple user names on America Online are causally implicated in the dramatic increase of people who exhibit symptoms of multiple-personality disorder (MPD), or that people on MUDs have MPD, or that MUDding (or online chatting) is like having MPD. I am saying that the many manifestations of multiplicity in our culture, including the adoption of online personae, are contributing to a general reconsideration of traditional, unitary notions of identity. Online experiences with "parallel lives" are part of the significant cultural context that supports new theorizing about nonpathological, indeed healthy, multiple selves.

In thinking about the self, *multiplicity* is a term that carries with it several centuries of negative associations, but such authors as Kenneth Gergen, Emily Martin, and Robert Jay Lifton speak in positive terms of an adaptive, "flexible" self. The flexible self is not unitary, nor are its parts stable entities. A person cycles through its aspects, and these are themselves ever-changing and in constant communication with each other. Daniel Dennett speaks of the flexible self by using the metaphor of consciousness as multiple drafts, analogous to the experience of several versions of a document open on a computer screen, where the user is able to move between them at will. For Dennett, knowledge of these drafts encourages a respect for the many different versions, while it imposes a certain distance from them. Donna Haraway, picking up on this theme of how a distance between self states may be salutory, equates a "split and contradictory self" with a "knowing self." She is optimistic about its possibilities: "The knowing self is partial in all its guises, never finished, whole, simply there and original; it is always constricted and stitched together imperfectly; and therefore able to join with another, to see together without claiming to be another." What most characterizes Haraway's and Dennett's models of a knowing self is that the lines of communication between its various aspects are open. The open communication encourages an attitude of respect for the many within us and the many within others.

24   Increasingly, social theorists and philosophers are being joined by psychoanalytic theorists in efforts to think about healthy selves whose resilience and capacity for joy comes from having access to their many aspects. For example, Philip Bromberg insists that our ways of describing "good parenting" must now shift away from an emphasis on confirming a child in a "core self" and onto helping a child develop the capacity to negotiate fluid transitions between self states. The healthy individual knows how to be many but to smooth out the moments of transition between states of self. Bromberg says: "Health is when you are multiple but feel a unity. Health is when different aspects of self can get to know each other and reflect upon each other." Here, within the psychoanalytic tradition, is a model of multiplicity as a state of easy traffic across selves, a conscious, highly articulated "cycling through."

FROM A PSYCHOANALYTIC TO A COMPUTER CULTURE?

25 Having literally written our online personae into existence, they can be a kind of Rorschach test. We can use them to become more aware of what we project into everyday life. We can use the virtual to reflect constructively on the real. Cyberspace opens the possibility for identity play, but it is very serious play. People who cultivate an awareness of what stands behind their screen personae are the ones most likely to succeed in using virtual experience for personal and social transformation. And the people who

make the most of their lives on the screen are those who are able to approach it in a spirit of self-reflection. What does my behavior in cyberspace tell me about what I want, who I am, what I may not be getting in the rest of my life?

As a culture, we are at the end of the Freudian century. 26 Freud, after all, was a child of the nineteenth century; of course, he was carrying the baggage of a very different scientific sensibility than our own. But faced with the challenges of cyberspace, our need for a practical philosophy of self-knowledge, one that does not shy away from issues of multiplicity, complexity, and ambivalence, that does not shy away from the power of symbolism, from the power of the word, from the power of identity play, has never been greater as we struggle to make meaning from our lives on the screen. It is fashionable to think that we have passed from a psychoanalytic culture to a computer culture—that we no longer need to think in terms of Freudian slips but rather of information processing errors. But the reality is more complex. It is time to rethink our relationship to the computer culture and psychoanalytic culture as a proudly held joint citizenship.

REFERENCES

Bromberg, Philip. 1994. "Speak that I May See You: Some Reflections on Dissociation, Reality, and Psychoanalytic Listening." *Psychoanalytic Dialogues* 4 (4): 517–47.

Dennett, Daniel. 1991. *Consciousness Explained.* Boston: Little, Brown.

Erikson, Erik. [1950] 1963. *Childhood and Society.* 2nd Ed. New York: Norton.

Gergen, Kenneth. 1991. *The Saturated Self-Dilemmas of Identity in Contemporary Life.* New York: Basic Books.

Haraway, Donna. 1991. "The Actors are Cyborg, Nature is Coyote, and the Geography is Elsewhere: Postscript to 'Cyborgs at Large.'" In Constance Penley and Andrew Ross (Eds.), Technoculture. Minneapolis: University of Minnesota Press.

Lifton, Robert Jay. 1993. *The Protean Self: Human Resilience in an Age of Fragmentation.* New York: Basic Books.

Martin, Emily. 1994. *Flexible Bodies: Tracking Immunity in American Culture from the Days of Polio to the Days of AIDS.* Boston: Beacon Press.

Minsky, Martin. 1987. *The Society of Mind*. New York: Simon & Schuster.

Turkle, Sherry. [1978] 1990. *Psychoanalytic Politics: Jacques Lacan and Freud's French Revolution*. 2nd Ed. New York: Guilford Press.

———.1984. *The Second Self: Computers and the Human Spirit*. New York: Simon & Schuster.

———.1995. *Life on the Screen: Identity in the Age of the Internet*. New York: Simon & Schuster.

Cyberspace: If You Don't Love It, Leave It

Esther Dyson

1 Something in the American psyche loves new frontiers. We hanker after wide-open spaces; we like to explore; we like to make rules instead of follow them. But in this age of political correctness and other intrusions on our national cult of independence, it's hard to find a place where you can go and be yourself without worrying about the neighbors.

2 There is such a place: cyberspace. Lost in the furor over porn on the Net is the exhilarating sense of freedom that this new frontier once promised—and still does in some quarters. Formerly a playground for computer nerds and techies, cyberspace now embraces every conceivable constituency: schoolchildren, flirtatious singles, Hungarian-Americans, accountants—along with pederasts and porn fans. Can they all get along? Or will our fear of kids surfing for cyberporn behind their bedroom doors provoke a crackdown?

3 The first order of business is to grasp what cyberspace *is*. It might help to leave behind metaphors of highways and frontiers and to think instead of real estate. Real estate, remember, is an intellectual, legal, artificial environment constructed *on top of* land. Real estate recognizes the difference between parkland and shopping mall, between red-light zone and school district, between church, state and drugstore.

In the same way, you could think of cyberspace as a giant 4
and unbounded world of virtual real estate. Some property is
privately owned and rented out; other property is common land;
some places are suitable for children, and others are best
avoided by all but the kinkiest citizens. Unfortunately, it's those
places that are now capturing the popular imagination: places
that offer bomb-making instructions, pornography, advice on
how to procure stolen credit cards. They make cyberspace sound
like a nasty place. Good citizens jump to a conclusion: Better
regulate it.

The most recent manifestation of this impulse is the Exon- 5
Coats Amendment, a well-meaning but misguided bill drafted by
Senators Jim Exon, Democrat of Nebraska, and Daniel R. Coats,
Republican of Indiana, to make cyberspace "safer" for children.
Part of the telecommunications reform bill passed by the Senate
and awaiting consideration by the House, the amendment would
outlaw making "indecent communication" available to anyone
under 18.[1] Then there's the Amateur Action bulletin board case,
in which the owners of a porn service in Milpitas, Calif., were convicted in a Tennessee court of violating "community standards"
after a local postal inspector requested that the material be transmitted to him.

Regardless of how many laws or lawsuits are launched, 6
regulation won't work.

Aside from being unconstitutional, using censorship to 7
counter indecency and other troubling "speech" fundamentally
misinterprets the nature of cyberspace. Cyberspace isn't a frontier
where wicked people can grab unsuspecting children, nor is it a
giant television system that can beam offensive messages at
unwilling viewers. In this kind of real estate, users have to *choose*
where they visit, what they see, what they do. It's optional, and
it's much easier to bypass a place on the Net than it is to avoid
walking past an unsavory block of stores on the way to your local
7-Eleven.

---

[1]The Communications Decency Act (CDA) was passed by Congress, but the
Supreme Court ruled that it was unconstitutional in 1996. [This note is the author's.]

8   Put plainly, cyberspace is a voluntary destination—in reality, many destinations. You don't just get "onto the net"; you have to go someplace in particular. That means that people can choose where to go and what to see. Yes, community standards should be enforced, but those standards should be set by cyberspace communities themselves, not by the courts or by politicians in Washington. What we need isn't Government control over all these electronic communities: We need self-rule.

9   What makes cyberspace so alluring is precisely the way in which it's *different* from shopping malls, television, highways and other terrestrial jurisdictions. But let's define the territory:

10   First, there are private e-mail conversations, akin to the conversations you have over the telephone or voice mail. These are private and consensual and require no regulation at all.

11   Second, there are information and entertainment services, where people can download anything from legal texts and lists of "great new restaurants" to game software or dirty pictures. These places are like bookstores, malls and movie houses—places where you go to buy something. The customer needs to request an item or sign up for a subscription; stuff (especially pornography) is not sent out to people who don't ask for it. Some of these services are free or included as part of a broader service like Compuserve or America Online; others charge and may bill their customers directly.

12   Third, there are "real" communities—groups of people who communicate among themselves. In real-estate terms, they're like bars or restaurants or bathhouses. Each active participant contributes to a general conversation, generally through posted messages. Other participants may simply listen or watch. Some are supervised by a moderator; others are more like bulletin boards—anyone is free to post anything. Many of these services started out unmoderated but are now imposing rules to keep out unwanted advertising, extraneous discussions or increasingly rude participants. Without a moderator, the decibel level often gets too high.

13   Ultimately, it's the rules that determine the success of such places. Some of the rules are determined by the supplier of content; some of the rules concern prices and membership fees. The rules may be simple: "Only high-quality content about oil-industry

liability and pollution legislation: $120 an hour." Or: "This forum is unmoderated, and restricted to information about copyright issues. People who insist on posting advertising or unrelated material will be asked to desist (and may eventually be barred)." Or: "Only children 8 to 12, on school-related topics and only clean words. The moderator will decide what's acceptable."

Cyberspace communities evolve just the way terrestrial 14 communities do: people with like-minded interests band together. Every cyberspace community has its own character. Overall, the communities on Compuserve tend to be more techy or professional; those on America Online, affluent young singles; Prodigy, family oriented. Then there are independents like Echo, a hip, downtown New York service, or Women's Wire, targeted to women who want to avoid the male culture prevalent elsewhere on the Net. There's SurfWatch, a new program allowing access only to locations deemed suitable for children. On the Internet itself, there are lots of passionate noncommercial discussion groups on topics ranging from Hungarian politics (Hungary-Online) to copyright law.

And yes, there are also porn-oriented services, where people 15 share dirty pictures and communicate with one another about all kinds of practices, often anonymously. Whether these services encourage the fantasies they depict is subject to debate—the same debate that has raged about pornography in other media. But the point is that no one is forcing this stuff on anybody.

What's unique about cyberspace is that it liberates us from the 16 tyranny of government, where everyone lives by the rule of the majority. In a democracy, minority groups and minority preferences tend to get squeezed out, whether they are minorities of race and culture or minorities of individual taste. Cyberspace allows communities of any size and kind to flourish; in cyberspace, communities are chosen by the users, not forced on them by accidents of geography. This freedom gives the rules that preside in cyberspace a moral authority that rules in terrestrial environments don't have. Most people are stuck in the country of their birth, but if you don't like the rules of a cyberspace community, you can just sign off. Love it or leave it. Likewise, if parents don't like the rules of a given cyberspace community, they can restrict their children's access to it.

17   What's likely to happen in cyberspace is the formation of new communities, free of the constraints that cause conflict on earth. Instead of a global village, which is a nice dream but impossible to manage, we'll have invented another world of self-contained communities that cater to their own members' inclinations without interfering with anyone else's. The possibility of a real market-style evolution of governance is at hand. In cyberspace, we'll be able to test and evolve rules governing what needs to be governed—intellectual property, content and access control, rules about privacy and free speech. Some communities will allow anyone in; others will restrict access to members who qualify on one basis or another. Those communities that prove self-sustaining will prosper (and perhaps grow and split into subsets with ever-more-particular interests and identities). Those that can't survive—either because people lose interest or get scared off—will simply wither away.

18   In the near future, explorers in cyberspace will need to get better at defining and identifying their communities. They will need to put in place—and accept—their own local governments, just as the owners of expensive real estate often prefer to have their own security guards rather than call in the police. But they will rarely need help from any terrestrial government.

19   Of course, terrestrial governments may not agree. What to do, for instance, about pornography? The answer is labeling—not banning—questionable material. In order to avoid censorship and lower the political temperature, it makes sense for cyberspace participants themselves to agree on a scheme for questionable items, so that people or automatic filters can avoid them. In other words, posting pornography in "alt.sex.bestiality" would be OK; it's easy enough for software manufacturers to build an automatic filter that would prevent you—or your child—from ever seeing that item on a menu. (It's as if all the items were wrapped with labels on the wrapper.) Someone who posted the same material under the title "Kid-Fun" could be sued for mislabeling.

20   Without a lot of fanfare, private enterprises and local groups are already producing a variety of labeling and ranking services, along with kid-oriented sites like Kidlink, EdWeb and Kids' Space. People differ in their tastes and values and can find services or reviewers on the Net that suit them in the same way they select

books and magazines. Or they can wander freely if they prefer, making up their own itinerary.

In the end, our society needs to grow up. Growing up means 21 understanding that there are no perfect answers, no all-purpose solutions, no government-sanctioned safe havens. We haven't created a perfect society on earth and we won't have one in cyberspace either. But at least we can have individual choice—and individual responsibility.

Virtual Students, Digital Classrooms

Neil Postman

If one has a trusting relationship with one's students (let us say, 1 graduate students), it is not altogether gauche to ask them if they believe in God (with a capital G). I have done this three or four times and most students say they do. Their answer is preliminary to the next question: If someone you love were desperately ill, and you had to choose between praying to God for his or her recovery or administering an antibiotic (as prescribed by a competent physician), which would you choose?

Most say the question is silly since the alternatives are not 2 mutually exclusive. Of course. But suppose they were—which would you choose? God helps those who help themselves, some say in choosing the antibiotic, therefore getting the best of two possible belief systems. But if pushed to the wall (e.g., God does not always help those who help themselves; God helps those who pray and who believe), most choose the antibiotic, after noting that the question is asinine and proves nothing. Of course, the question was not asked, in the first place, to prove anything but to begin a discussion of the nature of belief. And I do not fail to inform the students, by the way, that there has recently emerged evidence of a "scientific" nature that when sick people are prayed for they do better than those who aren't.

As the discussion proceeds, important distinctions are made 3 among the different meanings of "belief," but at some point it becomes far from asinine to speak of the god of Technology—

in the sense that people believe technology works, that they rely on it, that it makes promises, that they are bereft when denied access to it, that they are delighted when they are in its presence, that for most people it works in mysterious ways, that they condemn people who speak against it, that they stand in awe of it and that, in the "born again" mode, they will alter their life-styles, their schedules, their habits, and their relationships to accommodate it. If this be not a form of religious belief, what is?

4   In all strands of American cultural life, you can find so many examples of technological adoration that it is possible to write a book about it. And I would if it had not already been done so well. But nowhere do you find more enthusiasm for the god of Technology than among educators. In fact, there are those, like Lewis Perelman, who argue (for example, in his book, *School's Out*) that modern information technologies have rendered schools entirely irrelevant since there is now much more information available outside the classroom than inside it. This is by no means considered an outlandish idea. Dr. Diane Ravitch, former Assistant Secretary of Education, envisions, with considerable relish, the challenge that technology presents to the tradition that "children (and adults) should be educated in a specific place, for a certain number of hours, and a certain number of days during the week and year." In other words, that children should be educated in school. Imagining the possibilities of an information superhighway offering perhaps a thousand channels, Dr. Ravitch assures us that:

> In this new world of pedagogical plenty, children and adults will be able to dial up a program on their home television to learn whatever they want to know, at their own convenience. If Little Eva cannot sleep, she can learn algebra instead. At her home-learning station, she will tune in to a series of interesting problems that are presented in an interactive medium, much like video games. . . .
>
>   Young John may decide that he wants to learn the history of modern Japan, which he can do by dialing up the greatest authorities and teachers on the subject, who will not only use dazzling graphs and illustrations, but will narrate a historical video that excites his curiosity and imagination.

In this vision there is, it seems to me, a confident and typi- 5
cal sense of unreality. Little Eva can't sleep, so she decides to
learn a little algebra? Where does Little Eva come from? Mars?
If not, it is more likely she will tune in to a good movie. Young
John decides that he wants to learn the history of modern Japan?
How did young John come to this point? How is it that he never
visited a library up to now? Or is that he, too, couldn't sleep and
decided that a little modern Japanese history was just what he
needed?

What Ravitch is talking about here is not a new technology 6
but a new species of child, one who, in any case, no one has seen
up to now. Of course, new technologies do make new kinds of
people, which leads to a second objection to Ravitch's conception of the future. There is a kind of forthright determinism
about the imagined world described in it. The technology is here
or will be; we must use it because it is there; we will become
the kind of people the technology requires us to be, and whether
we like it or not, we will remake our institutions to accommodate technology. All of this must happen because it is good for
us, but in any case, we have no choice. This point of view is present in very nearly every statement about the future relationship
of learning to technology. And, as in Ravitch's scenario, there
is always a cheery, gee-whiz tone to the prophecies. Here is
one produced by the National Academy of Sciences, written by
Hugh McIntosh:

> School for children of the Information Age will be vastly differ-
> ent than it was for Mom and Dad.
>
> Interested in biology? Design your own life forms with
> computer simulation.
>
> Having trouble with a science project? Teleconference about
> it with a research scientist.
>
> Bored with the real world? Go into a virtual physics lab and
> rewrite the laws of gravity.
>
> These are the kinds of hands-on learning experiences
> schools could be providing right now. The technologies that
> make them possible are already here, and today's youngsters,
> regardless of economic status, know how to use them. They
> spend hours with them every week—not in the classroom, but
> in their own homes and in video game centers at every shop-
> ping mall.

7   It is always interesting to attend to the examples of learning, and the motivations that ignite them, in the songs of love that technophiles perform for us. It is, for example, not easy to imagine research scientists all over the world teleconferencing with thousands of students who are having difficulty with their science projects. I can't help thinking that most research scientists would put a stop to this rather quickly. But I find it especially revealing that in the scenario above we have an example of a technological solution to a psychological problem that would seem to be exceedingly serious. We are presented with a student who is "bored with the real world." What does it mean to say someone is bored with the real world, especially one so young? Can a journey into virtual reality cure such a problem? And if it can, will our troubled youngster want to return to the real world? Confronted with a student who is bored with the real world, I don't think we can solve the problem so easily by making available a virtual reality physics lab.

8   The role that new technology should play in schools or anywhere else is something that needs to be discussed without the hyperactive fantasies of cheerleaders. In particular, the computer and its associated technologies are awesome additions to a culture, and are quite capable of altering the psychic, not to mention the sleeping, habits of our young. But like all important technologies of the past, they are Faustian bargains, giving and taking away, sometimes in equal measure, sometimes more in one way than the other. It is strange—indeed, shocking—that with the twenty-first century so close, we can still talk of new technologies as if they were unmixed blessings—gifts, as it were, from the gods. Don't we all know what the combustion engine has done for us and against us? What television is doing for us and against us? At the very least, what we need to discuss about Little Eva, Young John, and McIntosh's trio is what they will lose, and what we will lose, if they enter a world in which computer technology is their chief source of motivation, authority, and, apparently, psychological sustenance. Will they become, as Joseph Weizenbaum warns, more impressed by calculation than human judgment? Will speed of response become, more than ever, a defining quality of intelligence? If, indeed, the idea of a school will be dramatically altered, what kinds of learning will be neglected, perhaps

made impossible? Is virtual reality a new form of therapy? If it is, what are its dangers?

These are serious matters, and they need to be discussed by those 9 who know something about children from the planet Earth, and whose vision of children's needs, and the needs of society, go beyond thinking of school mainly as a place for the convenient distribution of information. Schools are not now and have never been largely about getting information to children. That has been on the schools' agenda, of course, but has always been way down on the list. For technological utopians, the computer vaults information access to the top. This reshuffling of priorities comes at a most inopportune time. The goal of giving people greater access to more information faster, more conveniently, and in more diverse forms was the main technological thrust of the nineteenth century. Some folks haven't noticed it but that problem was largely solved, so that for almost a hundred years there has been more information available to the young outside the school than inside. That fact did not make the schools obsolete, nor does it now make them obsolete. Yes, it is true that Little Eva, the insomniac from Mars, could turn on an algebra lesson, thanks to the computer, in the wee hours of the morning. She could also, if she wished, read a book or magazine, watch television, turn on the radio or listen to music. All of this she could have done before the computer. The computer does not solve any problem she has but does exacerbate one. For Little Eva's problem is not how to get access to a well-structured algebra lesson but what to do with all the information available to her during the day, as well as during sleepless nights. Perhaps this is why she couldn't sleep in the first place. Little Eva, like the rest of us, is overwhelmed by information. She lives in a culture that has 260,000 billboards, 17,000 newspapers, 12,000 periodicals, 27,000 video outlets for renting tapes, 400 million television sets, and well over 500 million radios, not including those in automobiles. There are 40,000 new book titles published every year, and each day 41 million photographs are taken. And thanks to the computer, more than 60 billion pieces of advertising junk come into our mailboxes every year. Everything from telegraphy and photography in the nineteenth century to the silicon chip in the twentieth has amplified the din of information intruding on Little Eva's consciousness.

From millions of sources all over the globe, through every possible channel and medium—light waves, air waves, ticker tape, computer banks, telephone wires, television cables, satellites, and printing presses—information pours in. Behind it in every imaginable form of storage—on paper, on video, on audiotape, on disks, film, and silicon chips—is an even greater volume of information waiting to be retrieved. In the face of this we might ask: What can schools do for Little Eva besides making still more information available? If there is nothing, then new technologies will indeed make schools obsolete. But in fact, there is plenty.

10   One thing that comes to mind is that schools can provide her with a serious form of technology education. Something quite different from instruction in using computers to process information, which, it strikes me, is a trivial thing to do, for two reasons. In the first place, approximately 35 million people have already learned how to use computers without the benefit of school instruction. If the schools do nothing, most of the population will know how to use computers in the next ten years, just as most of the population learns how to drive a car without school instruction. In the second place, what we needed to know about cars—as we need to know about computers, television, and other important technologies—is not how to use them but how they use *us*. In the case of cars, what we needed to think about in the early twentieth century was not how to drive them but what they would do to our air, our landscape, our social relations, our family life, and our cities. Suppose in 1946 we had started to address similar questions about television: What will be its effects on our political institutions, our psychic habits, our children, our religious conceptions, our economy? Would we be better positioned today to control TV's massive assault on American culture? I am talking here about making technology itself an object of inquiry so that Little Eva and Young John are more interested in asking questions about the computer than getting answers from it.

11   I am not arguing against using computers in school. I am arguing against our sleepwalking attitudes toward it, against allowing it to distract us from important things, against making a god of it. This is what Theodore Roszak warned against in *The Cult of Information:* "Like all cults," he wrote, "this one also has the intention of enlisting mindless allegiance and acquiescence. People who

have no clear idea of what they mean by information or why they should want so much of it are nonetheless prepared to believe that we live in an Information Age, which makes every computer around us what the relics of the True Cross were in the Age of Faith: emblems of salvation." To this, I would add the sage observation of Alan Kay of Apple Computer. Kay is widely associated with the invention of the personal computer, and certainly has an interest in schools using them. Nonetheless, he has repeatedly said that any problems the schools cannot solve without computers, they cannot solve with them. What are some of those problems? There is, for example, the traditional task of teaching children how to behave in groups. One might even say that schools have never been essentially about individualized learning. It is true, of course, that groups do not learn, individuals do. But the idea of a school is that individuals must learn in a setting in which individual needs are subordinated to group interests. Unlike other media of mass communication, which celebrate individual response and are experienced in private, the classroom is intended to tame the ego, to connect the individual with others, to demonstrate the value and necessity of group cohesion. At present, most scenarios describing the uses of computers have children solving problems alone; Little Eva, Young John, and the others are doing just that. The presence of other children may, indeed, be an annoyance.

Like the printing press before it, the computer has a powerful bias 12 toward amplifying personal autonomy and individual problem-solving. That is why educators must guard against computer technology's undermining some of the important reasons for having the young assemble (to quote Ravitch) "in a specific place, for a certain number of hours, and a certain number of days during the week and year."

Although Ravitch is not exactly against what she calls "state 13 schools," she imagines them as something of a relic of a pretech-nological age. She believes that the new technologies will offer all children equal access to information. Conjuring up a hypothetical Little Mary who is presumably from a poorer home than Little Eva, Ravitch imagines that Mary will have the same opportunities as Eva "to learn any subject, and to learn it from the same master teachers as children in the richest neighborhood." For all of its liberalizing spirit, this scenario makes some important omissions. One is that though new technologies may be a solution to the learning of "subjects," they work against the learning of what are called "social values," including an understanding of democratic processes. If one reads the first chapter of Robert Fulghum's *All I Really Need to Know I Learned in Kindergarten,* one will find an elegant summary of a few things Ravitch's scenario has left out. They include learning the following lessons: Share everything, play fair, don't hit people, put things back where you found them, clean up your own mess, wash your hands before you eat, and, of course, flush. The only thing wrong with Fulghum's book is that no one has learned all these things at kindergarten's end. We have ample evidence that it takes many years of teaching these values in school before they have been accepted and internalized. That is why it won't do for children to learn in "settings of their own choosing." That is also why schools require children to be in a certain place at a certain time and to follow certain rules, like raising their hands when they wish to speak, not talking when others are talking, not chewing gum, not leaving until the bell rings, exhibiting patience toward slower learners, etc. This process is called making civilized people. The god of Technology does not appear interested in this function of schools. At least, it does not come up much when technology's virtues are enumerated.

14   The god of Technology may also have a trick or two up its sleeve about something else. It is often asserted that new technologies will equalize learning opportunities for the rich and poor. It is devoutly to be wished for, but I doubt it will happen. In the first place, it is generally understood by those who have studied the history of technology that technological change always produces winners and losers. There are many reasons for this, among them economic differences. Even in the case of the automobile, which is a commodity most people can buy (although not all), there are wide differences between the rich and poor in the quality of what is available to them. It would be quite astonishing if computer technology equalized all learning opportunities, irrespective of economic differences. One may be delighted that Little Eva's parents could afford the technology and software to make it possible for her to learn algebra at midnight. But Little Mary's parents may not be able to, may not even know such things are

available. And if we say that the school could make the technology available to Little Mary (at least during the day), there may [be] something else Little Mary is lacking.

It turns out, for example, that Little Mary may be having sleep- 15 less nights as frequently as Little Eva but not because she wants to get a leg up on her algebra. Maybe because she doesn't know who her father is, or, if she does, where he is. Maybe we can understand why McIntosh's kid is bored with the real world. Or is the child confused about it? Or terrified? Are there educators who seriously believe that these problems can be addressed by new technologies?

I do not say, of course, that schools can solve the problems 16 of poverty, alienation, and family disintegration, but schools can *respond* to them. And they can do this because there are people in them, because these people are concerned with more than algebra lessons or modern Japanese history, and because these people can identify not only one's level of competence in math but one's level of rage and confusion and depression. I am talking here about children as they really come to us, not children who are invented to show us how computers may enrich their lives. Of course, I suppose it is possible that there are children who, waking at night, want to study algebra or who are so interested in their world that they yearn to know about Japan. If there be such children, and one hopes there are, they do not require expensive computers to satisfy their hunger for learning. They are on their way, with or without computers. Unless, of course, they do not care about others or have no friends, or little respect for democracy or are filled with suspicion about those who are not like them. When we have machines that know how to do something about these problems, that is the time to rid ourselves of the expensive burden of schools or to reduce the function of teachers to "coaches" in the uses of machines (as Ravitch envisions). Until then, we must be more modest about this god of Technology and certainly not pin our hopes on it.

We must also, I suppose, be empathetic toward those who 17 search with good intentions for technological panaceas. I am a teacher myself and know how hard it is to contribute to the making of a civilized person. Can we blame those who want to find an easy way, through the agency of technology? Perhaps not. After all, it is an old quest. As early as 1918, H. L. Mencken (although completely devoid of empathy) wrote, "There is no sure-cure so idiotic that some superintendent of schools will not swallow it. The aim seems to be reduce the whole teaching process to a sort of automatic reaction, to discover some master formula that will not only take the place of competence and resourcefulness in the teacher but that will also create an artificial receptivity in the child."

18   Mencken was not necessarily speaking of technological panaceas but he may well have been. In the early 1920s a teacher wrote the following poem:

> Mr. Edison says
> That the radio will supplant the teacher.
> Already one may learn languages by means of
>   Victrola records.
> The moving picture will visualize
> What the radio fails to get across.
> Teachers will be relegated to the backwoods,
> With fire-horses,
> And long-haired women;
> Or, perhaps shown in museums.
> Education will become a matter
> Of pressing the button.
> Perhaps I can get a position at the switchboard.

19   I do not go as far back as the radio and Victrola, but I am old enough to remember when 16-millimeter film was to be the sure-cure. Then closed-circuit television. Then 8-millimeter film. Then teacher-proof textbooks. Now computers.

20   I know a false god when I see one.

The Intimacy of Blogs

Michael Snider

1 When Plain Layne suddenly pulled her site down in early June, a little corner of the blogosphere went nuts. Instead of the 26-year-old Minnesotan's poignant daily entries on her Weblog, an on-line journal, a blunt one-line message greeted visitors: "Take very good care of you." No more honestly introspective narratives of her life. No more unbridled entries detailing the search for her birth

parents, sessions with her therapist or her disappointing love affair with Violet, the stubby-tongued Dragon Lady. Comments flooded cyberspace. "Her surprising, unannounced departure is sending me and my overactive imagination into a frenzy of worry," wrote Gudy Two Shoes on his own Weblog. "If she's gone then I wish her well," posted Intellectual Poison. "She got me started with this whole blogging thing, something that I am truly grateful for." And Daintily Dirty asked, "Are the relationships we create by our blogging of any value?"

That's a good question. It turned out that Plaine Layne, aka 2 Layne Johnson, wasn't gone for good. She'd just had a week during which she moved into a new house and witnessed the birth of her surrogate little sister's baby before getting her site back up (*http://plainlayne.dreamhost.com*). But the reaction from her readers was genuine. One of the prime reasons people blog is to make connections with others, and when Plain Layne went missing, it was like a neighbour had just up and moved in the middle of the night, with no forwarding address.

Weblogs are independent Web sites usually operated by a 3 single person or by a small group of people. They serve as frequently updated forums to discuss whatever the blogger wants to discuss. Unmonitored, each blogger is author, editor and publisher, beholden solely to his or her own whims and desires. There are political blogs, media blogs, gay blogs, sports blogs, war blogs, antiwar blogs, tech blogs, photo blogs—hundreds of thousands of blogs, actually (estimates are as high as two million). "Blogging is not people wasting other people's time talking about the minutiae of their lives," says Joe Clark, 38, a Toronto author who operates several blogs. "The thing that's attractive about reading Weblogs is that you know there is one human being or a group of human beings behind them."

Free and easy-to-use publishing programs with names like 4 Blogger, Movable Type and Live Journal spurred the phenomenon. Now, anyone with a computer and an Internet connection can set up their own blog with relative ease. Paul Martin blogs, journalists blog, pundits, critics and social misfits blog. And what can you find there? Well, imagine standing in front of a library of gargantuan magazine racks loaded with glossy covers with everything from newsweeklies to girlie mags.

5   Blogs break down into two very general groups: linking blogs and personal online journals. Political blogs like Glenn Reynolds' *Instapundit.com*, media blogs like Jim Romenesko's Poynter Online (*www.poynter.org/medianews*), or tech blogs like *slashdot.com* are of the former kind. They're link-driven sites that connect readers to theme-related news stories and sometimes add a little commentary along with it. A personal blog is more like a diary entry or column in a daily newspaper, *a la* Rebecca Eckler of the *National Post* or Leah McLaren of the *Globe and Mail*—all about "me and what I think." Writers recount events in their lives—sometimes very private ones—and air their thoughts to a public audience.

6   Reasons vary. Sometimes, the practice is therapeutic. For some, like Ryan Rhodes, who runs Rambling Rhodes (*http://ramblingrhodes.blogspot.com*), blogging has some functional purposes. Rhodes, from Rochester, Minn., is news editor for an IBM publication called *eServer Magazine* but also writes humour columns for some local newspapers. He figured blogging would be a good writing exercise that might offer him instant feedback from readers. "I like knowing the stuff I write is being read," says Rhodes, "and I like it when it hits someone in a positive way and they tell me, so I can use it later for my column."

7   Personal blogs are famous for breaking usual standards of disclosure, revealing details considered by some to be very private. Dan Gudy, a 29-year-old Berliner, kept a diary when he was a teenager but gave it up, unhappy with the results. "My first experience was a total failure," says Gudy. "It was only myself talking about myself and I do that enough." But last year, when he created his site, Gudy Two Shoes (*http://gudy.blogspot.com*), the self-described introvert discovered that blogging opened a release valve. "I had to deal with some problems at the time and somehow needed to let it out. Part of me asked, why not use a blog for that?" Now, Gudy blogs about the books he reads and bike-riding through the German countryside. He also blogs about his sex life with his wife. "People can talk about what a nice bike ride they had or what a nice meal they had, but why can't they talk about what a nice f—they had last night?"

8   For many, that very willingness to discuss intimate details is one of the most alluring facets of blogging. "Your Weblog becomes an exterior part of you," says Clark, "so you can have some

distance from your feelings, even though you're putting them out for everyone to read. But then all your readers are right up close and they know you because you're writing directly to them." In turn, readers can offer their own feedback: personal blogs frequently allow them to comment after each post, with something as easy as clicking a link that opens a pop-up box where they can add their own two cents' worth. "When I first started blogging," writes Daintily Dirty (*http://www.blogdreams.blogspot.com*), an anonymous 32-year-old blogger who chatted with *Macleans* via instant messenger, "I had no idea what I was getting into with the personal nature of the interactions. But the connections you find are what keep you coming back."

Layne Johnson's readers can attest to that. An excellent narra- 9 tive writer who opens her soul to her readers, Plain Layne's daily entries regularly receive dozens of comments. "I hopped from one blog to the next and somewhere found Plain Layne," says Gudy. "What made me stay was her brutal honesty and intimacy of sharing, her very beautiful way of writing." Rhodes echoes the sentiment. "Layne is digital crack," he says. "Hands down, as far as I've read, she's got the best personal blog. I have to read her every day."

Johnson politely turned down a request for an interview, 10 explaining her blogging is a personal exercise that's meant to be cathartic. And somehow, that's the way it should be. Plain Layne does her talking, or typing, on her blog. "I think the hardest thing about sharing your life on-line is that at some point you discover people know you," Johnson wrote in a June post. "They know you from the inside out, the way your mind works, what makes you laugh or cry, your hopes and fears." It's clear to see she uses her blog as an outlet, a place to dump her anxiety and frustration in a search for identity and understanding. It's also a place of amusement and mirth, with stories of stupefying office meetings and uproarious golf outings, all told with a flair and talent that would make some "me" columnists envious.

Blogs might seem too revealing for people who prefer their 11 diaries to remain private. But more and more strangers are inviting millions of other strangers into their lives, with a willingness to share just about anything, finding their own shelf space on the world's most accessible magazine rack, open to anyone who cares to pick up a copy. Welcome to the blogosphere.

Chapter 12

Ethical Issues in Medicine: When Does Life Begin and End?

A New Look, an Old Battle

Anna Quindlen

1 Public personification has always been the struggle on both sides of the abortion battle lines. That is why the people outside clinics on Saturday mornings carry signs with photographs of infants rather than of zygotes, why they wear lapel pins fashioned in the image of tiny feet and shout, "Don't kill your baby," rather than, more accurately, "Don't destroy your embryo." Those who support the legal right to an abortion have always been somewhat at a loss in the face of all this. From time to time women have come forward to speak about their decision to have an abortion, but when they are prominent, it seems a bit like grandstanding, and when they are not, it seems a terrible invasion of privacy when privacy is the point in the first place. Easier to marshal the act of presumptive ventriloquism practiced by the opponents, pretending to speak for those unborn unknown to them by circumstance or story.

2 But the battle of personification will assume a different and more sympathetic visage in the years to come. Perhaps the change in the weather was best illustrated when conservative Senator Strom Thurmond invoked his own daughter to explain a position opposed by the anti-abortion forces. The senator's daughter has diabetes. The actor Michael J. Fox has Parkinson's

disease. Christopher Reeve is in a wheelchair because of a spinal-cord injury, Ronald Reagan locked in his own devolving mind by Alzheimer's. In the faces of the publicly and personally beloved lies enormous danger for the life-begins-at-conception lobby.

The catalytic issue is research on stem cells. These are versa- 3 tile building blocks that may be coaxed into becoming any other cell type; they could therefore hold the key to endless mysteries of human biology, as well as someday help provide a cure for ailments as diverse as diabetes, Parkinson's, spinal-cord degeneration, and Alzheimer's. By some estimates, more than 100 million Americans have diseases that scientists suspect could be affected by research on stem cells. Scientists hope that the astonishing potential of this research will persuade the federal government to help fund it and allow the National Institutes of Health to help oversee it. This is not political, researchers insist. It is about science, not abortion.

And they are correct. Stem-cell research is typically done by 4 using frozen embryos left over from in vitro fertilization. If these embryos were placed in the womb, they might eventually implant, become a fetus, then a child. Unused, they are the earliest undifferentiated collection of cells made by the joining of the egg and sperm, no larger than the period at the end of this sentence. One of the oft-used slogans of the anti-abortion movement is "abortion stops a beating heart." There is no heart in this preimplantation embryo, but there are stem cells that, in the hands of scientists, might lead to extraordinary work affecting everything from cancer to heart disease.

All of which leaves the anti-abortion movement trying des- 5 perately to hold its hard line, and failing. Judie Brown of the American Life League can refer to these embryos as "the tiniest person," and the National Right to Life organization can publish papers that refer to stem-cell research as the "destruction of life." But ordinary people with family members losing their mobility or their grasp on reality will be able to be more thoughtful and reasonable about the issues involved.

The anti-abortion activists know this, because they have 6 already seen the defections. Some senators have abandoned them to support fetal-tissue research, less promising than stem-cell work but still with significant potential for treating various ailments. Elected officials who had voted against abortion rights found themselves able to support procedures that used tissue from aborted fetuses; perhaps they were men who had fathers with heart disease, who had mothers with arthritis and whose hearts resonated with the possibilities for alleviating pain and prolonging life. Senator Thurmond was one, Senator McCain another. Former senator Connie Mack of Florida recently sent a letter to the president, who must decide the future role of the federal government in this area, describing himself "as a conservative pro-life now former member" of Congress, and adding that there "were those of us identified as such who supported embryonic stem-cell research."

7   When a recent test of fetal tissue in patients with Parkinson's had disastrous side effects, the National Right to Life Web site ran an almost gloating report: "horrific," "rips to shreds," "media cheerleaders," "defy description." The tone is a reflection of fear. It's the fear that the use of fetal tissue to produce cures for debilitating ailments might somehow launder the process of terminating a pregnancy, a positive result from what many people still see as a negative act. And it's the fear that thinking—really thinking—about the use of the earliest embryo for lifesaving research might bring a certain long-overdue relativism to discussions of abortion across the board.

8   The majority of Americans have always been able to apply that relativism to these issues. They are more likely to accept early abortions than later ones. They are more tolerant of a single abortion under exigent circumstances than multiple abortions. Some who disapprove of abortion in theory have discovered that they can accept it in fact if a daughter or a girlfriend is pregnant.

9   And some who believe that life begins at conception may look into the vacant eyes of an adored parent with Alzheimer's or picture a paralyzed child walking again, and take a closer look at what an embryo really is, at what stem-cell research really does, and then consider the true cost of a cure. That is what Senator Thurmond obviously did when he looked at his daughter and broke ranks with the true believers. It may be an oversimplification to say that real live loved ones trump the imagined unborn, that a cluster of undifferentiated cells due to be discarded anyway

is a small price to pay for the health and welfare of millions. Or perhaps it is only a simple commonsensical truth.

Active and Passive Euthanasia

James Rachels

The distinction between active and passive euthanasia is thought 1 to be crucial for medical ethics. The idea is that it is permissible, at least in some cases, to withhold treatment and allow a patient to die, but it is never permissible to take any direct action designed to kill the patient. This doctrine seems to be accepted by most doctors, and it is endorsed in a statement adopted by the House of Delegates of the American Medical Association on December 4, 1973:

> The intentional termination of the life of one human being by another—mercy killing—is contrary to that for which the medical profession stands and is contrary to the policy of the American Medical Association. The cessation of the employment of extraordinary means to prolong the life of the body when there is irrefutable evidence that biological death is imminent is the decision of the patient and/or his immediate family. The advice and judgment of the physician should be freely available to the patient and/or his immediate family.

However, a strong case can be made against this doctrine. In what follows I will set out some of the relevant arguments, and urge doctors to reconsider their views on this matter.

To begin with a familiar type of situation, a patient who is 2 dying of incurable cancer of the throat is in terrible pain, which can no longer be satisfactorily alleviated. He is certain to die within a few days, even if present treatment is continued, but he does not want to go on living for those days since the pain is unbearable. So he asks the doctor for an end to it, and his family joins in the request.

Suppose the doctor agrees to withhold treatment, as the con- 3 ventional doctrine says he may. The justification for his doing so is that the patient is in terrible agony, and since he is going to die anyway, it would be wrong to prolong his suffering needlessly. But now notice this. If one simply withholds treatment, it may take the patient longer to die, and so he may suffer more than he would if more direct action were taken and a lethal injection given. This fact provides strong reason for thinking that, once the initial decision not to prolong his agony has been made, active euthanasia is actually preferable to passive euthanasia, rather than the reverse. To say otherwise is to endorse the option that leads to more suffering rather than less, and is contrary to the humanitarian impulse that prompts the decision not to prolong his life in the first place.

4   Part of my point is that the process of being "allowed to die" can be relatively slow and painful, whereas being given a lethal injection is relatively quick and painless. Let me give a different sort of example. In the United States about one in six hundred babies is born with Down's syndrome. Most of these babies are otherwise healthy—that is, with only the usual pediatric care, they will proceed to an otherwise normal infancy. Some, however, are born with congenital defects such as intestinal obstructions that require operations if they are to live. Sometimes, the parents and the doctor will decide not to operate, and let the infant die. Anthony Shaw describes what happens then:

> When surgery is denied [the doctor] must try to keep the infant from suffering while natural forces sap the baby's life away. As a surgeon whose natural inclination is to use the scalpel to fight off death, standing by and watching a salvageable baby die is the most emotionally exhausting experience I know. It is easy at a conference, in a theoretical discussion to decide that such infants should be allowed to die. It is altogether different to stand by in the nursery and watch as dehydration and infection wither a tiny being over hours and days. This is a terrible ordeal for me and the hospital staff—much more so than for the parents who never set foot in the nursery.[1]

I can understand why some people are opposed to all euthanasia, and insist that such infants must be allowed to live. I think

---

[1]Anthony Shaw, "Doctor, Do We Have a Choice?" *New York Times Magazine,* January 30, 1972, p. 54. [Author's note.]

I can also understand why other people favor destroying these babies quickly and painlessly. But why should anyone favor letting "dehydration and infection wither a tiny being over hours and days"? The doctrine that says that a baby may be allowed to dehydrate and wither, but may not be given an injection that would end its life without suffering, seems so patently cruel as to require no further refutation. The strong language is not intended to offend, but only to put the point in the clearest possible way.

My second argument is that the conventional doctrine leads to decisions concerning life and death made on irrelevant grounds. 5

Consider again the case of the infants with Down's syndrome who need operations for congenital defects unrelated to the syndrome to live. Sometimes, there is no operation, and the baby dies, but when there is no such defect, the baby lives on. Now, an operation such as that to remove an intestinal obstruction is not prohibitively difficult. The reason why such operations are not performed in these cases is, clearly, that the child has Down's syndrome and the parents and the doctor judge that because of that fact it is better for the child to die. 6

But notice that this situation is absurd, no matter what view one takes of the lives and potentials of such babies. If the life of such an infant is worth preserving, what does it matter if it needs a simple operation? Or, if one thinks it better that such a baby should not live on, what difference does it make that it happens to have an unobstructed intestinal tract? In either case, the matter of life and death is being decided on irrelevant grounds. It is the Down's syndrome, and not the intestines, that is the issue. The matter should be decided, if at all, on that basis, and not be allowed to depend on the essentially irrelevant question of whether the intestinal tract is blocked. 7

What makes this situation possible, of course, is the idea that when there is an intestinal blockage, one can "let the baby die," but when there is no such defect there is nothing that can be done, for one must not "kill" it. The fact that this idea leads to such results as deciding life or death on irrelevant grounds is another good reason why the doctrine would be rejected. 8

One reason why so many people think that there is an important moral difference between active and passive euthanasia is that they think killing someone is morally worse than letting 9 someone die. But is it? Is killing, in itself, worse than letting die? To investigate this issue, two cases may be considered that are exactly alike except that one involves killing whereas the other involves letting someone die. Then, it can be asked whether this difference makes any difference to the moral assessments. It is important that the cases be exactly alike, except for this one difference, since otherwise one cannot be confident that it is this difference and not some other that accounts for any variation in the assessments of the two cases. So, let us consider this pair of cases:

10   In the first, Smith stands to gain a large inheritance if anything should happen to his six-year-old cousin. One evening while the child is taking his bath, Smith sneaks into the bathroom and drowns the child, and then arranges things so that it will look like an accident.

11   In the second, Jones also stands to gain if anything should happen to his six-year-old cousin. Like Smith, Jones sneaks in planning to drown the child in his bath. However, just as he enters the bathroom Jones sees the child slip and hit his head, and fall face down in the water. Jones is delighted; he stands by, ready to push the child's head back under if it is necessary, but it is not necessary. With only a little thrashing about, the child drowns all by himself, "accidentally," as Jones watches and does nothing.

12   Now Smith killed the child, whereas Jones "merely" let the child die. That is the only difference between them. Did either man behave better, from a moral point of view? If the difference between killing and letting die were in itself a morally important matter, one should say that Jones's behavior was less reprehensible than Smith's. But does one really want to say that? I think not. In the first place, both men acted from the same motive, personal gain, and both had exactly the same end in view when they acted. It may be inferred from Smith's conduct that he is a bad man, although the judgment may be withdrawn or modified if certain further facts are learned about him—for example, that he is mentally deranged. But would not the very same thing be inferred about Jones from his conduct? And would not the same further considerations also be relevant to any modification of this judgment? Moreover, suppose Jones pleaded, in his own defense, "After all, I didn't do anything except just stand there and watch

the child drown. I didn't kill him; I only let him die." Again, if letting die were in itself less bad than killing, this defense should have at least some weight. But it does not. Such a "defense" can only be regarded as a grotesque perversion of moral reasoning. Morally speaking, it is no defense at all.

Now, it may be pointed out, quite properly, that the cases 13 of euthanasia with which doctors are concerned are not like this at all. They do not involve personal gain or the destruction of normal healthy children. Doctors are concerned only with cases in which the patient's life is of no further use to him, or in which the patient's life has become or will soon become a terrible burden. However, the point is the same in these cases: The bare difference between killing and letting die does not, in itself, make a moral difference. If a doctor lets a patient die, for humane reasons, he is in the same moral position as if he had given the patient a lethal injection for humane reasons. If his decision was wrong—if, for example, the patient's illness was in fact curable—the decision would be equally regrettable no matter which method was used to carry it out. And if the doctor's decision was the right one, the method used is not in itself important.

The AMA policy statement isolates the crucial issue very well; 14 the crucial issue is "the intentional termination of the life of one human being by another." But after identifying this issue, and forbidding "mercy killing," the statement goes on to deny that the cessation of treatment is the intentional termination of life. This is where the mistake comes in, for what is the cessation of treatment, in these circumstances, if it is not "the intentional termination of life of one human being by another"? Of course it is exactly that, and if it were not, there would be no point to it.

Many people will find this judgment hard to accept. One 15 reason, I think, is that it is very easy to conflate the question of whether killing is, in itself, worse than letting die, with the very different question of whether most actual cases of killing are more reprehensible than most actual cases of letting die. Most actual cases of killing are clearly terrible (think, for example, of all the murders reported in the newspapers), and one hears of such cases every day. On the other hand, one hardly ever hears of a case of letting die, except for the actions of doctors who are motivated by humanitarian reasons. So one learns to think of killing in a much worse light than of letting die. But this does not mean that there is something about killing that makes it in itself worse than letting die, for it is not the bare difference between killing and letting die that makes the difference in these cases. Rather, the other factors—the murderer's motive of personal gain, for example, contrasted with the doctor's humanitarian motivation—account for different reactions to the different cases.

16   I have argued that killing is not in itself any worse than letting die; if my contention is right, it follows that active euthanasia is not any worse than passive euthanasia. What arguments can be given on the other side? The most common, I believe, is the following:

> The important difference between active and passive euthanasia is that, in passive euthanasia, the doctor does not do anything to bring about the patient's death. The doctor does nothing, and the patient dies of whatever ills already afflict him. In active euthanasia, however, the doctor does something to bring about the patient's death: He kills him. The doctor who gives the patient with cancer a lethal injection has himself caused his patient's death; whereas if he merely ceases treatment, the cancer is the cause of the death.

A number of points need to be made here. This first is that it is not exactly correct to say that in passive euthanasia the doctor does nothing, for he does do one thing that is very important: He lets the patient die. "Letting someone die" is certainly different, in some respects, from other types of action—mainly in that it is a kind of action that one may perform by way of not performing certain other actions. For example, one may let a patient die by way of not giving medication, just as one may insult someone by way of not shaking his hand. But for any purpose of moral assessment, it is a type of action nonetheless. The decision to let a patient die is subject to moral appraisal in the same way that a decision to kill him would be subject to moral appraisal: It may be assessed as wise or unwise, compassionate or sadistic, right or wrong. If a doctor deliberately let a patient die who was suffering from a routinely curable illness, the doctor would certainly be to blame for what he had done, just as he would be to blame if he had needlessly killed the patient. Charges against him would then be appropriate. If so, it would be no defense at all for him to insist that he didn't "do anything." He would have done something very serious indeed, for he let his patient die.

Fixing the cause of death may be very important from a legal point of view, for it may determine whether criminal charges are brought against the doctor. But I do not think that this notion can be used to show a moral difference between active and passive euthanasia. The reason why it is considered bad to be the cause of someone's death is that death is regarded as a great evil—and so it is. However, if it has been decided that euthanasia—even passive euthanasia—is desirable in a given case, it has also been decided that in this instance death is not greater an evil than the patient's continued existence. And if this is true, the usual reason for not wanting to be the cause of someone's death simply does not apply. 17

Finally, doctors may think that all of this is only of academic interest—the sort of thing that philosophers may worry about but that has no practical bearing on their own work. After all, doctors must be concerned about the legal consequences of what they do, and active euthanasia is clearly forbidden by the law. But even so, doctors should also be concerned with the fact that the law is forcing upon them a moral doctrine that may be indefensible, and has a considerable effect on their practices. Of course, most doctors are not now in the position of being coerced in this matter, for they do not regard themselves as merely going along with what the law requires. Rather, in statements such as the AMA policy statement that I have quoted, they are endorsing this doctrine as a central point of medical ethics. In that statement, active euthanasia is condemned not merely as illegal but as "contrary to that for which the medical profession stands," whereas passive euthanasia is approved. However, the preceding considerations suggest that there is really no moral difference between the two, considered in themselves (there may be important moral differences in some cases in their *consequences*, but, as I pointed out, these differences may make active euthanasia, and not passive euthanasia, the morally preferable option). So, whereas doctors may have to discriminate between active and 18 passive euthanasia to satisfy the law, they should not do any more than that. In particular, they should not give the distinction any added authority and weight by writing it into official statements of medical ethics.

We Do Abortions Here

Sallie Tisdale

1 We do abortions here; that is all we do. There are weary, grim moments when I think I cannot bear another basin of bloody remains, utter another kind phrase of reassurance. So I leave the procedure room in the back and reach for a new chart. Soon I am talking to an eighteen-year-old woman pregnant for the fourth time. I push up her sleeve to check her blood pressure and find row upon row of needle marks, neat and parallel and discolored. She has been so hungry for her drug for so long that she has taken to using the loose skin of her upper arms; her elbows are already a permanent ruin of bruises. She is surprised to find herself nearly four months pregnant. I suspect she is often surprised, in a mild way, by the blows she is dealt. I prepare myself for another basin, another brief and chafing loss.

2   "How can you stand it?" Even the clients ask. They see the machine, the strange instruments, the blood, the final stroke that wipes away the promise of pregnancy. Sometimes I see that too: I watch a woman's swollen abdomen sink to softness in a few stuttering moments and my own belly flip-flops with sorrow. But all it takes for me to catch my breath is another interview, one more story that sounds so much like the last one. There is a numbing sameness lurking in this job: the same questions, the same answers, even the same trembling tone in the voices. The worst is the sameness of human failure, of inadequacy in the face of each day's dull demands.

3   In describing this work, I find it difficult to explain how much I enjoy it most of the time. We laugh a lot here, as friends and as professional peers. It's nice to be with women all day. I like the sudden, transient bonds I forge with some clients: moments when

I am in my strength, remembering weakness, and a woman in weakness reaches out for my strength. What I offer is not power, but solidness, offered almost eagerly. Certain clients waken in me every tender urge I have—others make me wince and bite my tongue. Both challenge me to find a balance. It is a sweet brutality we practice here, a stark and loving dispassion.

I look at abortion as if I am standing on a cliff with a tele- 4
scope, gazing at some great vista. I can sweep the horizon with both eyes, survey the scene in all its distance and size. Or I can put my eye to the lens and focus on the small details, suddenly so close. In abortion the absolute must always be tempered by the contextual, because both are real, both valid, both hard. How can we do this? How can we refuse? Each abortion is a measure of our failure to protect, to nourish our own. Each basin I empty is a promise—but a promise broken a long time ago.

I grew up on the great promise of birth control. Like many 5
women my age, I took the pill as soon as I was sexually active. To risk pregnancy when it was so easy to avoid seemed stupid, and my contraceptive success, as it were, was part of the promise of social enlightenment. But birth control fails, far more frequently than laboratory trials predict. Many of our clients take the pill; its failure to protect them is a shocking realization. We have clients who have been sterilized, whose husbands have had vasectomies; each one is a statistical misfit, fine print come to life. The anger and shame of these women I hold in one hand, and the basin in the other. The distance between the two, the length I pace and try to measure, is the size of an abortion.

The procedure is disarmingly simple. Women are surprised, 6
as though the mystery of conception, a dark and hidden genesis, requires an elaborate finale. In the first trimester of pregnancy, it's a mere few minutes of vacuuming, a neat tidying up. I give a woman a small yellow Valium, and when it has begun to relax her, I lead her into the back, into bareness, the stirrups. The doctor reaches in her, opening the narrow tunnel to the uterus with a succession of slim, smooth bars of steel. He inserts a plastic tube and hooks it to a hose on the machine. The woman is framed against white paper that crackles as she moves, the light bright in her eyes. Then the machine rumbles low and loud in the small windowless room; the doctor moves the tube back and forth with

an efficient rhythm, and the long tail of it fills with blood that spurts and stumbles along into a jar. He is usually finished in a few minutes. They are long minutes for the woman; her uterus frequently reacts to its abrupt emptying with a powerful, unceasing cramp, which cuts off the blood vessels and enfolds the irritated, bleeding tissue.

7   I am learning to recognize the shadows that cross the faces of the women I hold. While the doctor works between her spread legs, the paper drape hiding his intent expression, I stand beside the table. I hold the woman's hands in mine, resting them just below her ribs. I watch her eyes, finger her necklace, stroke her hair. I ask about her job, her family; in a haze she answers me; we chatter, faces close, eyes meeting and sliding apart.

8   I watch the shadows that creep up unnoticed and suddenly darken her face as she screws up her features and pushes a tear out each side to slide down her cheeks. I have learned to anticipate the quiver of chin, the rapid intake of breath and the surprising sobs that rise soon after the machine starts to drum. I know this is when the cramp deepens, and the tears are partly the tears that follow pain—the sharp, childish crying when one bumps one's head on a cabinet door. But a well of woe seems to open beneath many women when they hear that thumping sound. The anticipation of the moment has finally come to fruit; the moment has arrived when the loss is no longer an imagined one. It has come true.

9   I am struck by the sameness and I am struck every day by the variety here—how this commonplace dilemma can so display the differences of women. A twenty-one-year-old woman, unemployed, uneducated, without family, in the fifth month of her fifth pregnancy. A forty-two-year-old mother of teenagers, shocked by her condition, refusing to tell her husband. A twenty-three-year-old mother of two having her seventh abortion, and many women in their thirties having their first. Some are stoic, some hysterical, a few giggle uncontrollably, many cry.

10   I talk to a sixteen-year-old uneducated girl who was raped. She has gonorrhea. She describes blinding headaches, attacks of breathlessness, nausea. "Sometimes I feel like two different people," she tells me with a calm smile, "and I talk to myself."

11   I pull out my plastic models. She listens patiently for a time, and then holds her hands wide in front of her stomach.

"When's the baby going to go up into my stomach?" she asks. 12
I blink. "What do you mean?"

"Well," she says, still smiling, "when women get so big, 13
isn't the baby in your stomach? Doesn't it hatch out of an egg 14
there?"

My first question in an interview is always the same. As I 15
walk down the hall with the woman, as we get settled in chairs
and I glance through her files, I am trying to gauge her, to get a
sense of the words, and the tone, I should use. With some I joke,
with others I chat, sometimes I fall into a brisk, business-like pat-
ter. But I ask every woman, "Are you sure you want to have an
abortion?" Most nod with grim knowing smiles. "Oh yes," they
sigh. Some seek forgiveness, offer excuses. Occasionally a woman
will flinch and say, "Please don't use that word."

Later I describe the procedure to come, using care with my 16
language. I don't say "pain" any more than I would say "baby."
So many are afraid to ask how much it will hurt. "My sister told
me—" I hear. "A friend of mine said—" and the dire expectations
unravel. I prick the index finger of a woman for a drop of blood
to test, and as the tiny lancet approaches the skin she averts her
eyes, holding her trembling hand out to me and jumping at my
touch.

It is when I am holding a plastic uterus in one hand, a suc- 17
tion tube in the other, moving them together in imitation of the
scrubbing to come, that women ask the most secret question. I am
speaking in a matter-of-fact voice about "the tissue" and "the
contents" when the woman suddenly catches my eye and asks,
"How big is the baby now?" These words suggest a quiet need
for a definition of the boundaries being drawn. It isn't so odd,
after all, that she feels relief when I describe the growing bud's
bulbous shape, its miniature nature. Again I gauge, and sometimes lie a little, weaseling around its infantile features until its
clinging power slackens.

But when I look in the basin, among the curdlike blood clots, 18
I see an elfin thorax, attenuated, its pencilline ribs all in parallel
rows with tiny knobs of spine rounding upwards. A translucent
arm and hand swim beside.

A sleepy-eyed girl, just fourteen, watched me with a slight 19
and goofy smile all through her abortion. "Does it have little feet

and little fingers and all?" she'd asked earlier. When the suction was over she sat up woozily at the end of the table and murmured, "Can I see it?" I shook my head firmly.

20   "It's not allowed," I told her sternly, because I knew she didn't really want to see what was left. She accepted this statement of authority, and a shadow of confused relief crossed her plain, pale face.

21 Privately, even grudgingly, my colleagues might admit the power of abortion to provoke emotion. But they seem to prefer the broad view and disdain the telescope. Abortion is a matter of choice, privacy, control. Its uncertainty lies in specific cases: retarded women and girls too young to give consent for surgery, women who are ill or hostile or psychotic. Such common dilemmas are met with both compassion and impatience: they slow things down. We are too busy to chew over ethics. One person might discuss certain concerns, behind closed doors, or describe a particularly disturbing dream. But generally there is to be no ambivalence.

22   Every day I take calls from women who are annoyed that we cannot see them, cannot do their abortion today, this morning, now. They argue the price, demand that we stay after hours to accommodate their job or class schedule. Abortion is so routine that one expects it to be like a manicure: quick, cheap, and painless.

23   Still, I've cultivated a certain disregard. It isn't negligence, but I don't always pay attention. I couldn't be here if I tried to judge each case on its merits; after all, we do over a hundred abortions a week. At some point each individual in this line of work draws a boundary and adheres to it. For one physician the boundary is a particular week of gestation; for another, it is a certain number of repeated abortions. But these boundaries can be fluid too: one physician overruled his own limit to abort a mature but severely malformed fetus. For me, the limit is allowing my clients to carry their own burden, shoulder the responsibility themselves. I shoulder the burden of trying not to judge them.

24   This city has several "crisis pregnancy centers" advertised in the Yellow Pages. They are small offices staffed by volunteers,

and they offer free pregnancy testing, glossy photos of dead fetuses, and movies. I had a client recently whose mother is active in the anti-abortion movement. The young woman went to the local crisis center and was told that the doctor would make her touch her dismembered baby, that the pain would be the most horrible she could imagine, and that she might, after an abortion, never be able to have children. All lies. They called her at home and at work, over and over and over, but she had been wise enough to give a false name. She came to us a fugitive. We who do abortions are marked, by some, as impure. It's dirty work.

When a deliveryman comes to the sliding glass window by the reception desk and tilts a box toward me, I hesitate. I read the packing slip, assess the shape and weight of the box in light of its supposed contents. We request familiar faces. The doors are carefully locked; I have learned to half glance around at bags and boxes, looking for a telltale sign. I register with security when I arrive, and I am careful not to bang a door. We are all a little on edge here. 25

Concern about size and shape seems to be natural, and so is the relief that follows. We make the powerful assumption that the fetus is different from us, and even when we admit the similarities, it is too simplistic to be seduced by form alone. But the form is enormously potent—humanoid, powerless, palm-sized, and pure, it evokes an almost fierce tenderness when viewed simply as what it appears to be. But appearance, and even potential, aren't enough. The fetus, in becoming itself, can ruin others; its utter dependence has a sinister side. When I am struck in the moment by the contents in the basin, I am careful to remember the context, to note the tearful teenager and the woman sighing with something more than relief. One kind of question, though, I find considerably trickier. 26

"Can you tell what it is?" I am asked, and this means gender. This question is asked by couples, not women alone. Always couples would abort a girl and keep a boy. I have been asked about twins, and even if I could tell what race the father was. 27

An eighteen-year-old woman with three daughters brought her husband to the interview. He glared first at me, then at his 28 wife, as he sank lower and lower in the chair, picking his teeth with a toothpick. He interrupted a conversation with his wife to ask if I could tell whether the baby would be a boy or a girl. I told him I could not.

29   "Good," he replied in a slow and strangely malevolent voice, "'cause if it was a boy I'd wring her neck."

30   In a literal sense, abortion exists because we are able to ask such questions, able to assign a value to the fetus which can shift with changing circumstances. If the human bond to a child were as primitive and unflinchingly narrow as that of other animals, there would be no abortion. There would be no abortion because there would be nothing more important than caring for the young and perpetuating the species, no reason for sex but to make babies. I sense this sometimes, this wordless organic duty, when I do ultrasounds.

31   We do ultrasound, a sound-wave test that paints a faint, gray picture of the fetus, whenever we're uncertain of gestation. Age is measured by the width of the skull and confirmed by the length of the femur or thighbone; we speak of a pregnancy as being a certain "femur length" in weeks. The usual concern is whether a pregnancy is within the legal limit for an abortion. Women this far along have bellies which swell out round and tight like trim muscles. When they lie flat, the mound rises softly above the hips, pressing the umbilicus upward.

32   It takes practice to read an ultrasound picture, which is grainy and etched as though in strokes of charcoal. But suddenly a rapid rhythmic motion appears—the beating heart. Nearby is a soft oval, scratched with lines—the skull. The leg is harder to find, and then suddenly the fetus moves, bobbing in the surf. The skull turns away, an arm slides across the screen, the torso rolls. I know the weight of a baby's head on my shoulder, the whisper of lips on ears, the delicate curve of a fragile spine in my hand. I know how heavy and correct a newborn cradled feels. The creature I watch in secret requires nothing from me but to be left alone, and that is precisely what won't be done.

33   These inadvertently made beings are caught in a twisting web of motive and desire. They are at least inconvenient, some- times quite literally dangerous in the womb, but most often they fall somewhere in between—consequences never quite believed

in come to roost. Their virtue rises and falls outside their own nature: they become only what we make them. A fetus created by accident is the most absolute kind of surprise. Whether the blame lies in a failed IUD, a slipped condom, or a false impression of safety, that fetus is a thing whose creation has been actively worked against. Its existence is an error. I think this is why so few women, even late in a pregnancy, will consider giving a baby up for adoption. To do so means making the fetus real—imagining it as something whole and outside oneself. The decision to terminate a pregnancy is sometimes so difficult and confounding that it creates an enormous demand for immediate action. The decision is a rejection; the pregnancy has become something to be rid of, a condition to be ended. It is a burden, a weight, a thing separate.

Women have abortions because they are too old, and too 34 young, too poor, and too rich, too stupid, and too smart. I see women who berate themselves with violent emotions for their first and only abortion, and others who return three times, five times, hauling two or three children, who cannot remember to take a pill or where they put the diaphragm. We talk glibly about choice. But the choice for what? I see all the broken promises in lives lived like a series of impromptu obstacles. There are the sweet, light promises of love and intimacy, the glittering promise of education and progress, the warm promise of safe families, long years of innocence and community. And there is the promise of freedom: freedom from failure, from faithlessness. Freedom from biology. The early feminist defense of abortion asked many questions, but the one I remember is this: Is biology destiny? And the answer is yes, sometimes it is. Women who have the fewest choices of all exercise their right to abortion the most.

Oh, the ignorance. I take a woman to the back room and 35 ask her to undress; a few minutes later I return and find her positioned discreetly behind a drape, still wearing underpants. "Do I have to take these off too?" she asks, a little shocked. Some swear they have not had sex, many do not know what a uterus is, how sperm and egg meet, how sex makes babies. Some late seekers do not believe themselves pregnant; they believe themselves *impregnable.* I was chastised when I began this job for referring to some clients as girls: it is a feminist heresy. They come so young, snapping gum, sockless and sneakered, and their shakily applied eyeliner smears when they cry. I call them girls with maternal benignity. I cannot imagine them as mothers.

36   The doctor seats himself between the woman's thighs and reaches into the dilated opening of a five-month pregnant uterus. Quickly he grabs and crushes the fetus in several places, and the room is filled with a low clatter and snap of forceps, the click of the tanaculum, and a pulling, sucking sound. The paper crinkles as the drugged and sleepy woman shifts, the nurse's low, honey-brown voice explains each step in delicate words.

37   I have fetus dreams, we all do here: dreams of abortions one after the other; of buckets of blood splashed on the walls; trees full of crawling fetuses. I dreamed that two men grabbed me and began to drag me away. "Let's do an abortion," they said with a sickening leer, and I began to scream, plunged into a vision of sucking, scraping pain, of being spread and torn by impartial instruments that do only what they are bidden. I woke from this dream barely able to breathe and thought of kitchen tables and coat hangers, knitting needles striped with blood, and women all alone clutching a pillow in their teeth to keep the screams from piercing the apartment-house walls. Abortion is the narrowest edge between kindness and cruelty. Done as well as it can be, it is still violence—merciful violence, like putting a suffering animal to death.

38   Maggie, one of the nurses, received a call at midnight not long ago. It was a woman in her twentieth week of pregnancy; the necessarily gradual process of cervical dilation begun the day before had stimulated labor, as it sometimes does. Maggie and one of the doctors met the woman at the office in the night. Maggie helped her onto the table, and as she lay down the fetus was delivered into Maggie's hands. When Maggie told me about it the next day, she cupped her hands into a small bowl—"It was just like a little kitten," she said softly, wonderingly. "Everything was still attached."

39   At the end of the day I clean out the suction jars, pouring blood into the sink, splashing the sides with flecks of tissue. From the sink rises a rich and humid smell, hot, earthy, and moldering;

it is the smell of something recently alive beginning to decay. I take care of the plastic tub on the floor, filled with pieces too big to be trusted to the trash. The law defines the contents of the bucket I hold protectively against my chest as "tissue." Some would say my complicity in filling that bucket gives me no right to call it anything else. I slip the tissue gently into a bag and place it in the freezer, to be burned at another time. Abortion requires of me an entirely new set of assumptions. It requires a willingness to live with conflict, fearlessness, and grief. As I close the freezer door, I imagine a world where this won't be necessary, and then return to the world where it is.

Remarks by the President on Stem Cell Research

George W. Bush

Good evening. I appreciate you giving me a few minutes of your 1 time tonight so I can discuss with you a complex and difficult issue, an issue that is one of the most profound of our time.

The issue of research involving stem cells derived from 2 human embryos is increasingly the subject of a national debate and dinner table discussions. The issue is confronted every day in laboratories as scientists ponder the ethical ramifications of their work. It is agonized over by parents and many couples as they try to have children, or to save children already born.

The issue is debated within the church, with people of differ- 3 ent faiths, even many of the same faith coming to different conclusions. Many people are finding that the more they know about stem cell research, the less certain they are about the right ethical and moral conclusions.

My administration must decide whether to allow federal 4 funds, your tax dollars, to be used for scientific research on stem cells derived from human embryos. A large number of these embryos already exist. They are the product of a process called in vitro fertilization, which helps so many couples conceive children.

When doctors match sperm and egg to create life outside the womb, they usually produce more embryos than are planted in the mother. Once a couple successfully has children, or if they are unsuccessful, the additional embryos remain frozen in laboratories.

5   Some will not survive during long storage; others are destroyed. A number have been donated to science and used to create privately funded stem cell lines. And a few have been implanted in an adoptive mother and born, and are today healthy children.

6   Based on preliminary work that has been privately funded, scientists believe further research using stem cells offers great promise that could help improve the lives of those who suffer from many terrible diseases—from juvenile diabetes to Alzheimer's, from Parkinson's to spinal cord injuries. And while scientists admit they are not yet certain, they believe stem cells derived from embryos have unique potential.

7   You should also know that stem cells can be derived from sources other than embryos—from adult cells, from umbilical cords that are discarded after babies are born, from human placenta. And many scientists feel research on these types of stem cells is also promising. Many patients suffering from a range of diseases are already being helped with treatments developed from adult stem cells.

8   However, most scientists, at least today, believe that research on embryonic stem cells offer the most promise because these cells have the potential to develop in all of the tissues in the body.

9   Scientists further believe that rapid progress in this research will come only with federal funds. Federal dollars help attract the best and brightest scientists. They ensure new discoveries are widely shared at the largest number of research facilities and that the research is directed toward the greatest public good.

10   The United States has a long and proud record of leading the world toward advances in science and medicine that improve human life. And the United States has a long and proud record of upholding the highest standards of ethics as we expand the limits of science and knowledge. Research on embryonic stem cells raises profound ethical questions, because extracting the

stem cell destroys the embryo, and thus destroys its potential for life. Like a snowflake, each of these embryos is unique, with the unique genetic potential of an individual human being.

As I thought through this issue, I kept returning to two fundamental questions: First, are these frozen embryos human life, and therefore, something precious to be protected? And second, if they're going to be destroyed anyway, shouldn't they be used for a greater good, for research that has the potential to save and improve other lives?

I've asked those questions and others of scientists, scholars, bioethicists, religious leaders, doctors, researchers, members of Congress, my Cabinet, and my friends. I have read heartfelt letters from many Americans. I have given this issue a great deal of thought, prayer and considerable reflection. And I have found widespread disagreement.

On the first issue, are these embryos human life—well, one researcher told me he believes this five-day-old cluster of cells is not an embryo, not yet an individual, but a pre-embryo. He argued that it has the potential for life, but it is not a life because it cannot develop on its own.

An ethicist dismissed that as a callous attempt at rationalization. Make no mistake, he told me, that cluster of cells is the same way you and I, and all the rest of us, started our lives. One goes with a heavy heart if we use these, he said, because we are dealing with the seeds of the next generation.

And to the other crucial question, if these are going to be destroyed anyway, why not use them for good purpose—I also found different answers. Many argue these embryos are by-products of a process that helps create life, and we should allow couples to donate them to science so they can be used for good purpose instead of wasting their potential. Others will argue there's no such thing as excess life, and the fact that a living being is going to die does not justify experimenting on it or exploiting it as a natural resource.

At its core, this issue forces us to confront fundamental questions about the beginnings of life and the ends of science. It lies at a difficult moral intersection, juxtaposing the need to protect life in all its phases with the prospect of saving and improving life in all its stages.

17   As the discoveries of modern science create tremendous hope, they also lay vast ethical mine fields. As the genius of science extends the horizons of what we can do, we increasingly confront complex questions about what we should do. We have arrived at that brave new world that seemed so distant in 1932, when Aldous Huxley wrote about human beings created in test tubes in what he called a "hatchery."

18   In recent weeks, we learned that scientists have created human embryos in test tubes solely to experiment on them. This is deeply troubling, and a warning sign that should prompt all of us to think through these issues very carefully.

19   Embryonic stem cell research is at the leading edge of a series of moral hazards. The initial stem cell researcher was at first reluctant to begin his research, fearing it might be used for human cloning. Scientists have already cloned a sheep. Researchers are telling us the next step could be to clone human beings to create individual designer stem cells, essentially to grow another you, to be available in case you need another heart or lung or liver.

20   I strongly oppose human cloning, as do most Americans. We recoil at the idea of growing human beings for spare body parts, or creating life for our convenience. And while we must devote enormous energy to conquering disease, it is equally important that we pay attention to the moral concerns raised by the new frontier of human embryo stem cell research. Even the most noble ends do not justify any means.

21   My position on these issues is shaped by deeply held beliefs. I'm a strong supporter of science and technology, and believe they have the potential for incredible good—to improve lives, to save life, to conquer disease. Research offers hope that millions of our loved ones may be cured of a disease and rid of their suffering. I have friends whose children suffer from juvenile diabetes. Nancy Reagan has written me about President Reagan's struggle with Alzheimer's. My own family has confronted the tragedy of child-hood leukemia. And, like all Americans, I have great hope for cures.

22   I also believe human life is a sacred gift from our Creator. I worry about a culture that devalues life, and believe as your President I have an important obligation to foster and encour-age respect for life in America and throughout the world. And while we're all hopeful about the potential of this research, no

one can be certain that the science will live up to the hope it has generated.

Eight years ago, scientists believed fetal tissue research 23 offered great hope for cures and treatments—yet, the progress to date has not lived up to its initial expectations. Embryonic stem cell research offers both great promise and great peril. So I have decided we must proceed with great care.

As a result of private research, more than 60 genetically 24 diverse stem cell lines already exist. They were created from embryos that have already been destroyed, and they have the ability to regenerate themselves indefinitely, creating ongoing opportunities for research. I have concluded that we should allow federal funds to be used for research on these existing stem cell lines, where the life and death decision has already been made.

Leading scientists tell me research on these 60 lines has great 25 promise that could lead to breakthrough therapies and cures. This allows us to explore the promise and potential of stem cell research without crossing a fundamental moral line, by providing taxpayer funding that would sanction or encourage further destruction of human embryos that have at least the potential for life.

I also believe that great scientific progress can be made 26 through aggressive federal funding of research on umbilical cord placenta, adult and animal stem cells which do not involve the same moral dilemma. This year, your government will spend $250 million on this important research.

I will also name a President's council to monitor stem cell 27 research, to recommend appropriate guidelines and regulations, and to consider all of the medical and ethical ramifications of bio-medical innovation. This council will consist of leading scientists, doctors, ethicists, lawyers, theologians and others, and will be chaired by Dr. Leon Kass, a leading biomedical ethicist from the University of Chicago.

This council will keep us apprised of new developments and 28 give our nation a forum to continue to discuss and evaluate these important issues. As we go forward, I hope we will always be guided by both intellect and heart, by both our capabilities and our conscience.

I have made this decision with great care, and I pray it is the 29 right one.

Thank you for listening. Good night, and God bless America. 30

Of SNPS, TRIPS, and Human Dignity: Ethics and Gene Patenting

Miriam Schulman

1 If you bring up the topic of gene patenting with a group of scientists, they are likely to talk about what impact limiting access to DNA sequences will have on research. A similar conversation with lawyers may provoke debate about the utility or inventiveness of particular patent applications. But raise the question of granting intellectual property rights over pieces of the human genome in any gathering of regular folks, and the initial response is probably going to be, "Yuck."

2 Intellectual property attorney William L. Anthony Jr., a partner at Orrick, Herrington & Sutcliffe LLP, frequently discusses these issues with jury focus groups. At a recent conference, "Patenting Human Life," held at Santa Clara University, Anthony described his experience: "Almost invariably, if I talk about patenting something that has to do with human beings, the first reaction is revulsion."

3 While it may be tempting for people in the biotechnology field to dismiss this response as untutored, it points to a significant ethical issue that should be of concern to people at all levels of scientific and legal understanding: There is something about the human genome that is different from other subjects of patent application, and the difference is encapsulated in the adjective. Human DNA symbolizes something essential about humans themselves, and, as such, raises the issue of human dignity. While we may be able to respect that dignity and still offer the intellectual property protections crucial to drug development, it is unwise to ignore widespread public concern about how we deal with the building blocks of human life.

4 Dignity was just one of the ethical issues raised at the "Patenting Human Life" conference, sponsored by SCU's High Tech Law Institute and Markkula Center for Applied Ethics and the Bay Area Bioscience Center. Other ethical questions included: What system of intellectual property protection would produce the best therapeutics and so improve human well-being? And

what system would come closest to ensuring that these discoveries are accessible to all who need them?

DIGNITY

When the average person expresses reservations about patenting DNA, they are often reacting to the idea of owning something fundamental to human personhood. A lawyer would probably respond that a patent doesn't confer ownership. John Barton, professor of law at Stanford University, described intellectual property protections as "a set of statutory exclusion rights." In other words, the holder of a DNA patent does not own the gene sequence; he or she simply has the right, for a limited period of time, to prevent others from using it.

True, but not enough to entirely moot the concern over dignity. Patenting DNA still suggests to many that human genes are commodities. It's an equation that troubled Suzanne Holland, associate professor of religion at University of Puget Sound and affiliate associate professor in medical history and ethics at the University of Washington School of Medicine. "Biotechnology products are not widgets," she said. Holland worried that patenting genes may "erode our dignity, as the process results in increasing acceptance that it's okay to buy and sell things that speak to us of our humanity."

Of course, there are those who believe that humans don't deserve any specially protected status and that such dignity concerns reveal a sort of hubris. In his conference keynote, Rigel Pharmaceuticals President Brian Cunningham sounded this note: "It seems to be okay to patent every animal in the zoo but us, a reflection of our need to believe that we are special—not part of the continuum of nature."

Margaret R. McLean, director of biotechnology and health care ethics at the Markkula Center for Applied Ethics, took a middle view. While accepting the basic notion that humans "ought not to be used," she allowed that patenting DNA "doesn't necessarily imply commodification of human persons." The trick, McLean argued, is to distinguish between genetic identity and personal identity. "A human is more than the sum of his or her genes," she said. In discussing the patent issue, we must be careful not to suggest that humans can be reduced to a piece of code, she continued, which would indeed be an assault on dignity.

PROMOTING HUMAN HEALTH

9   While patenting DNA runs the risk of diminishing respect for human dignity, some risk might be acceptable if the end result were an increase in human well-being. Most people in the biotechnology industry start with this understanding and proceed to the instrumental ethical question: If the goal is to improve human health by the creation of diagnostics and therapeutics, does the patent system help to achieve that goal?

10   There was almost universal agreement among lawyers and biotech professionals at the conference that some form of intellectual property protection was necessary to encourage investment in the development of new drugs. Investors will not put money into a company without evidence that the firm has secured protection for its intellectual property, Sue Markland Day, president of the Bay Area Bioscience Center, argued. As an example, she cited the plunge in biotech stock prices when Former President Bill Clinton and British Prime Minister Tony Blair issued a joint statement March 14, 2000, which was interpreted to advocate limits on gene patenting. "Patents," Markland Day said, "are the lifeblood of biotechnology."

11   That does not mean that people in the biotech industry want to ignore the ethical dimension of gene patenting, simply that their ethical questions tend to be not "Whether to?" but "How to?" Thane Kreiner, vice president for corporate affairs at Affymetrix, posed the issue this way, "It's not a question of whether patents are right or wrong, but where to set the bar."

12   Kreiner was referring to the guidelines for patentability and how they are applied to biotechnology. There are three key criteria in this regard: novelty, inventiveness, and usefulness. As the United States and other signatories to the Agreement on Trade-Related Aspects of Intellectual Property Rights (TRIPS) evaluate whether to grant patents on gene sequences, they must decide whether to apply these standards stringently (that is, to

set the bar high) or loosely (to set the bar low). A high bar might require, for example, that applicants state the specific utility of a sequence and include evidence that the gene actually does what the applicant claims. A low bar might allow applications to rest on the theoretical possibility that a gene might have a certain utility.

The issue is complicated by the fact that the science is in such 13 rapid flux. The discovery of a sequence that might have represented considerable novelty and inventiveness in the 1990s—such as the connection of the BRCA1 gene with breast cancer—might be less impressive now that technology has made it much easier to identify disease susceptibility genes.

Another complication has to do with the scope of the patents. 14 Many applications have been filed for fragments of genes—ESTs and SNPs—and it is unclear whether patents on these fragments extend to uses of the entire gene.

These were among the issues that troubled Stanford's Barton, 15 who was a member of the roundtable that produced the Nuffield Council on Bioethics report on the ethics of patenting DNA. That roundtable concluded:

> In general, the law has, in our view, tended to be generous in granting patents in relation to DNA sequences. Not only are many of the patents broad in scope, but they have been granted when the criteria for inventiveness and utility were weakly applied. Many of these patents are broad because an inventor who successfully makes a claim in relation to a DNA sequence will, in effect, obtain broad protection on all uses of the DNA, and sometimes the proteins which the DNA produces.

What does all this have to do with ethics? If the bar for patentabil- 16 ity is set too low, it will pervert the incentive structures of the patent system, which should reward new inventions that increase human well-being. Patent holders who may have contributed very little to the understanding of the gene or its function will have too much control over its use in research and development. Especially in the area of genetics, where more than one gene may control a disease process, a company that wants to develop therapeutics may need to buy licenses from multiple patent holders. That, Kreiner argued, could make research prohibitively expensive.

17   If the bar is set too high, on the other hand, pharmaceutical and biotechnology companies will not put the vast sums necessary into research because they will have no way of protecting their investment. "The patent system doesn't exist to pin a badge of appreciation on the inventor," Anthony said, "but to encourage ordinary people to invest in something that might do some good."

ACCESSIBILITY

18   Proper setting of the bar may promote the creation of therapeutics that have the potential to improve human lives. But the ethical story does not end there. Sometimes, our patent policies produce good medicines that are simply too expensive to reach all of the people who need them.

19   Many who work in biotech agree this is a problem but argue it is not their problem. A company, they point out, is not a philanthropic institution. It exists to make profits. But to raise the issue of accessibility is not to suggest that industry should solve the problem on its own. Industry, however, needs to be part of the discussion, which might begin with an exploration of distributive justice: How can benefits—in this context, therapeutics—be allocated fairly.

20   One criterion of fairness says that those who have contributed to the creation of the benefit should have a share in it. Usually, there has been some public contribution to successful drug discovery. Of the 50 best-selling drugs in this country, 48 benefited from public money, according to Holland. In the case of genes, the public has certainly contributed to the knowledge base that is producing innovations through government funding of the Human Genome Project and other scientific endeavors. By that measure, the public is entitled to expect some access to the fruits of genetic research.

21   Can the patent system be adjusted to spread the fruits more widely? Not without tradeoffs, said June Carbone, Presidential Professor of Ethics and the Common Good at SCU and one of the conference organizers:

> The real public question is whether we want:
> a) the existing system, which places a premium on the

development of life-saving drugs, even if they are so costly they cannot realistically be made available to everyone;

b) greater redirection of government-subsidized research toward products of more general utility or accessibility, even if that means the development of some life-saving drugs will be delayed or discouraged; or

c) dramatically higher overall public health expenditures.

These public health decisions have important implications for the common good. Physical well-being is not solely an individual matter. For example, we all rely on the public provision of clean water and sewage systems to protect our health. We handle serious infectious disease risks by offering vaccines to everyone because a policy that provided protection only for those who could afford it might eventually harm everyone. [22]

Gene patenting needs to be seen within this common good context, McLean argued. If, as a society, we develop patent policies that direct research only to the development of expensive drugs, we may ultimately bankrupt the health care infrastructure on which we all rely. [23]

Finally, as we think about patents and access, we must invoke the old-fashioned virtue of compassion. Do we really want to be the kind of people who restrict the access of the poor and the uninsured to life-saving therapies? Holland proposes this litmus test for patenting DNA: "What does it do for the most vulnerable members of society?" [24]

These ethical issues might be addressed in any number of ways. We could support government programs that provide DNA-based therapeutics to the underserved. We could support industry efforts, such as the Genentech policy described by Brian Cunningham, through which the company put aside a portion of its profits from Human Growth Hormone to provide the therapy for any child whose family could not afford it. We could force companies to license patents so that research could be expanded and cheaper therapeutics developed. [25]

The resolution of all these ethical dilemmas is limited only by our moral imagination. The only thing we can't do is ignore the ethical dimension of patenting human life. [26]

Index

Notes

Notes

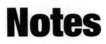

Notes

Notes

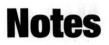

Notes

Notes